STUDENT WORKBOOK TO ACCOMPANY

NURSING ASSISTANT

A Nursing Process Approach

12th Edition

Barbara Acello, MS, RN
Independent Nurse Consultant and Educator

Barbara R. Hegner
(deceased)

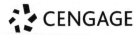

CENGAGE

Australia • Brazil • Japan • Korea • Mexico • Singapore • Spain • United Kingdom • United States

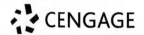

Workbook to Accompany Nursing Assistant: A Nursing Process Approach, **12th Edition,**
Barbara Acello and Barbara R. Hegner

SVP, Higher Education & Skills Product:
Erin Joyner

Senior Product Director: Matthew Seeley

Senior Product Team Manager: Laura Stewart

Director, Learning Design: Rebecca von Gillern

Senior Manager, Learning Design: Leigh Hefferon

Senior Learning Designer: Deborah Bordeaux

Marketing Director: Michele McTighe

Marketing Manager: Courtney Cozzy

Director, Content Creation: Juliet Steiner

Senior Content Creation Manager: Patty Stephan

Senior Content Manager: Kenneth McGrath

Digital Delivery Lead: Allison Marion

Art Director: Felicia Bennett

Text Designer: Angela Sheehan

Cover Designer: Angela Sheehan

Cover images:
Monkey Business Images/ShutterStock.com
Rawpixel.com/ShutterStock.com
Monkey Business Images/ShutterStock.com
iStockPhoto.com/monkeybusinessimages

© 2022, 2016 Cengage Learning, Inc.

Unless otherwise noted, all content is © Cengage.

ALL RIGHTS RESERVED. No part of this work covered by the copyright herein may be reproduced or distributed in any form or by any means, except as permitted by U.S. copyright law, without the prior written permission of the copyright owner.

For product information and technology assistance, contact us at
Cengage Customer & Sales Support, 1-800-354-9706 or support.cengage.com.

For permission to use material from this text or product,
submit all requests online at **www.cengage.com/permissions.**

Library of Congress Control Number: 2020917872

ISBN-13: 978-0-357-37203-6

Cengage
200 Pier 4 Boulevard
Boston, MA 02210
USA

Cengage is a leading provider of customized learning solutions with employees residing in nearly 40 different countries and sales in more than 125 countries around the world. Find your local representative at **www.cengage.com.**

To learn more about Cengage platforms and services, register or access your online learning solution, or purchase materials for your course, visit **www.cengage.com.**

Notice to the Reader

Publisher does not warrant or guarantee any of the products described herein or perform any independent analysis in connection with any of the product information contained herein. Publisher does not assume, and expressly disclaims, any obligation to obtain and include information other than that provided to it by the manufacturer. The reader is expressly warned to consider and adopt all safety precautions that might be indicated by the activities described herein and to avoid all potential hazards. By following the instructions contained herein, the reader willingly assumes all risks in connection with such instructions. The publisher makes no representations or warranties of any kind, including but not limited to, the warranties of fitness for particular purpose or merchantability, nor are any such representations implied with respect to the material set forth herein, and the publisher takes no responsibility with respect to such material. The publisher shall not be liable for any special, consequential, or exemplary damages resulting, in whole or part, from the readers' use of, or reliance upon, this material.

Printed at CLDPC, USA, 05-21

CONTENTS

© 2022 Cengage Learning. All Rights Reserved. May not be scanned, copied or duplicated, or posted to a publicly accessible website, in whole or in part.

© 2022 Cengage Learning. All Rights Reserved. May not be scanned, copied or duplicated, or posted to a publicly accessible website, in whole or in part.

© 2022 Cengage Learning. All Rights Reserved. May not be scanned, copied or duplicated, or posted to a publicly accessible website, in whole or in part.

The content of this workbook follows a basic organizational plan. Each lesson in the workbook includes:

- Behavioral objectives.
- A summary of the related unit in the *Nursing Assistant* text.
- Exercises to help you review, recall, and reinforce concepts that have been taught.
- Nursing Assistant Alerts, which are key points to remember about each unit.
- Opportunities to apply nursing assistant care to the nursing process and expand your horizons.

It has been shown that students who complete a special guide as they learn new materials perform better, have greater confidence, and are more secure in the basic concepts than those who do not. You may wish to complete the workbook activities in preparation for your class, or after class, while the information is fresh in your mind. In either case, the workbook and classwork will reinforce each other.

You can make the best use of the workbook if you:

- Read and study the related chapter in the text.
- Observe and listen carefully to your instructor's explanations and demonstrations.
- Read over the behavioral objectives before you start the workbook and then check to be sure you have met them after you complete the lesson exercises.
- Use the summary to review the chapter content.
- Complete the activities in the workbook. Circle any questions you are unable to finish to discuss with your instructor at the next class meeting.

You have chosen a special goal for yourself: You have decided to become a knowledgeable, skilled nursing assistant. Keep this goal in mind, but realize that to reach it, you need to take many small steps. Each step you master takes you closer to your ultimate goal. Best wishes as you embark on your journey!

Barbara Acello

© 2022 Cengage Learning. All Rights Reserved. May not be scanned, copied or duplicated, or posted to a publicly accessible website, in whole or in part.

THE LEARNING PROCESS

Students may feel anxious about learning. However, learning really can be very rewarding if you have an open mind, a desire to succeed, and a willingness to follow some simple steps.

You already have won half the battle, because you have entered an educational program. This shows your desire to accomplish a real-life goal: to become a nursing assistant.

Steps to Learning

There are three basic steps to learning:

- Active listening

- Effective studying

- Careful practicing

Active Listening

Listening actively is not easy, natural, or passive. It is, however, a skill that can be learned and must be practiced.

Good listeners are not born, they are made. Studies show that the average listening efficiency in this culture is only about 25 percent. That means that although you may hear (a passive action) all that is said, you actually listen to and process only about one-quarter of the material. Effective listening requires a conscious effort by the listener. The most neglected communication skill is listening.

An important part of your work as a nursing assistant involves active listening to patients and co-workers. Begin to listen actively to your instructor or supervisor. Hearing but not processing information puts you and your patient in jeopardy.

Active listening is listening with personal involvement. There are three actions in active listening:

- Hearing what is said (passive action)

- Processing the information (active action)

- Using the information (active action)

Hearing What Is Said

People speak at an average rate of 125 words per minute. Pay close attention to the speaker to hear what is said. This is not difficult if you focus and do not let other thoughts and sounds interfere with your thinking. If you sit up straight and lean forward in the classroom or stand erect in the clinical area, your whole body is more receptive. Position yourself where you can adequately see or hear and keep your attention focused on the speaker. Make eye contact if possible and remain alert.

Many distractions can break your concentration unless you actively prevent them from doing so. For example, distractions may be:

- Interruptions, such as other activities in the classroom or in the patient's unit that catch your attention or create noise.

- Using the smartphone or answering texts during class.

vii

© 2022 Cengage Learning. All Rights Reserved. May not be scanned, copied or duplicated, or posted to a publicly accessible website, in whole or in part.

- Daydreaming and thinking about personal activities or problems.

- Physical fatigue. Adequate sleep and rest are powerful aids to the ability to concentrate.

- Lack of interest, because you cannot immediately see the importance of the information.

To be an effective listener, you must actively work at eliminating these distractions. You must put energy into staying focused.

Processing the Information

Remember that hearing the words is not enough. You must actively process (make sense of) the words in your brain by putting meaning to them, and that takes effort. Other things can also help the process, including:

- Interacting with the speaker using eye contact, smiles, and nods.

- Asking meaningful questions; contribute your own comments if it is a discussion.

- Taking notes.

These actions allow your memory to establish relationships with previously learned knowledge and to make new connections.

Taking notes gives you another way to imprint what you are processing. You are not only hearing the sounds of the words, but also seeing the important words on paper. Note-taking helps you recall points that you may have forgotten.

Note-taking is a skill that can be learned. If used, it will greatly improve your learning process. You may need to take notes in class, during demonstrations, and when your supervisor or instructor gives you a clinical assignment. Here are some hints to make developing this skill easier:

- Come prepared with a pencil and paper.

- Don't try to write down every word.

- Write down only the important points or key words.

- Learn to take notes in an outline form.

- Listen with particular care to the beginning sentence. It usually reveals the primary purpose.

- Pay special attention to the final statement. It is often a summary.

Outlines include the important points summarized in a meaningful way. Be sure to leave room so that you can add material.

There are different ways of outlining. One way is to use letters and numbers to designate important points. Another is to draw a pattern of lines to show relationships. Use either way or one of your own design, but be consistent. Practice helps you master the skill of outlining.

As you make notes of material that is not clear, add a star or some other mark next to the material. When the speaker asks for questions, you can quickly find yours.

If the speaker stresses a point, underline the information to call attention to important points to study.

After class, you can reorganize your notes and compare them with your text.

GENERAL TIPS

Here are some general tips to help you study better.

- Feel certain that each lesson you master is important to add to your knowledge and skills. The workbook, text, and instructor materials have been carefully coordinated to meet the objectives. Review the objectives before you begin to study. They are like a road map that will take you to your goal.

- Remember that you are the learner, so you can take credit for your success. The instructor is an important guide and the workbook, text, and clinical experiences are tools, but you are the learner and whether you use the tools wisely is up to you in the end.

© 2022 Cengage Learning. All Rights Reserved. May not be scanned, copied or duplicated, or posted to a publicly accessible website, in whole or in part.

- Take an honest look at yourself and your study habits. Take positive steps to avoid habits that could limit your success. For example, do you let family responsibilities or social opportunities interfere with study times? If so, sit down with your family and plan a schedule for study that they will support and to which you will adhere. Find a special place to study that is free from distraction. If the telephone interferes, turn it off.

The Study Plan

Plan a schedule for study. Actually, sit down and write out a weekly schedule hour by hour so that you know exactly how your time is being spent. Then plan specific study time, but be realistic. Study must be balanced with the other activities of your life. Learn to budget your time so that you have time to study. Block in extra time when tests are scheduled. Don't forget to block in time for fun as well! Look back over the week to see how well you have managed your schedule. If you have had difficulty, try to adjust the schedule to better meet your needs. If you have been successful, pat yourself on the back. You have done very well.

Make your study area special. It need not be elaborate, but make sure there is ample light. You should have a desk to work on and a supply of paper and pencils. Sharpen your pencils at the end of each study period and leave papers readily at hand. You may think this sounds strange, but often time is wasted at the beginning of a study session finding paper and sharpening pencils. If these things are ready when you first sit down, you can get started without distractions or delay. Keep your medical dictionary and other references in your work area. When you get home, put your text and workbook there also. In other words, your work area should be designed for study. When you treat it this way, you will find that as soon as you sit down there, you will be psychologically prepared to study.

Class Study

Now that you have your study area and work schedule organized, you need to think about how you can get the most out of your class experience.

- Come prepared. Read the behavioral objectives and the lesson before class. This introduces you to the focus of the lesson and the vocabulary.

- Listen actively as the instructor explains the lesson. Pay close attention. Refocus immediately if your thoughts start to wander.

- Take notes on the special points to use for study at home.

- Participate in class discussions. Remember that discussion subjects are chosen because they relate to the lesson. You can learn much from hearing the comments of others and by contributing your own. Pay attention to slides, films, and overhead transparencies, because these offer a visual approach to the subject matter. You might even take notes on important points during a film or jot down questions you would like the instructor to answer.

- Ask intelligent and pertinent questions. Make sure your questions are simple and centered on the topic. Focus on one point at a time and write down the answers for later review.

- Use any models and charts that are available. Study them and see how they apply to the lesson.

- Carefully observe the demonstrations your instructor gives. Note in your book any change that may have been made in the procedure steps to conform with the policy of your facility.

- Perform return demonstrations carefully in the classroom. Remember, you are learning skills that will be used with real patients in the clinical situation.

After Class

When class is over and you have had a break, you are ready to settle down and study. You can gain the most from the experience by:

- Studying in your prepared study area. Everything will be ready and waiting for you if you followed the first part of this plan.

© 2022 Cengage Learning. All Rights Reserved. May not be scanned, copied or duplicated, or posted to a publicly accessible website, in whole or in part.

- Read over the lesson, beginning with the behavioral objectives.
- Read with a highlighter or pencil in hand so you can underline or highlight important material.
- Answer the questions at the end of the unit. Check any you found difficult by reviewing that section of the text.
- Complete the related workbook unit.
- Review the behavioral objectives at the beginning of the unit. Ask yourself if you have met them. If not, go back and review. Prepare the next day's lesson by reading over the next day's unit.
- Use the medical dictionary for words you may learn that are not in the text glossary. The dictionary provides pronunciations.

Study Groups

Studying with someone else who is trying to learn the same material can be very helpful and supportive, but there are some pitfalls you must avoid. If studying with someone else is to be effective and productive:

- Limit the number of people studying to a maximum of three; one other person is best.
- Keep focused on the subject. Don't begin to talk about classmates or the day's social events.
- Come prepared for the study session. Have your work completed. Use the study session to reinforce your learning and explore deeper understanding of the material.
- Ask each other questions about the materials.
- Make a list of ideas to ask your instructor.
- Limit the study session to a specific length. Follow the plan and you will succeed!

© 2022 Cengage Learning. All Rights Reserved. May not be scanned, copied or duplicated, or posted to a publicly accessible website, in whole or in part.

PART 1

Student Activities

© 2022 Cengage Learning. All Rights Reserved. May not be scanned, copied or duplicated, or posted to a publicly accessible website, in whole or in part.

Introduction to Nursing Assisting

C H A P T E R **1**

Community Health Care

OBJECTIVES

After completing this chapter, you will be able to:

1-1 Spell and define terms.

1-2 List the five basic functions that all health care facilities have in common.

1-3 Describe four changes that have taken place in health care in the past few decades.

1-4 State the functions of hospitals, long-term care facilities, home health care, hospices, and other types of health care facilities.

1-5 Name at least five departments within a hospital and describe their functions.

1-6 List at least five ways by which health care costs are paid.

1-7 State the purpose of health care facility surveys.

1-8 Describe patient-focused care.

1-9 Explain why transitional care is important.

VOCABULARY BUILDER

Definitions

Define the words in the spaces provided.

1. facility

© 2022 Cengage Learning. All Rights Reserved. May not be scanned, copied or duplicated, or posted to a publicly accessible website, in whole or in part.

2. hospice

_____

3. patient

_____

4. transitional care

_____

5. community

_____

Matching

Match each term to the correct definition.

1. _____ chronic illness

2. _____ accreditation

3. _____ physical therapy

4. _____ postpartum

5. _____ license

a. treatable but has no cure and requires life-long care

b. assists patients to regain mobility skills

c. care unit for people who have given birth to babies

d. permits a facility to conduct business

e. recognizes a facility as meeting quality standards and other criteria

CHAPTER REVIEW

Short Answer

Complete the assessment in the space provided.

1. List five basic functions of all health care facilities.

   a. _____

   b. _____

   c. _____

   d. _____

   e. _____

2. Patient-focused care means

_____

3. The cost of health care has increased because of demand for services as a result of

_____

4. The person receiving care in an acute care hospital is called a

_____

© 2022 Cengage Learning. All Rights Reserved. May not be scanned, copied or duplicated, or posted to a publicly accessible website, in whole or in part.

5. List three examples of health care facilities.

   a. _____

   b. _____

   c. _____

6. Three names applied to the person receiving care are

   a. _____

   b. _____

   c. _____

7. Explain what activities take place in each of the following departments.

   a. pharmacy

   _____

   b. medical

   _____

   c. radiology

   _____

   d. pediatric

   _____

   e. physical therapy

   _____

8. Explain the activities of each of the following departments.

   a. dietary

   _____

   b. housekeeping

   _____

   c. maintenance

   _____

   d. business

   _____

9. List four ways volunteers help patients.

   a. _____

   b. _____

   c. _____

   d. _____

10. The majority of health care is paid for with

   _____

© 2022 Cengage Learning. All Rights Reserved. May not be scanned, copied or duplicated, or posted to a publicly accessible website, in whole or in part.

11. The purpose of diagnosis-related groups is to

_____

12. A health care facility survey is done to

_____

13. The Occupational Safety and Health Administration is a governmental agency that

_____

True/False

Mark the following true or false by circling T or F.

1. T F A multiskilled worker is cross-trained to perform additional skills.
2. T F Managed care means that insurance companies pay for all costs of care.
3. T F One important function of the nursing assistant is to prevent infection.
4. T F One function of a community is to keep the residents safe.
5. T F Preventive care is given to treat a disease.
6. T F Emergency care is used to treat a sudden injury or illness.
7. T F A resident receives care in their own home.
8. T F Adult day care is a type of long-term care.
9. T F The goal of rehabilitation is to restore a patient to the highest level of functioning.
10. T F Orthopedic care focuses on kidney disease.

CERTIFICATION REVIEW

Complete the following multiple-choice assessments.

1. Which is a characteristic of patient-focused care?
    a. Is a place where health care is given
    b. Provides a full range of health care services
    c. Respects the needs, values, and beliefs of patients
    d. Promotes research in medicine and nursing

2. Which statement is true about health care today?
    a. Patients are discharged earlier from hospitals to reduce the cost of care.
    b. Patients are refusing to go to the hospital for care.
    c. Families use hospitals to provide care to older family members.
    d. Insurance companies pay for all services provided in the hospital.

© 2022 Cengage Learning. All Rights Reserved. May not be scanned, copied or duplicated, or posted to a publicly accessible website, in whole or in part.

3. What type of care is provided in a special facility or arrangement to a terminally ill patient?

    a. Acute

    b. Chronic

    c. Palliative

    d. Hospice

4. Which is a type of short-term care?

    a. Subacute facility

    b. Assisted-living facility

    c. Home care

    d. Hospital

5. Which of the following is true of transitional care?

    a. Provides current medical treatment

    b. Diagnoses a health problem

    c. Educates the patient and family

    d. Supports the nutritional needs of the patient

6. Which hospital department provides diagnostic services?

    a. Pathology

    b. Physical therapy

    c. Occupational therapy

    d. Respiratory therapy

7. On what is payment to hospitals based?

    a. Age of the patient

    b. Diagnosis-related groups

    c. Federal government programs

    d. Type of health insurance

8. How are costs contained when providing care?

    a. Achieve maximum benefit for every dollar spent

    b. Reuse supplies between patients

    c. Limit the type of care provided in the hospital

    d. Discharge the patient to a lesser level of care as soon as possible

9. Which person inspects a facility for compliance with regulations?

    a. Nurse manager

    b. Physician

    c. Social worker

    d. Surveyor

© 2022 Cengage Learning. All Rights Reserved. May not be scanned, copied or duplicated, or posted to a publicly accessible website, in whole or in part.

10. On what is the Magnet Program for Excellence in Nursing Services based?

    a. Number of staff with licenses

    b. Ratio of care providers to patients

    c. Average number of days a patient is in the facility

    d. Quality indicators and standards of nursing practice

CHAPTER APPLICATION

Answer the following questions in the space provided.

1. What response will you make when a co-worker says that they does not want to get a flu vaccination?

2. Why should you attend continuing education classes?

3. What is the value in being cross-trained?

4. What is the difference between a patient and a client?

5. What is the criteria for admission to a long-term care hospital?

6. Which type of unit provides care to a patient after surgery?

7. What type of care is given in an orthopedic unit?

8. Which activities are completed by people in environmental services?

9. What is Medicare?

10. What type of care is provided by the Veterans Administration?

© 2022 Cengage Learning. All Rights Reserved. May not be scanned, copied or duplicated, or posted to a publicly accessible website, in whole or in part.

DEVELOPING GREATER INSIGHT

1. Visit a local community health agency such as a city or county health department and learn about its services. Report back to the class.

2. Accompany a volunteer in a hospital. Learn about the volunteer's work and see how many departments you can identify.

3. Make a list of the health care facilities within your immediate vicinity and identify the type of care provided in each.

4. Invite a nursing assistant who is currently employed by a health care facility to visit the class and discuss the care provided by nursing assistants in that facility. An alternative activity is to prepare a list of questions about the roles and responsibilities of the nursing assistant. Interview a nursing assistant, then discuss the responses with your class.

© 2022 Cengage Learning. All Rights Reserved. May not be scanned, copied or duplicated, or posted to a publicly accessible website, in whole or in part.

CHAPTER 2

On the Job: Being a Nursing Assistant

OBJECTIVES

After completing this chapter, you will be able to:

2-1 Spell and define terms.

2-2 Identify the members of the interdisciplinary health care team and the nursing team.

2-3 List the job responsibilities of the nursing assistant.

2-4 Explain how the Nurse Practice Act affects nursing assistant practice.

2-5 Discuss the importance of working within the established scope of nursing assistant practice.

2-6 List the federal requirements for nursing assistants working in long-term care facilities.

2-7 State the purpose of evidence-based practice.

2-8 Identify common nursing care delivery systems and briefly describe each.

2-9 Describe your facility's lines of authority.

2-10 Discuss the five rights of delegation.

2-11 Explain why good time management is a key to nursing assistant success.

2-12 Describe methods of organizing assignments to make the best use of your time.

2-13 State the purpose of shift report and handoff communication.

2-14 Explain why critical thinking is an essential skill for nursing assistants.

2-15 Describe the importance of good human relations.

2-16 List ways of building good relationships with patients, families, and staff.

2-17 Explain why projecting a professional image is important.

2-18 List the rules of personal hygiene and appropriate dress.

2-19 Explain why a healthy mental attitude is important.

2-20 Describe ways of relieving stress and preventing illness.

© 2022 Cengage Learning. All Rights Reserved. May not be scanned, copied or duplicated, or posted to a publicly accessible website, in whole or in part.

VOCABULARY BUILDER

Definitions

Define the words in the spaces provided.

1. attitude

   _____

2. burnout

   _____

3. nursing team

   _____

4. scope of practice

   _____

5. nursing assistant

   _____

6. partners in practice

   _____

CHAPTER REVIEW

Short Answer

Complete the statements in the spaces provided.

1. Write four terms used to describe a nursing assistant.

   a. _____

   b. _____

   c. _____

   d. _____

2. List three members of the nursing team.

   a. _____

   b. _____

   c. _____

3. Explain what is meant by the "line of authority."

   _____

   _____

© 2022 Cengage Learning. All Rights Reserved. May not be scanned, copied or duplicated, or posted to a publicly accessible website, in whole or in part.

4. What should you do if you have any doubts about your assignment?

   _____

5. Give a brief explanation of the three primary ways in which nursing care is organized.

   a. primary nursing _____

   _____

   b. case management _____

   _____

   c. team nursing _____

   _____

6. List three goals of patient-focused care.

   a. _____

   b. _____

   c. _____

7. Name three characteristics of a successful nursing assistant.

   a. _____

   b. _____

   c. _____

8. List three activities you could carry out to ensure good personal hygiene.

   a. _____

   b. _____

   c. _____

9. Explain why wearing jewelry is unwise when you are on duty.

   _____

   _____

10. What jewelry is part of your uniform?

    _____

11. The main concern of every nursing assistant should be the well-being and

    _____

12. List four reasons a patient might be irritable, complaining, or uncooperative.

    a. _____

    b. _____

    c. _____

    d. _____

© 2022 Cengage Learning. All Rights Reserved. May not be scanned, copied or duplicated, or posted to a publicly accessible website, in whole or in part.

13. List three dimensions in which patients have needs.

    a. _____

    b. _____

    c. _____

14. List five ways you can ensure good working relationships.

    a. _____

    b. _____

    c. _____

    d. _____

    e. _____

15. Check the positive and negative grooming traits of a nursing assistant.

Trait	Positive	Negative
a. long hair		
b. clean shoelaces		
c. cigarette odor		
d. bright nail polish		
e. unpolished shoes		
f. dangling earrings		
g. light lipstick		
h. long fingernails		
i. use of antiperspirant/deodorant		

16. Explain why stress is an issue for all nursing assistants and how you can reduce its effects.

    _____

    _____

    _____

17. Define the following terms.

    a. palliative care

    _____

    b. cross-training

    _____

© 2022 Cengage Learning. All Rights Reserved. May not be scanned, copied or duplicated, or posted to a publicly accessible website, in whole or in part.

18. Complete the chart to show the proper lines of communication.

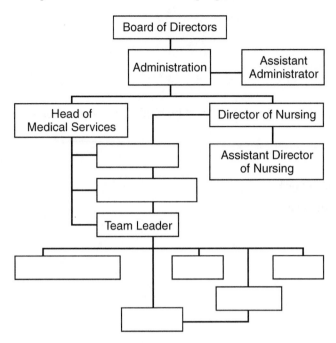

Matching

Match each specialist with the type of care provided.

Type of Care

1. _____ care of the aging person
2. _____ treats and diagnoses disorders of the eye
3. _____ treats disorders of the skin
4. _____ treats disorders of the digestive system
5. _____ treats disorders of the heart and blood vessels
6. _____ treats and diagnoses disorders of the nervous system
7. _____ treats disorders of the blood
8. _____ cares for women during pregnancy
9. _____ diagnoses and treats with X-rays
10. _____ treats disorders of the mind

Specialist

a. cardiologist
b. gastroenterologist
c. neurologist
d. radiologist
e. obstetrician
f. hematologist
g. psychiatrist
h. ophthalmologist
i. gerontologist
j. dermatologist

CERTIFICATION REVIEW

Complete the following multiple-choice assessments.

1. Which statement explains the role of a licensed practical nurse (LPN)?

    a. A person who provides care under the supervision of an RN

    b. A certified nursing assistant who can provide medications

    c. A nurse who can diagnose and manage illnesses

    d. A person who works with physician supervision

© 2022 Cengage Learning. All Rights Reserved. May not be scanned, copied or duplicated, or posted to a publicly accessible website, in whole or in part.

2. Which federal law regulates the education and certification of nursing assistants?

   a. Affordable Care Act (ACA)

   b. Omnibus Budget Reconciliation Act (OBRA)

   c. Health Insurance Portability and Accountability Act (HIPAA)

   d. Social Security Act of 1962

3. Which action should be taken if you are asked to perform something that is beyond your scope of practice?

   a. Complete the task

   b. Ask someone to watch you complete the task

   c. State that training was not provided to complete the task

   d. Ask another nursing assistant to help complete the task

4. Which is a characteristic of professionalism?

   a. Arriving late to work

   b. Wearing a dirty uniform

   c. Completing work on time

   d. Adopting an attitude of completing a job

5. Which action related to hair would be appropriate?

   a. Making sure hair is off of the face

   b. Wearing a current style to express individuality

   c. Using different hair colors to complement your uniform color

   d. Avoiding using barrettes or headbands

6. Which approach to care is task-oriented?

   a. Team

   b. Primary

   c. Case

   d. Functional

7. To which person will the nursing assistant give end-of-shift report?

   a. Nurse manager

   b. The nurse who is supervising the work

   c. The physician

   d. The director of nursing

8. Which is a "right" of delegation?

   a. Right meal

   b. Right activity

   c. Right person

   d. Right nurse

© 2022 Cengage Learning. All Rights Reserved. May not be scanned, copied or duplicated, or posted to a publicly accessible website, in whole or in part.

9. Which action helps with time management?

    a. Focusing on tasks

    b. Setting an alarm on a watch

    c. Completing a task every hour

    d. Making rounds

10. Which action helps to reduce personal stress?

    a. Having a drink with friends after work

    b. Lying in bed on a day off from work

    c. Skipping meals when at work to reduce weight

    d. Avoiding using drugs

CHAPTER APPLICATION

Answer the following questions in the space provided.

1. Who are the members of an interdisciplinary team?

2. List at least three specialty services.

3. Which facility needs to adhere to OBRA requirements?

4. What is the purpose of the Nurse Practice Act?

5. Why is a first impression important?

6. Why should hoop earrings be avoided in the clinical area?

7. What is the goal of evidence-based practice?

8. What is the partners in practice method of providing care?

9. What is the purpose of an organizational chart?

10. For which reasons would you refuse a delegated task?

© 2022 Cengage Learning. All Rights Reserved. May not be scanned, copied or duplicated, or posted to a publicly accessible website, in whole or in part.

DEVELOPING GREATER INSIGHT

1. With other students, role-play a properly dressed and improperly dressed nursing assistant. State your first impressions about each assistant based on how they are dressed. Discuss how this influences your feelings about the person. Divide the class into teams and assign points for each positive or negative finding.

2. With the class, discuss ways you have personally found to relieve stress. Discuss why alcohol and other drugs are a poor solution to stress.

3. Discuss burnout, what it feels like, and how people behave when they experience it. Try to learn what effect it might have on the burned-out individual, co-workers, and patients.

© 2022 Cengage Learning. All Rights Reserved. May not be scanned, copied or duplicated, or posted to a publicly accessible website, in whole or in part.

CHAPTER 3

Consumer Rights and Responsibilities in Health Care

OBJECTIVES

After completing this chapter, you will be able to:

3-1 Spell and define terms.

3-2 Explain the purpose of health care consumer rights.

3-3 Describe six items that are common to the Patient Care Partnership booklet, the Residents' Rights, and the Clients' Rights in Home Care documents.

3-4 List three specific rights from each of the three documents.

3-5 State the purpose of the Affordable Care Act and review the new Patient's Bill of Rights under that law.

3-6 Describe eight responsibilities of health care consumers.

3-7 List at least three responsibilities of the ombudsman.

VOCABULARY BUILDER

Definitions

Write the terms in the spaces provided.

1. given to patients upon admission to a hospital

   _____

2. relates to people receiving care at home

   _____

© 2022 Cengage Learning. All Rights Reserved. May not be scanned, copied or duplicated, or posted to a publicly accessible website, in whole or in part.

3. given to people before admission to a long-term care facility

_____

4. gives instructions about consumers' wishes regarding care when they are unable to make their wishes known

_____

CHAPTER REVIEW

True/False

Mark the following true or false by circling T or F.

1. T   F   All citizens in the United States have certain rights that are guaranteed by law.

2. T   F   Consumers have no rights once they enter a health care facility.

3. T   F   The Omnibus Budget Reconciliation Act of 1987 was enacted by the federal government to ensure the rights of patients in acute care facilities.

4. T   F   Informed consent means that the person gives permission for care, even if they does not fully understand the purpose of the care.

5. T   F   A consumer with a grievance feels there are grounds for a complaint.

6. T   F   Both caregiver and consumer have responsibilities that help ensure quality health care.

7. T   F   Patients have the right to know the cost of care.

8. T   F   All personal and clinical records pertaining to a patient must be kept confidential.

9. T   F   An experimental procedure may not be performed without the consumer's consent.

10. T   F   Long-term care facility visitors may be restricted against the resident's wishes.

11. T   F   Patients have a role in making treatment choices and planning care.

12. T   F   Patients have the right to open and honest communication with caregivers.

13. T   F   A patient who feels that they have been injured must keep this information to themselves.

14. T   F   A long-term care facility resident has the right to choose an attending physician.

15. T   F   A long-term care facility resident has the right to freedom from corporal punishment.

16. T   F   Patients must accept the treatment prescribed by their physicians.

17. T   F   Patients do not have the right to examine their medical bills as long as the insurance company is paying those bills.

18. T   F   Continuity of care is important only in the acute care hospital.

© 2022 Cengage Learning. All Rights Reserved. May not be scanned, copied or duplicated, or posted to a publicly accessible website, in whole or in part.

Identification

Determine the appropriateness of a nursing assistant's behavior by indicating C for correct or I for incorrect.

1. _____ listening to visitors' conversations with patients and residents.

2. _____ discussing a resident's physical status with one of the resident's relatives.

3. _____ making shift reports so that patients cannot hear.

4. _____ reading a patient's record to satisfy one's curiosity.

5. _____ sharing information from the medical records with the resident's minister.

6. _____ telling a patient that their roommate has a terminal condition.

7. _____ telling another nursing assistant that a resident eats best when fed from the right side.

8. _____ informing another staff member that the resident is incontinent.

9. _____ telling another resident that a roommate has dirty toenails.

10. _____ mentioning that a patient has beautiful white hair to the patient's roommate.

11. _____ treating patients with dignity and respect.

12. _____ handling a patient's personal items carefully.

13. _____ not telling the client your name before beginning care.

14. _____ letting a client know that someone else will be making the next visit.

15. _____ not allowing the client to assist with a bath when she is able to do so.

16. _____ explaining restrictions on the number of visitors each patient may have while in intensive care.

17. _____ referring the patient's question about their blood pressure to the nurse.

18. _____ telling the patient's daughter that her father does not have long to live.

Matching

Match each term with the definition provided.

1. _____ law that gives consumers control of care

2. _____ document that states wishes for end-of-life care

3. _____ care given on a continuing basis

4. _____ giving permission for care after learning benefits and risks

5. _____ booklet given to patients at the time of hospital admission

A. Informed consent

B. Affordable Care Act

C. Patient Care Partnership

D. Advance directive

E. Continuity of care

© 2022 Cengage Learning. All Rights Reserved. May not be scanned, copied or duplicated, or posted to a publicly accessible website, in whole or in part.

CERTIFICATION REVIEW

Complete the following multiple-choice assessments.

1. Which action will be taken if a patient is unable to read or understand the Patient Care Partnership booklet?
   a. Read the booklet to the patient
   b. Give the booklet to a family member
   c. Place it in the patient's bedside stand
   d. Document that the patient refused the booklet

2. Which term describes a situation in which a health care consumer feels the need to make a complaint?
   a. Damage
   b. Grievance
   c. Unfairness
   d. Disservice

3. Which statement is true based on the Residents' Rights document?
   a. The resident cannot leave the facility.
   b. The resident is assigned an attending physician.
   c. The resident should expect corporal punishment.
   d. The resident has the right to manage personal funds.

4. Which is a right of a person receiving home care services?
   a. Provide the agency with a complete health history
   b. Sign the required consents and releases for insurance billing
   c. Be treated with dignity, consideration, and respect
   d. Accept responsibility for any refusal of treatment

5. Which is a responsibility of a person receiving home care services?
   a. Have property treated with respect
   b. Participate in planning care
   c. Know how to make a complaint
   d. Provide a safe home environment

6. Which document is used to ensure continuity of care?
   a. Plan of care
   b. Graphic sheet
   c. Nurse's notes
   d. Medication administration record

7. Which legislation provides consumers with control over their own health care?
   a. Social Security
   b. Affordable Care Act
   c. American's with Disabilities Act
   d. Health Insurance Portability and Accountability Act

© 2022 Cengage Learning. All Rights Reserved. May not be scanned, copied or duplicated, or posted to a publicly accessible website, in whole or in part.

8. Which is a provision of the Affordable Care Act?

    a. Treatment choices are to be provided.

    b. Changes in care are to be communicated.

    c. Patients have the right to know their caregivers.

    d. Preexisting conditions are covered by insurance.

9. Which is a responsibility of a health care consumer?

    a. Complete an advance directive

    b. Identify a health care power of attorney

    c. Access records through a health care portal

    d. Live a healthy lifestyle by avoiding risks of illness

10. Which professional advocates for patients and residents of health care facilities?

    a. Physician

    b. Ombudsman

    c. Social worker

    d. Registered nurse

CHAPTER APPLICATION

Complete the following statements by using the correct term(s) from the list provided. Some may be used more than once.

accept	clarification	Clients' Rights	federal
financial	honestly	medications	past
Patient Care Partnership	responsibility	will not	

1. The Omnibus Budget Reconciliation Act of 1987 a _____ legislation.

2. A copy of the _____ is given to a person upon admission to a hospital.

3. A copy of the _____ is given to consumers during the first home health care visit.

4. Consumers have a _____ to maintain personal health care records.

5. Consumers are responsible for communicating _____ with the physician and other caregivers.

6. It is important for consumers to provide accurate information regarding _____ hospitalizations and _____.

7. Consumers are responsible for informing health care providers if they _____ be able to carry out prescribed treatment.

8. Consumers must _____ responsibility for learning how to manage their own health.

9. Consumers are responsible for asking for _____ if they do not fully understand instructions.

10. Consumers must assume _____ responsibility to pay for health care.

© 2022 Cengage Learning. All Rights Reserved. May not be scanned, copied or duplicated, or posted to a publicly accessible website, in whole or in part.

DEVELOPING GREATER INSIGHT

1. In groups of two, practice reading a copy of a bill of rights to each other. Brainstorm what you would do if a patient were to have any questions about any of the rights.

2. You are taking care of two residents who share a room. The residents are of different religions and do not want the other to have their religious articles out for all to see. What would you do, considering that both residents have the same right to keep religious items in the room?

3. While measuring vital signs, a new resident tells you of a health problem but then asks you to not tell the nurse. Discuss what you would do.

© 2022 Cengage Learning. All Rights Reserved. May not be scanned, copied or duplicated, or posted to a publicly accessible website, in whole or in part.

CHAPTER 4

Ethical and Legal Issues Affecting the Nursing Assistant

OBJECTIVES

After completing this chapter, you will be able to:

4-1 Spell and define terms.

4-2 Discuss ethical and legal situations in health care.

4-3 Describe the legal and ethical responsibilities of the nursing assistant.

4-4 Describe how to protect the patients' right to privacy.

4-5 Define abuse and give examples.

4-6 Define neglect and give examples.

4-7 Define sexual harassment and give examples.

4-8 Identify professional boundaries in relationships with patients and families.

4-9 Explain why working in a virtual world affects patient boundaries.

4-10 Give examples of boundary violations using the Internet and wireless media.

4-11 State the purpose of the HIPAA laws.

4-12 Explain why most facilities prohibit employees from posting work-related information on social networking sites.

VOCABULARY BUILDER

Definitions

Define the words in the spaces provided.

1. confidential

© 2022 Cengage Learning. All Rights Reserved. May not be scanned, copied or duplicated, or posted to a publicly accessible website, in whole or in part.

2. assault

_____

3 negligence

_____

4. verbal abuse

_____

5. slander

_____

6. malpractice

_____

7. neglect

_____

CHAPTER REVIEW

Short Answer

Complete the assessment in the space provided.

1. Ethical standards are a _____ code rather than a legal code.

2. List five ways to ensure that the patient receives the proper treatment.

   a. _____

   b. _____

   c. _____

   d. _____

   e. _____

3. The patient offers you a tip for going to the lobby to get him a newspaper from the machine. Describe and explain your response.

   _____

4. You have not stolen something belonging to a patient yourself, but you observed someone else do so and failed to report it. Of what crime are you guilty?

   _____

5. A visitor asks you if her father really has cancer. How should you respond?

   _____

6. Restraining a patient without proper permission is _____

   _____

7. Abuse is any act that is not _____ and caused harm to the patient.

© 2022 Cengage Learning. All Rights Reserved. May not be scanned, copied or duplicated, or posted to a publicly accessible website, in whole or in part.

8. A door that is shut against a patient's will when the patient is confined to bed is a form of

_____

9. Define the Golden Rule.

_____

_____

10. Define the Platinum Rule.

_____

_____

11. You are in the _____ when you get too close to a boundary.

True/False

Mark the following true or false by circling T or F.

1. T F It is the responsibility of a nursing assistant to determine whether a patient has been abused.
2. T F A nursing assistant who reports seeing bruises or injuries on a patient is acting properly.
3. T F Self-abuse may occur when a person with a disability is unable to adequately carry out ADLs and will not accept help.
4. T F Signs of poor personal hygiene and a change in personality may indicate abuse.
5. T F Most abuse originates in feelings of frustration and fatigue.
6. T F An employee assistance program has resources to help reduce stress.
7. T F Involuntary seclusion is permitted when it is part of a patient's care plan to reduce agitation.
8. T F A nursing assistant may independently decide to isolate a patient.
9. T F In some states, a person who does not report abuse is considered as guilty as the person doing the abusing.
10. T F You may write about patients on your blog as long as you alter their names.
11. T F Employee behavior reflects upon the employer, even if the employee is not on duty.
12. T F Whenever you use the Internet, you leave footprints that can be traced.
13. T F Loretta forgot to feed Mr. Locklear his lunch. This is a form of neglect.

CERTIFICATION REVIEW

Complete the following multiple-choice assessments.

1. Which facility employees handle difficult situation in which no single "right" decision is possible?

   a. Medical committee

   b. Ethics committee

   c. Department of nursing

   d. Environmental services

© 2022 Cengage Learning. All Rights Reserved. May not be scanned, copied or duplicated, or posted to a publicly accessible website, in whole or in part.

2. Which action supports the idea that information about patients is privileged and not be shared with others?

   a. Maintaining the patient's quality of life

   b. Ensuring the patient's culture is respected

   c. Treating the patient's religious articles with respect

   d. Refusing to talk about patients during breaks

3. Which statement is true about policies and procedures?

   a. They are the law.

   b. They are guiding principles.

   c. They are never to be broken.

   d. They are a substitute for judgment.

4. Which behavior encourages negligence?

   a. Rushing to complete a task

   b. Falsifying a medical record

   c. Using restraints without an order

   d. Touching a patient without permission

5. Which action should be taken to prevent reckless behavior?

   a. Following your conscience

   b. Questioning policies and procedures

   c. Reporting patient changes at the end of the shift

   d. Withholding information if requested by the patient

6. Which patient outcome occurs in cases of malpractice?

   a. Injury

   b. Stealing

   c. Threatening

   d. Loss of property

7. Which term describes forcing patients to do something against their wishes?

   a. Abuse

   b. Assault

   c. Battery

   d. Coercion

8. Which action is considered neglect?

   a. Assisting a patient with meals

   b. Helping a patient sit in a chair

   c. Bathing a patient every morning

   d. Failing to turn a patient as required

© 2022 Cengage Learning. All Rights Reserved. May not be scanned, copied or duplicated, or posted to a publicly accessible website, in whole or in part.

9. Which action prevents the invasion of a patient's privacy?

   a. Staying in the room when family members come to visit

   b. Encouraging a patient to go to religious service

   c. Leaving when a patient receives a telephone call

   d. Keeping the door open while providing a bed bath

10. Which action on social media violates a patient's privacy?

    a. Commenting about hours of work

    b. Posting a photo of the patient on Facebook

    c. Deleting place of employment on your profile

    d. Refusing to participate in a conversation about a patient

CHAPTER APPLICATION

Complete the Chart

Place an X in the appropriate space to show which type of abuse has taken place.

Action	Verbal Abuse	Sexual Abuse	Psychological Abuse	Physical Abuse
1. Touching a patient in a sexual way	—	—	—	—
2. Using obscene gestures	—	—	—	—
3. Raising your voice in anger	—	—	—	—
4. Teasing a patient	—	—	—	—
5. Handling a patient roughly	—	—	—	—
6. Making threats	—	—	—	—
7. Making fun of a patient	—	—	—	—
8. Ridiculing a patient's behavior	—	—	—	—
9. Suggesting that a patient engage in sexual acts with you	—	—	—	—
10. Hitting a patient	—	—	—	—
11. Leaving a patient in bed when they asks repeatedly to get up	—	—	—	—
12. Holding an alert patient down while the nurse performs a dressing change against their will	—	—	—	—
13. Seating an alert patient at a table with three confused patients, rather than seating him or her in an empty spot at a table with three alert patients	—	—	—	—

© 2022 Cengage Learning. All Rights Reserved. May not be scanned, copied or duplicated, or posted to a publicly accessible website, in whole or in part.

Action	Verbal Abuse	Sexual Abuse	Psychological Abuse	Physical Abuse
14. Wiping a female patient internally with a washcloth while doing routine perineal care	—	—	—	—
15. Turning a sleeping patient with no warning	—	—	—	—
16. Saying, "If you don't stop using the call signal so much, I am not going to bring your lunch tray."	—	—	—	—
17. Unplugging the patient's call signal because they are making too many minor requests	—	—	—	—
18. Deliberately arousing a confused male patient when applying a condom catheter	—	—	—	—

Complete the Diagram

Label the professional behaviors in the answer spaces outside the Zone of Helpfulness in the figure below.

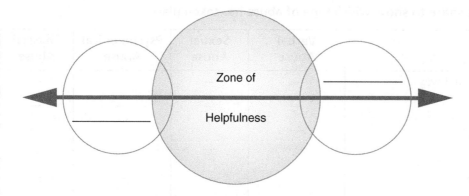

DEVELOPING GREATER INSIGHT

1. A resident that you are caring for shows you a bottle full of medications that the resident has faked taking and plans to take all at once to commit suicide. Discuss what action you would take.

2. When you are preparing to go home after work, you see that another employee dropped an envelop full of cash. While bending over to pick it up, the employee says, "Mrs. Smith gave me a birthday present." Discuss what you would say to the employee. Discuss what action you would take.

3. While going through Facebook at home after work, you see a friend that you work with has posted a picture with a resident and the family in the community dining room. Discuss what you would do after seeing this picture.

© 2022 Cengage Learning. All Rights Reserved. May not be scanned, copied or duplicated, or posted to a publicly accessible website, in whole or in part.

Scientific Principles

C H A P T E R **5**

Medical Terminology and Body Organization

OBJECTIVES

After completing this chapter, you will be able to:

5-1 Spell and define terms.

5-2 Recognize the meanings of common prefixes, suffixes, and root words.

5-3 Build medical terms from word parts.

5-4 Define the abbreviations commonly used in health care facilities.

5-5 Describe the organization of the body, from simple to complex.

5-6 Identify four types of tissues and describe their characteristics.

5-7 Name and locate major organs as parts of body systems, using proper anatomic terms.

VOCABULARY BUILDER

Definitions

Define each word in the space provided.

1. prefix

   _____

2. suffix

   _____

3. abbreviation

   _____

© 2022 Cengage Learning. All Rights Reserved. May not be scanned, copied or duplicated, or posted to a publicly accessible website, in whole or in part.

4. combining form

_____

5. word root

_____

Matching

Match each set of letters with the correct medical diagnosis.

1. AIDS		a.	fracture
2. CHF		b.	transient ischemic attack
3. CVA		c.	hepatitis C virus
4. Fx		d.	multiple sclerosis
5. TIA		e.	acquired immune deficiency syndrome
6. MI		f.	nonspecific urethritis
7. HCV		g.	sexually transmitted disease
8. KS		h.	cerebrovascular accident
9. STD		i.	Kaposi's sarcoma
10. MS		j.	myocardial infarction
		k.	congestive heart failure

CHAPTER REVIEW

Short Answer

Complete the statements in the spaces provided.

1. Name the book, other than your text, that would be most helpful in studying medical terms.

2. Underline the *root* in each of the following words and give a definition of the word.

   Example: <u>abdomin</u>al   pertaining to the abdomen

   a. adenoma _____

   b. colectomy _____

   c. craniotomy _____

   d. dentist _____

   e. hysterectomy _____

   f. myalgia _____

   g. nephrolithiasis _____

   h. pneumonectomy _____

   i. thoracotomy _____

   j. urinometer _____

© 2022 Cengage Learning. All Rights Reserved. May not be scanned, copied or duplicated, or posted to a publicly accessible website, in whole or in part.

3. Underline the *prefix* in each of the following words and give a definition of the prefix.

    Example: <u>neo</u>plasm   new

    a. asepsis _____

    b. bradycardia _____

    c. dysuria _____

    d. hypertension _____

    e. hypotension _____

    f. pandemic _____

    g. polyuria _____

    h. gerontology _____

    i. premenstrual _____

    j. tachycardia _____

4. Underline the *suffix* in each of the following words and give a definition of the suffix.

    Example: acro<u>megaly</u>   great

    a. appendectomy _____

    b. hepatitis _____

    c. electrocardiogram _____

    d. anemia _____

    e. tracheotomy _____

    f. hematology _____

    g. hemiplegia _____

    h. apnea _____

    i. otoscope _____

    j. proctoscopy _____

5. Listed below are five words that are not in your text. Define each and then check your accuracy with a medical dictionary.

    a. adenitis

    _____

    b. cardiopathy

    _____

    c. leucopenia

    _____

    d. arthroscope

    _____

    e. cytomegaly

    _____

© 2022 Cengage Learning. All Rights Reserved. May not be scanned, copied or duplicated, or posted to a publicly accessible website, in whole or in part.

6. Substitute one word for the underlined words in each of the following statements.

   Example: The patient experienced <u>pus in the urine</u>. pyuria

   a. There was <u>sugar in the urine</u>. _____

   b. The patient made an appointment with a <u>physician who specializes in female diseases</u>.

   _____

   c. The nurse performed a <u>puncture in a vein</u> and drew blood.

   _____

   d. The patient has an <u>incision made into the trachea</u> to ease breathing.

   _____

   e. The patient had a <u>tumor composed mainly of fibrous tissue</u> removed from her uterus.

   _____

   f. The patient was receiving chemotherapy for cancer, which caused <u>depression of all the cell levels</u>.

   _____

   g. The nursing assistant listened with the stethoscope to the patient's heart. It was found that <u>the heart rate was slow</u>.

   _____

   h. The medication did not seem to help the patient's <u>high blood pressure</u>.

   _____

   i. The postoperative diagnosis was <u>removal of a lung</u>. _____

   j. The patient complained of pain <u>below the stomach</u>. _____

7. Explain the following diagnoses.

   a. thrombosis

   _____

   b. pyogenic infection

   _____

   c. pneumonitis

   _____

   d. cystitis

   _____

   e. mastitis

   _____

8. Write the name of the body part indicated by the abbreviation.

   a. abd _____

   b. bld _____

   c. G.I. _____

   d. AX _____

   e. GU _____

   f. Vag _____

   g. Sh _____

© 2022 Cengage Learning. All Rights Reserved. May not be scanned, copied or duplicated, or posted to a publicly accessible website, in whole or in part.

Abbreviations

The following is a list of abbreviations you will see relating to orders and patient care. Write your understanding of each abbreviation.

1. a. amb. ad lib. _____

   b. urine to lab ASAP _____

   c. BR only _____

   d. ✔ drsg freq _____

   e. OOB daily _____

   f. position HOB 45° _____

   g. d/c cl liq diet _____

   h. SSE prn _____

   i. CBC in AM _____

   j. NPO preop _____

2. Write the names of the following hospital departments.

   a. CS _____

   b. EENT _____

   c. PT _____

   d. ICCU _____

   e. ED _____

   f. PAR _____

   g. Peds _____

   h. DR _____

   i. OR _____

   j. Lab _____

3. Write the appropriate abbreviation for each time indicated.

   a. before meals _____

   b. twice daily _____

   c. morning _____

   d. three times daily _____

   e. after meals _____

   f. immediately _____

   g. four times a day _____

   h. while awake _____

   i. every hour _____

   j. night _____

© 2022 Cengage Learning. All Rights Reserved. May not be scanned, copied or duplicated, or posted to a publicly accessible website, in whole or in part.

4. Write the word for each of the following measurements.

a. cm _____

b. mL _____

c. lb _____

d. kg _____

e. L _____

Short Answer

Answer the following questions in the space provided.

1. Write the Roman numeral for each of the following numbers.

a. one _____

b. twelve _____

c. six _____

d. nine _____

e. four _____

2. Complete the organizational pattern of the body.

cells $\rightarrow$ _____ $\rightarrow$ _____ $\rightarrow$ systems

3. There are four tissue types. Write their names and list their functions.

a. _____

_____

b. _____

_____

c. _____

_____

d. _____

_____

4. Select the correct term (anterior/posterior) to identify the relationships of the body parts listed and write the correct answer in the space provided.

a. breasts	(anterior)	(posterior)	_____
b. heels	(anterior)	(posterior)	_____
c. toes	(anterior)	(posterior)	_____
d. buttocks	(anterior)	(posterior)	_____
e. abdomen	(anterior)	(posterior)	_____
f. breast related to legs	(superior)	(inferior)	_____

© 2022 Cengage Learning. All Rights Reserved. May not be scanned, copied or duplicated, or posted to a publicly accessible website, in whole or in part.

g. ankles related to legs   (superior)   (inferior)   _____

h. head related to toes   (superior)   (inferior)   _____

i. hips related to breasts   (superior)   (inferior)   _____

j. thumb related to little finger   (medial)   (lateral)   _____

5. Another term for anterior is _____

6. Another term for posterior is _____

Matching

Match each body part with the proper system.

Body Part
1. _____ spleen
2. _____ brain
3. _____ breasts
4. _____ kidneys
5. _____ ureters
6. _____ vagina
7. _____ bones
8. _____ heart
9. _____ pituitary gland
10. _____ joints

System
a. cardiovascular
b. endocrine
c. digestive
d. integumentary
e. skeletal
f. muscular
g. nervous
h. reproductive
i. respiratory
j. urinary

Match each function with the correct system.

Function
1. _____ transports, absorbs food
2. _____ regulates body processes through hormones
3. _____ fulfils sexual needs
4. _____ brings in oxygen
5. _____ forms walls of some organs
6. _____ eliminates liquid wastes
7. _____ acts as levers in movement
8. _____ produces hormones to regulate body functions
9. _____ carries oxygen and nutrients to cells
10. _____ coordinates body activities through nervous impulses

System
a. cardiovascular
b. endocrine
c. digestive
d. integumentary
e. skeletal
f. muscular
g. nervous
h. reproductive
i. respiratory
j. urinary

CERTIFICATION REVIEW

Complete the following multiple-choice assessments.

1. What is a word for *cyte*?

    a. Cell

    b. Spore

    c. Cardiac

    d. Centimeter

© 2022 Cengage Learning. All Rights Reserved. May not be scanned, copied or duplicated, or posted to a publicly accessible website, in whole or in part.

2. Which term is defined as a state of well-being?

    a. Health

    b. Disease

    c. Independence

    d. Medical science

3. Which is a characteristic of the anatomic position?

    a. Face the observer

    b. Above the midline

    c. Close to the midline

    d. Away from the midline

4. What term is defied as being the furthest away from the midline?

    a. Medial

    b. Lateral

    c. Inferior

    d. Superior

5. Which type of tissue forms the brain and spinal cord?

    a. Muscle

    b. Smooth

    c. Nervous

    d. Epithelial

6. Which type of tissue forms the blood and bone?

    a. Smooth

    b. Cardiac

    c. Skeletal

    d. Connective

7. Which is a characteristic of the synovial membrane?

    a. Produces mucus

    b. Covers the organs

    c. Lines joint cavities

    d. Surrounds the heart

8. Which term refers to the skin?

    a. Pleural

    b. Cutaneous

    c. Peritoneum

    d. Pericardium

© 2022 Cengage Learning. All Rights Reserved. May not be scanned, copied or duplicated, or posted to a publicly accessible website, in whole or in part.

9. Which body system includes the thyroid gland?

    a. Urinary

    b. Skeletal

    c. Muscular

    d. Endocrine

10. Which cavity contains the adrenal glands?

    a. Pelvic

    b. Cranial

    c. Thoracic

    d. Retroperitoneal

CHAPTER APPLICATION

Answer the following questions in the space provided.

1. Select the proper directional term from the list provided for each area indicated. Then color the organs as specified in the list.

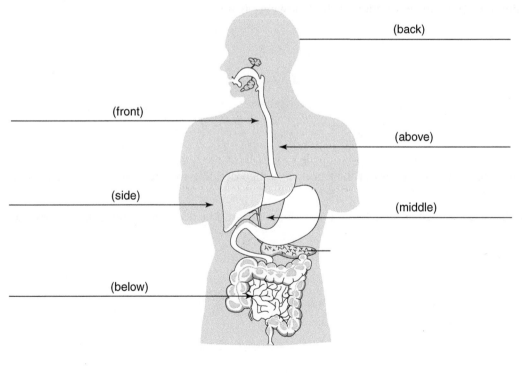

(back)

(front)

(above)

(side)

(middle)

(below)

anterior   medial
inferior   posterior
lateral   superior

© 2022 Cengage Learning. All Rights Reserved. May not be scanned, copied or duplicated, or posted to a publicly accessible website, in whole or in part.

Organ Colors

Appendix—brown
Liver—green
Small intestine—red
Pancreas—yellow
Stomach—orange

2. Write the proper abbreviations for abdominal regions.

   a. Patient a is complaining of pain in an area of the appendix. You properly identify this area as the

   _____

   b. Patient b is complaining of discomfort in an area of the stomach. You properly identify this area as the

   _____

   c. Patient c is complaining of pain over the region of the liver. You properly identify this area as the

   _____

   d. Patient d is complaining of pain over the region where the lower descending colon is located. You properly identify this area as the _____

DEVELOPING GREATER INSIGHT

1. With a partner, find the approximate location of the following organs.

   a. brain

   b. heart

   c. lung

   d. stomach

   e. liver

   f. appendix

2. Have a partner indicate pain in some part of their body and then describe the area using proper anatomic terms.

3. If available, examine models such as a skeleton, torso, or wall chart. Practice naming the major bones and organs.

© 2022 Cengage Learning. All Rights Reserved. May not be scanned, copied or duplicated, or posted to a publicly accessible website, in whole or in part.

CHAPTER 6

Classification of Disease

OBJECTIVES

After completing this chapter, you will be able to:

6-1 Spell and define terms.

6-2 Define disease and list some possible causes.

6-3 Distinguish between signs and symptoms.

6-4 List six major health problems.

6-5 Identify disease-related terms.

6-6 List ways in which a diagnosis is made.

6-7 Describe malignant and benign tumors.

VOCABULARY BUILDER

Fill-in-the-Blank

Complete each term by filling in the missing letters of words found in this unit. Use the definitions to help you determine the correct words.

1. naming the disease process	1. D _ _ _ _ _ _ _ _
2. protective body chemicals	2. — — — — — — I — —
3. seen by others	3. S — — — —
4. abnormalities present at birth	4. — — — E — — — —
5. injury	5. — — A — — —
6. new growth	6. — — — — — S —
7. treatment	7. — — E — — —

8. Define disease.

_____

9. Define etiology.

_____

© 2022 Cengage Learning. All Rights Reserved. May not be scanned, copied or duplicated, or posted to a publicly accessible website, in whole or in part.

Matching

Match each clinical condition with the proper pathological classification.

Condition

1. _____ fractured femur
2. _____ pneumonia
3. _____ spina bifida
4. _____ rectal abscess
5. _____ diabetes
6. _____ lupus erythematosus
7. _____ osteoma
8. _____ thrombosis

Classification

a. ischemia
b. congenital abnormality
c. infection
d. neoplasia
e. trauma
f. inflammation
g. metabolic imbalance
h. obstruction
i. autoimmune reaction

CHAPTER REVIEW

Matching

Match each clinical condition with the common cause or predisposing factor.

Condition

1. _____ trauma
2. _____ age
3. _____ malnutrition
4. _____ tumors
5. _____ microorganisms
6. _____ radiation
7. _____ heredity

Classification

a. external
b. internal
c. predisposing

Condition

8. _____ radiation
9. _____ rash
10. _____ nausea
11. _____ pain
12. _____ elevated temperature
13. _____ increased pulse rate
14. _____ vomiting
15. _____ flushed skin
16. _____ dizziness
17. _____ itching
18. _____ anxious feelings

Classification

a. sign
b. symptom

© 2022 Cengage Learning. All Rights Reserved. May not be scanned, copied or duplicated, or posted to a publicly accessible website, in whole or in part.

Short Answer

Complete the assessment in the space provided.

1. The body has special natural defenses. List five.

   a. _____

   b. _____

   c. _____

   d. _____

   e. _____

2. List four basic forms of therapy.

   a. _____

   b. _____

   c. _____

   d. _____

CERTIFICATION REVIEW

Complete the following multiple-choice assessments.

1. Which is an outcome related to poor nutrition?

   a. Osteoporosis

   b. Heart disease

   c. Skin breakdown

   d. High blood pressure

2. Which is an internal etiology that causes disease?

   a. Heredity

   b. Radiation

   c. Microorganisms

   d. Metabolic disorders

3. Which is a symptom of a health problem?

   a. Pain

   b. Rash

   c. Cyanosis

   d. Laceration

© 2022 Cengage Learning. All Rights Reserved. May not be scanned, copied or duplicated, or posted to a publicly accessible website, in whole or in part.

4. Which is a term related to a health problem becoming more serious?

    a. Complication

    b. Acute disease

    c. Chronic disease

    d. Acute exacerbation

5. Which term explains a localized protective reaction of tissue to irritation or injury?

    a. Infection

    b. Ischemia

    c. Complication

    d. Inflammation

6. Which situation blocks the flow of fluids in the body?

    a. Neoplasm

    b. Obstruction

    c. Autoimmune

    d. Hypersensitivity

7. Which diagnostic test uses a magnetic field to produce an image?

    a. X-ray

    b. Fluoroscopy

    c. Thermography

    d. Magnetic resonance imaging

8. Which type of therapy supports the body to return to health?

    a. Surgery

    b. Palliative

    c. Radiation

    d. Chemotherapy

9. Which is a characteristic of a benign tumor?

    a. Does not spread

    b. Causes death if untreated

    c. May have a specialized name

    d. Spreads through the bloodstream

10. What is used to prevent disease before exposure occurs?

    a. Therapy

    b. Dressings

    c. Medication

    d. Vaccination

© 2022 Cengage Learning. All Rights Reserved. May not be scanned, copied or duplicated, or posted to a publicly accessible website, in whole or in part.

CHAPTER APPLICATION

Answer the following questions in the space provided.

1. Your neighbor Elizabeth Simmons tells you she has a lump in her breast, but she has told no one else. Briefly describe how a nursing assistant should react to this situation.

_____

2. Mrs. Torres has a cerebral thrombus. Follow the maze to identify its location.

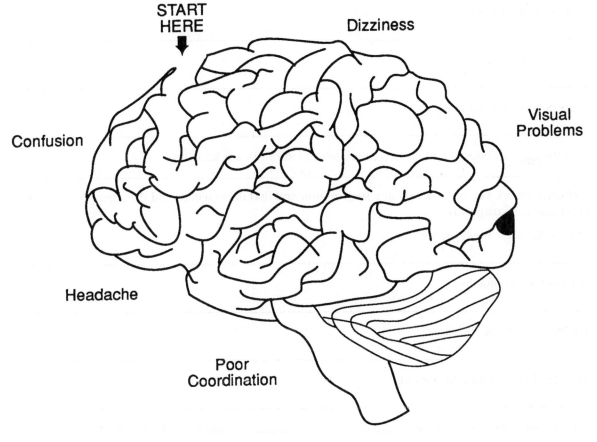

a. What part of the body is affected? _____

b. Define the words:

cerebral _____

thrombus _____

© 2022 Cengage Learning. All Rights Reserved. May not be scanned, copied or duplicated, or posted to a publicly accessible website, in whole or in part.

Short Answer

1. You are assigned to the pediatric unit and have five patients in your care. Briefly explain each of their diagnoses.

   a. Jessica R. has hemophilia.

   _____

   b Billy B. has sickle cell anemia.

   _____

   c. Jennifer F. has talipes.

   _____

   d. Casey B. has a cleft lip.

   _____

   e. Leslie S. has renal agenesis.

   _____

2. Each of the cases in question 1 falls into the classification of disease known as
   _____, or _____.

3. The following week you are working in a surgical unit and find these names and diagnoses on your assignment. Define each diagnosis.

   a. Mrs. McFarland—nephroptosis

   _____

   b. Ms. Horton—cholelithiasis

   _____

   c. Mr. Hughes—renal lithiasis

   _____

   d. Mrs. Ramirez—cerebral thrombosis

   _____

4. The conditions in question 3 involve _____ to the flow of body fluids.

5. Several of your other patients have diagnoses of metabolic imbalances. List four conditions you have learned that fall into this classification.

   a. _____

   b. _____

   c. _____

   d. _____

6. One of your patients has been admitted for surgery with a diagnosis of adenoma.
   You recognize this as a _____ involving a _____.

© 2022 Cengage Learning. All Rights Reserved. May not be scanned, copied or duplicated, or posted to a publicly accessible website, in whole or in part.

7. Mrs. Bolen has been admitted for tests because of a possible diagnosis of cancer. List six signs and symptoms of cancer you might note when caring for her.

a. _____

b. _____

c. _____

d. _____

e. _____

f. _____

DEVELOPING GREATER INSIGHT

1. Discuss the importance of mammograms with the class. Invite anyone who has had a mammogram to share her impressions of the experience, or ask a technician to discuss the procedure.

2. Review an unidentified case history of a person who suffered a stroke. Try to relate what you are hearing about the case to the material you have learned in this unit.

3. Discuss the use of ultrasound and MRI as diagnostic tools. Invite anyone who has undergone one of these tests to discuss their experience, or ask a technician to discuss the procedures.

© 2022 Cengage Learning. All Rights Reserved. May not be scanned, copied or duplicated, or posted to a publicly accessible website, in whole or in part.

Basic Human Needs and Communication

Communication Skills

OBJECTIVES

After completing this chapter, you will be able to:

7-1 Spell and define terms.

7-2 Explain types of verbal and nonverbal communication.

7-3 Demonstrate how to answer the telephone while on duty.

7-4 Describe four tools of communication for staff members.

7-5 Describe the guidelines for communicating with patients with impaired hearing.

7-6 Describe the guidelines for communicating with patients with impaired vision.

7-7 Describe the guidelines for communicating with patients with aphasia.

7-8 Describe the guidelines for communicating with patients with disorientation.

7-9 State the guidelines for working with interpreters.

VOCABULARY BUILDER

Definitions

Write each term next to the correct definition.

aphasia

communication

body language

disorientation

© 2022 Cengage Learning. All Rights Reserved. May not be scanned, copied or duplicated, or posted to a publicly accessible website, in whole or in part.

memo	nonverbal communication
eye contact	sign language
symbols	verbal communication

1. objects used to represent something else _____

2. a state of mental confusion _____

3. spoken words _____

4. inability to understand spoken or written language, or inability to express spoken or written language

_____

5. makes the greatest impression during communication and will be remembered the longest

_____

6. communicating through body movements _____

7. form of communication used by some persons with hearing impairment _____

8. communicating without oral speech _____

9. brief written communication that informs or reminds employees _____

10. exchanging information _____

Fill-in-the-Blank

Complete the following statements by selecting the correct term(s) from the list provided.

anger	articulate	caring	clearly	cues
cover	double	hand	happiness	hearing
identify	lengthy	lightly	loudness (volume)	objects
one	patronizing	sadness	see	slang
specific	substitutes	talking	tone	

1 When communicating verbally, remember to:

 a. Control the _____ of your voice.

 b. Control your voice _____.

 c. Be aware of the way you _____.

 d. Avoid _____ meanings or cultural meanings.

 e. Avoid using informal language or _____.

2. Loudness and the tone of your voice can convey a message of:

 a. _____

 b. _____

 c. _____

 d. _____

© 2022 Cengage Learning. All Rights Reserved. May not be scanned, copied or duplicated, or posted to a publicly accessible website, in whole or in part.

3. With a patient who is hard of hearing:

   a. Make sure the patient can _____ you clearly.

   b. Stand on the patient's _____ side.

   c. Do not _____ your mouth when speaking.

   d. Speak _____, distinctly, and naturally.

   e. Use _____ gestures and body language to help express your meanings.

2. With a patient who is visually impaired:

   a. Describe the environment and _____ around the patient to establish a frame of reference.

   b. Touch the patient _____ on the hand to avoid startling the patient.

   c. Be _____ when giving directions.

   d. When entering a room, _____ yourself and state your purpose.

   e. Make sure the patient is aware of the availability of _____ books.

3. With a disoriented patient:

   a. Ask the patient to do only _____ task at a time.

   b. Use word _____ if they have meaning for the patient.

   c. Be specific in speech and show respect for the patient by not being _____.

   d. Avoid _____ explanations.

   e. Use nonverbal _____ freely and respectfully.

CHAPTER REVIEW

Short Answer

Complete the assessment in the space provided.

1. Describe the purpose of each of the following.

   a. Employee's personnel handbook

   _____

   b. Disaster manual

   _____

   c. Procedure manual

   _____

   d. Nursing policy manual

   _____

   e. Assignment

   _____

© 2022 Cengage Learning. All Rights Reserved. May not be scanned, copied or duplicated, or posted to a publicly accessible website, in whole or in part.

2. List the types of information that might be learned in a staff development class.

    a. _____

    b. _____

    c. _____

    d. _____

3. List the four things needed for successful communication.

    a. _____

    b. _____

    c. _____

    d. _____

4. List six ways in which people communicate without using words.

    a. _____

    b. _____

    c. _____

    d. _____

    e. _____

    f. _____

5. State five ways you can improve communications with patients.

    a. _____

    b. _____

    c. _____

    d. _____

    e. _____

6. List three important activities that are part of active listening.

    a. _____

    b. _____

    c. _____

7. List six ways a message can be sent through body language.

    a. _____

    b. _____

    c. _____

    d. _____

    e. _____

    f. _____

© 2022 Cengage Learning. All Rights Reserved. May not be scanned, copied or duplicated, or posted to a publicly accessible website, in whole or in part.

Fill-in-the-Blank

Fill in the elements of communication.

_____ → _____ → _____ = **COMMUNICATION**

1. Your verbal message is interpreted like this:

_____% words

+ _____% tone of voice

+ _____% facial expression, body language, gestures
= 100% total communication

CERTIFICATION REVIEW

Complete the following multiple-choice assessments.

1. Which communication technique restates an understanding of what was said?

   a. Restate

   b. Interpret

   c. Repeat

   d. Paraphrase

2. Which communication technique makes the biggest impression and is remembered the best?

   a. Posture

   b. Appearance

   c. Eye contact

   d. Facial expression

3. For which reason is a memo used?

   a. Complete a performance appraisal

   b. Explain a change in unit procedure

   c. Compare changes made to policies

   d. Communicate an upcoming meeting

4. Which manual should be used if a chemical spills on the floor?

   a. Safety Data Sheet

   b. Procedure manual

   c. Personnel handbook

   d. Infection control manual

© 2022 Cengage Learning. All Rights Reserved. May not be scanned, copied or duplicated, or posted to a publicly accessible website, in whole or in part.

5. What information does the nursing assistant document in the medical record?

    a. Medications provided

    b. Response to treatments

    c. Activities of daily living

    d. Findings from an assessment

6. Which action is done when communicating with a patient who has impaired hearing?

    a. Speak loudly

    b. Shine a light on the face

    c. Cover the mouth while talking

    d. Stand on the side of the good ear

7. Which action is taken when communicating with all patients?

    a. Avoid eye contact

    b. Interrupt the patient

    c. Provide false reassurance

    d. Allow the patient to respond

8. Which action should be taken when communicating with a visually impaired patient?

    a. Move objects on the bedside stand

    b. Leave mail on the over-the-bed table

    c. Place the meal tray in front of the patient

    d. Offer to help with dressing if clothing is soiled

9. Which action helps when communicating with a patient who has aphasia?

    a. Speak loudly

    b. Face the patient

    c. Limit nonverbal cues

    d. Refrain from talking

10. Which action is taken when an interpreter is needed to communicate with a patient?

    a. Talk directly to the interpreter

    b. Address all communication to the patient

    c. Use another staff member as an interpreter

    d. Ask a family member to interpret for a patient

© 2022 Cengage Learning. All Rights Reserved. May not be scanned, copied or duplicated, or posted to a publicly accessible website, in whole or in part.

CHAPTER APPLICATION

Complete the Form.

1. Father Duchene, the priest at St. Gregory's Catholic Church, called at 10:00 a.m. on November 11 to ask how Mrs. Riley was feeling. He wanted to speak to the nurse manager, Mr. Burke, who was busy at the time and unavailable. Father Duchene asked that the nurse manager return his call. His telephone number is 555-4972. How do you communicate this information? Complete the following form to demonstrate your understanding of the proper way to do this task.

```
┌─────────────────────────────────────────┐
│  To                          ☐ URGENT    │
│  Date_____Time_____    A.M.     │
│                                  P.M.     │
│         WHILE YOU WERE OUT                │
│  From_____    │
│  Of_____    │
│  Phone_____    │
│        Area Code    Number         Ext.   │
│  ┌──────────────────┬──────────────────┐  │
│  │ Telephoned     │ │ Please call    │ │  │
│  ├──────────────────┼──────────────────┤  │
│  │ Came to see you│ │ Wants to see you│ │ │
│  ├──────────────────┼──────────────────┤  │
│  │ Returned your call│ │ Will call again│ │ │
│  └──────────────────┴──────────────────┘  │
│                                           │
│  Message _____     │
│  _____  │
│  _____  │
│  _____  │
│  _____  │
│  _____  │
│  _____  │
│                                           │
│  Signed _____     │
└─────────────────────────────────────────┘
```

Yes or No

Do the words and the body language send the same message? Circle Y for yes or N for no.

1. Y N Wendy rubs her head with her hand and tells you she does not have a headache.

2. Y N Ellen sits with her arms and legs crossed, has turned her wheelchair toward the window, and tells you she is happy to meet her new daughter-in-law.

3. Y N Aimee makes a face when you feed her and says she hates chocolate pudding.

4. Y N Mary appears on duty with dirty shoes and untidy hair, and says she is proud to be a nursing assistant.

5. Y N Chris keeps moving about the room and rubbing her hands together, and says she feels calm about her transfer to another facility.

6. Y N Nichole says she is interested in her patients. She often looks out the window and seldom makes eye contact when patients speak.

7. Y N Carrie and Terry claim to care about patients and often talk "over" them as they work together giving care.

© 2022 Cengage Learning. All Rights Reserved. May not be scanned, copied or duplicated, or posted to a publicly accessible website, in whole or in part.

8. Y   N   Tim describes himself as a caring nursing assistant. He often interrupts patients when they are talking.

9. Y   N   Fernando says he is sensitive to patients' feelings and stands about six feet away when conversing with them.

10. Y   N   Grace is careful to show caring by never discussing personal activities with other staff members in the presence of patients.

Clinical Situations

Read the following situations and answer the questions.

1. Pam Bradley has been hard of hearing since she was born. A hearing aid has helped, but she still occasionally uses sign language. Kate, the nursing assistant, likes to communicate with her this way.

    Refer to the following figures. Interpret each picture and write the message being communicated in the space provided.

    a. _____

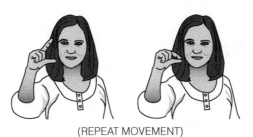

(REPEAT MOVEMENT)

    b. _____

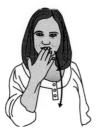 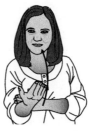

    c. _____

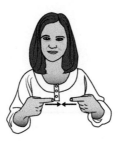

© 2022 Cengage Learning. All Rights Reserved. May not be scanned, copied or duplicated, or posted to a publicly accessible website, in whole or in part.

2. Mr. Baudine has aphasia. Communication with him has been particularly difficult for the staff. You are assigned to care for him.

a. Describe the condition of aphasia and state a common cause.

_____

_____

b. When he becomes frustrated, what action should you take?

_____

_____

c. Will raising your voice help Mr. Baudine understand?

_____

_____

d. What are two nonverbal communication techniques that speech therapists sometimes use to help patients with aphasia?

_____

_____

DEVELOPING GREATER INSIGHT

1. Check with your local college or deaf association and take a course in signing.
2. Practice taking messages over the telephone.
3. With your classmates, practice communicating the following messages without using words.

a. yes, no

b. happiness

c. pain in the abdomen

d. headache

e. depression

© 2022 Cengage Learning. All Rights Reserved. May not be scanned, copied or duplicated, or posted to a publicly accessible website, in whole or in part.

CHAPTER 8

Observation, Reporting, and Documentation

OBJECTIVES

After completing this chapter, you will be able to:

8-1 Spell and define terms.

8-2 Define each component of the nursing process.

8-3 Explain the responsibilities of the nursing assistant for each component of the nursing process.

8-4 Describe two observations to make for each body system.

8-5 State the purpose of the care plan conference.

8-6 List three times when oral reports are given.

8-7 Describe the information given when reporting.

8-8 State the purpose of the patient's medical record.

8-9 Explain the rules for documentation.

8-10 State the purpose of the HIPAA laws.

8-11 Describe the difference between an electronic medical record (EMR), an electronic patient record (EPR), an electronic health record (EHR), and a personal health record (PHR).

8-12 List at least 10 guidelines for computerized documentation.

© 2022 Cengage Learning. All Rights Reserved. May not be scanned, copied or duplicated, or posted to a publicly accessible website, in whole or in part.

VOCABULARY BUILDER

Spelling

Each line has four different spellings of a word from this unit. Circle the correctly spelled word.

1. assesment	ascesment	accessment	assessment
2. charing	charting	sharting	chartting
3. process	procese	prosess	processe
4. graphic	grephic	grafic	graffic
5. obsavation	obserbation	observation	observachian
6. communication	comunication	cummunication	communikation
7. planing	planning	planinng	pleanning
8. evaleation	evaloation	evaluation	eveluation

Matching

Match each observation on the left with the system on the right to which it most relates.

Observation

1.	_____	curled up in bed
2.	_____	disoriented as to time and place
3.	_____	regular pulse
4.	_____	elevated blood pressure
5.	_____	jaundiced skin
6.	_____	skin warm to touch
7.	_____	difficulty breathing
8.	_____	unable to respond with words
9.	_____	cloudy urine
10.	_____	site of injection hot and red
11.	_____	difficulty passing stool
12.	_____	belching frequently following a meal
13.	_____	vaginal discharge
14.	_____	drowsy, not responding well
15.	_____	nauseated, vomited small amount of clear fluid

System

a. circulatory
b. integumentary
c. muscular
d. skeletal
e. nervous
f. respiratory
g. digestive
h. endocrine
i. reproductive
j. urinary

© 2022 Cengage Learning. All Rights Reserved. May not be scanned, copied or duplicated, or posted to a publicly accessible website, in whole or in part.

CHAPTER REVIEW

Short Answer

Complete the assessment in the space provided.

1. The four steps of the nursing process and their definitions are:

   Step   **Definition**

   a. _____   _____

   b. _____   _____

   c. _____   _____

   d. _____   _____

2. What are the three types of information you will find on the care plan?

   a. _____

   b. _____

   c. _____

3. The nursing diagnosis is a statement of _____

   _____.

4. The nursing diagnosis reflects:

   a. _____

   b. _____

   c. _____

   d. _____

5. The nursing diagnosis provides the foundation for _____.

6. The nurse coordinates assessment with _____.

7. The care plan goals must be _____ in order to know if the plan is successful.

8. The intervention (approach) states:

   a. _____

   b. _____

   c. _____

9. Nursing assistants are responsible for knowing when and _____
   the approach is to be carried out and for implementing the approach _____.

10. The final step in the nursing process is the _____.

11. The nursing assistant is responsible for reporting to the nurse when _____.

12. Critical pathways detail the:

    a. _____

    b. _____

13. The critical pathway lists nursing actions to _____.

© 2022 Cengage Learning. All Rights Reserved. May not be scanned, copied or duplicated, or posted to a publicly accessible website, in whole or in part.

Matching

Name the sense used to determine each piece of information.

1. _____ body odor   a. eyes
2. _____ radial pulse   b. ears
3. _____ wheezing when the patient breathes   c. smell
4. _____ comments from the patient   d. touch
5. _____ blood in urine
6. _____ a change in the way a patient walks
7. _____ warmth of the patient's skin
8. _____ bruises
9. _____ lump under the patient's skin
10. _____ the patient crying

Matching

Match each regular time with its equivalent in international time.

Regular Time   **International Time**

1. _____ 12:30 AM   a. 1230
2. _____ 7:15 AM   b. 1915
3. _____ 2:30 PM   c. 0800
4. _____ 8 PM   d. 1430
5. _____ 4:30 PM   e. 2000
                                    f. 0030
                                    g. 0715
                                    h. 1630

Fill-in-the-Blank

Complete each statement as it relates to charting by selecting the proper word from those provided.

| blank | recommendation | background | completely | entry |
| SBAR | sequence | spell | title | cumulative |

1. Fill out new headings _____.
2. The _____ is a review of the circumstances leading up to a situation.
3. Date and time each _____.
4. Chart entries in correct _____.
5. Your _____ is what you think should to be done to correct a problem.

© 2022 Cengage Learning. All Rights Reserved. May not be scanned, copied or duplicated, or posted to a publicly accessible website, in whole or in part.

6. _____ each word correctly.

7. Leave no _____ spaces between entries.

8. Give report in _____ format.

9. Sign each entry with your first initial, last name, and _____.

10. _____ information is collected over a period of time.

Short Answer

Fill in brief answers in the spaces provided.

1. Your hospital uses a computerized documentation system. You learned how to use the computer in high school but have not used one since graduation. List four guidelines for using a computerized charting system:

   a. _____

   b. _____

   c. _____

   d. _____

2. The HIPAA laws protect all individually _____.

3. List four provisions of the HIPAA laws other than the one in question 2.

   a. _____

   b. _____

   c. _____

   d. _____

4. The _____ is a digital patient record for a single setting.

5. Information may be stored in a _____ and accessed via the Internet.

6. An _____ is an incomplete record containing information such as the patient's address, phone number, and insurance information.

7. The patient may elect to keep and control a(n) _____ to ensure that their medical information is accurate and readily available.

8. _____ is done at the patient's location at the time care is needed.

9. Personnel must use headsets if the facility uses a _____ documentation and information system.

CERTIFICATION REVIEW

Complete the following multiple-choice assessments

1. To find information about care to be given to an individual patient, you should consult the _____.

   a. patient's medical record

   b. procedure manual

   c. patient care plan

   d. nursing policy manual

© 2022 Cengage Learning. All Rights Reserved. May not be scanned, copied or duplicated, or posted to a publicly accessible website, in whole or in part.

2. For the most up-to-date information about the patient's condition, check the _____.

    a. patient's medical record

    b. nursing policy manual

    c. procedure manual

    d. patient care plan

3. The patient's medical record _____.

    a. is not a permanent document

    b. is a legal document

    c. is the nurses' responsibility

    d. may be used only while the patient is in the hospital facility

4. When you report off duty, your report should include _____.

    a. details on how your day went

    b. the care you gave each patient

    c. comments about patients not in your care

    d. observations on how well the staff got along

5. Nursing assistants may document on the _____.

    a. physician's order sheet

    b. consultant record

    c. dietary record

    d. flow sheet

6. Charting must _____.

    a. be about all the patients in one room

    b. address problems listed in the care plan

    c. include the wishes of the family

    d. be documented in subjective terms

7. When charting _____.

    a. use objective statements

    b. use complete sentences

    c. make up abbreviations to save space

    d. round off times to the closest hour

8. Your patient has a kidney condition. You should note _____.

    a. rate of respirations

    b. edema

    c. vaginal drainage

    d. appetite

© 2022 Cengage Learning. All Rights Reserved. May not be scanned, copied or duplicated, or posted to a publicly accessible website, in whole or in part.

9. Your patient has a digestive problem. You should note _____.

   a. color of sputum

   b. orientation to time

   c. belching

   d. lumps

10. Your patient has a heart problem. You should note _____.

    a. regularity of pulse

    b. mental status

    c. nasal drainage

    d. ability to walk

CHAPTER APPLICATION

Short Answer

1. Fill in the blanks in the diagram. Explain the difference between nursing diagnosis and medical diagnosis.

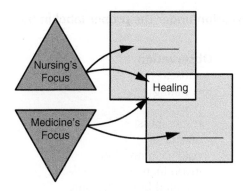

Clinical Situations

Answer the following questions in regard to this patient's care.

Robert Gonzales is 62 years of age. He has had a brain attack. He shows right-side weakness, alteration in cerebral tissue perfusion, and aphasia. The nurse has instructed you to assist with all ADLs. The patient showers. Vital signs are to be checked T.I.D.

1. How many times each day will you measure the patient's vital signs?

   _____

2. What kind of help might this patient need with ADLs?

   _____

3. What particular safety measure must you take during the shower?

   _____

© 2022 Cengage Learning. All Rights Reserved. May not be scanned, copied or duplicated, or posted to a publicly accessible website, in whole or in part.

4. What problem does the aphasia cause?

_____

5. Explain the meanings of the following conditions.

a. right-side weakness _____

_____

b. alteration in cerebral tissue perfusion _____

_____

6. Will raising your voice help Mr. Gonzales understand? Why, or why not?

_____

_____

7. What are two nonverbal communication techniques that speech therapists sometimes use to help a patient with aphasia?

a. _____

b. _____

Differentiation

Differentiate between signs and symptoms by writing each observation under the proper label in the spaces provided.

Sign	Symptom	Observation
1. _____	_____	nausea
2. _____	_____	vomiting
3. _____	_____	pain
4. _____	_____	restlessness
5. _____	_____	dizziness
6. _____	_____	cold, clammy skin
7. _____	_____	incontinence
8. _____	_____	elevated blood pressure
9. _____	_____	anxiety
10. _____	_____	cough

DEVELOPING GREATER INSIGHT

1. Examine care plans from unidentifiable patients. Try giving an oral report based on the information.

2. Select a partner. Use your senses to make observations, then describe the signs or symptoms you identify.

3. Using the unidentified care plans from question 1, document on facility flow sheets the nursing assistant care that is to be given on your shift.

© 2022 Cengage Learning. All Rights Reserved. May not be scanned, copied or duplicated, or posted to a publicly accessible website, in whole or in part.

CHAPTER **9**

Meeting Basic Human Needs

OBJECTIVES

After completing this chapter, you will be able to:

9-1 Spell and define terms.

9-2 Describe the stages of human growth and development.

9-3 Explain how the generation in which one is born affects the lives of its members.

9-4 List five physical needs of patients.

9-5 Define self-esteem.

9-6 Describe how the nursing assistant can meet the patient's emotional needs.

9-7 List nursing assistant actions to ensure that patients have the opportunity for intimacy.

9-8 Explain why cultural and spiritual beliefs influence patients' psychological responses.

9-9 Discuss methods of dealing with a fearful patient.

9-10 List guidelines to assist patients in meeting their spiritual needs.

VOCABULARY BUILDER

Matching

Match each word with the correct definition.

1. _____ period of time between newborn and the first two years of life

2. _____ introduction to the teen years for 12- to 14-year-olds

3. _____ a group of people born within the same period of time

4. _____ continuous related series of events or actions

© 2022 Cengage Learning. All Rights Reserved. May not be scanned, copied or duplicated, or posted to a publicly accessible website, in whole or in part.

5. _____ two- to three-year-olds

6. _____ physical changes that take place in the body during development

7. _____ 14- to 20-year-olds

8. _____ gradual growth

9. _____ feelings of closeness and familiarity

10. _____ person whose personal feelings about gender identity do not match the anatomical sex they were born with

11. _____ activity performed without conscious thought

12. _____ maleness or femaleness of an individual

a. continuum	b. growth	c. preadolescence	d. development
e. intimacy	f. sexuality	g. reflex	h. neonate
i. toddler	j. generation	k. transgender	l. adolescence

CHAPTER REVIEW

Matching

1. In the playroom for ambulatory patients, you find six children to check. Indicate which children are demonstrating behavior appropriate for their age group by marking A for appropriate or I for inappropriate.

   a. _____ Scott, 16, is receiving an IV and is talking to Patty, 17, who is two days postoperative following an appendectomy.

   b. _____ Bobbi, 13, is stringing beads to make a bracelet.

   c. _____ Felicia, 8, and Kimmie, 11, are playing Pokémon Monopoly.

   d. _____ Tommy, 14, and Brian, 15, are playing with the wooden cars and trucks.

   e. _____ Johnny, 2½, is playing with blocks near the older boys.

   f. _____ Doña, 3, is sitting near Joanie, pushing different-shaped blocks through the precut holes in a plastic ball.

2. Match each term with the correct explanation of sexual expression.

   a. _____ sexual attraction to members of both sexes   1. masturbation

   b. _____ self-stimulation for sexual pleasure   2. homosexuality

   c. _____ sexual attraction between members of the same sex   3. bisexuality

   d. _____ sexual attraction to members of the opposite sex   4. heterosexuality

© 2022 Cengage Learning. All Rights Reserved. May not be scanned, copied or duplicated, or posted to a publicly accessible website, in whole or in part.

Short Answer

Complete the statements in the spaces provided.

1. The stages of growth and development refer to the _____ that must be mastered before moving on to the next stage.

2. Jimmy Hinkle is 12 months old. He weighs 16 pounds and is 26 inches tall. You know this is _____ than average for his chronological age.

3. The average vocabulary of a two-year-old is about _____ words.

4. Members of each generation are affected by the same _____.

5. Five characteristics of early adulthood include the following:

   a. _____

   b. _____

   c. _____

   d. _____

   e. _____

6. The sandwich generation of middle age refers to _____
   _____

7. The time that elapses between the birth of a set of parents and the birth of their offspring is a _____
   _____

8. Later maturity is characterized by a period of _____
   _____

9. The first U.S. generation to be given a label was the _____
   _____

Short Answer

Briefly answer the following questions or directions.

1. Explain Erickson's belief regarding personality development.
   _____
   _____

2. Briefly explain Maslow's theory regarding human needs.
   _____
   _____
   _____

© 2022 Cengage Learning. All Rights Reserved. May not be scanned, copied or duplicated, or posted to a publicly accessible website, in whole or in part.

3. Complete the Chart

STAGES OF GROWTH AND DEVELOPMENT

Neonate	Birth to 1 month
Infancy	a.
b.	2–3 years
Preschool	3–5 years
School Age	5–12 years
Preadolescence	c.
Adolescence	14–20 years
d.	20–49 years
Middle Age	50–64 years
Later Maturity	e.
Old Age	75 years and beyond
f.	Category used by some experts to describe those age 85 and older

TASKS OF PERSONALITY DEVELOPMENT ACCORDING TO THE STAGES DEFINED BY ERIKSON

Physical Stage	Year of Occurrence	Tasks to Be Mastered
Oral-sensory	Birth–1 year (infant)	a.
Muscular-anal	1–3 years (toddler)	b.
Locomotor	3–5 years (preschool years)	To recognize self as a family member (Initiative)
c.	6–11 years (school-age years)	To demonstrate physical and mental skills/ abilities (Industry)
Adolescence	12–18 years	d.
e.	19–35 years	To establish intimate personal relationships with a mate (Intimacy)
Adulthood	f.	To live a satisfying and productive life
Maturity	50+ years	g.

CERTIFICATION REVIEW

Complete the following multiple-choice assessments.

1. Which is a characteristic of development?

    a. Change in height

    b. Change in weight

    c. Change in skin texture

    d. Change in psychological level

© 2022 Cengage Learning. All Rights Reserved. May not be scanned, copied or duplicated, or posted to a publicly accessible website, in whole or in part.

2. What is the developmental goal for people who are age 65 and older?

    a. Trust versus mistrust

    b. Integrity versus despair

    c. Industry versus inferiority

    d. Identity versus role confusion

3. Which is a characteristic of an infant?

    a. Can roll over

    b. Learns to control urination

    c. Becomes aware of right and wrong

    d. Becomes aware of being a separate person

4. Which characteristics identifies a school-age child?

    a. Develops rivalries with siblings

    b. Has developed fine motor skills

    c. Grows less reliant on the mother

    d. Develops a more active imagination

5. Which characteristic is common in a preadolescent patient?

    a. Gradual development of sexual maturity

    b. Conflict between independent and dependence

    c. Greater appreciation of identity as a male or female

    d. Arms and legs out of proportion to the rest of the body

6. Which is an age of optimal health?

    a. 20–49 years

    b. 50–64 years

    c. 65–75 years

    d. 75 years and older

7. Which is a basic physical need?

    a. Safety

    b. Friends

    c. Elimination

    d. Employment

8. Which action supports security and safety when caring for patients?

    a. Helping a patient with eating a meal

    b. Knowing how to respond in the event of a fire

    c. Covering a patient with a blanket during a bed bath

    d. Ensuring the temperature in the room is comfortable

© 2022 Cengage Learning. All Rights Reserved. May not be scanned, copied or duplicated, or posted to a publicly accessible website, in whole or in part.

9. Which term describes a sexual attraction to members of both sexes?

   a. Bisexuality

   b. Transgender

   c. Homosexuality

   d. Heterosexuality

10. In which way are social needs met?

    a. Giving and receiving care

    b. Daily bathing and grooming

    c. Achieving positive self-esteem

    d. Spending time in spiritual activities

CHAPTER APPLICATION

Clinical Situations

Briefly explain why you think the patient is acting this way and how you think the nursing assistant should react to the following situations.

1. Jeannie Hunt, age 16, has been diagnosed as suffering from osteosarcoma of her right tibia. Her prognosis is guarded and she has been scheduled for surgery to remove the right leg at mid-calf, to be followed by radiation. She asks to see the youth leader of her church.

   _____

   _____

2. Craig Martin, age 52, is recovering from a partial prostatectomy. He is complaining loudly about his care, the food, and the other patients in the room.

   _____

   _____

3. You are serving nourishments and find the door to Rudolph Baker's room closed.

   _____

   _____

4. You are assigned to care for the two male patients in Room 762. You have reason to believe that they may be lovers, and another nursing assistant asks you what you know about their relationship.

   _____

   _____

5. Every time you enter Belinda Mitchell's room, she makes sexual advances toward you and tries to find reasons to touch you.

   _____

   _____

© 2022 Cengage Learning. All Rights Reserved. May not be scanned, copied or duplicated, or posted to a publicly accessible website, in whole or in part.

Relating to the Nursing Process

Write the step of the nursing process that is related to each nursing assistant action.

Nursing Assistant Action	Nursing Process Step
1. The nursing assistant assists the mature adult to ambulate.	_____
2. The nursing assistant reports that the 18-month-old baby has difficulty sitting up.	_____
3. The nursing assistant reports that the teenager still appears to be having periods of depression.	_____
4. The nursing assistant pads the oxygen cannula to reduce irritation behind the patient's ears.	_____
5. The nursing assistant notifies the nurse that Mrs. Tsai has met her care plan goal for bathing two days in a row.	_____
6. The nursing assistant cleans Mr. Hernandez after he was incontinent.	_____
7. The nursing assistant notifies the nurse immediately when she finds that Kelly, age 4, has a rectal temperature of 104°F.	_____
8. The nursing assistant rocks the infant when she cries.	_____

DEVELOPING GREATER INSIGHT

1. Divide the class into pairs. Have the students in each pair identify their personal stage of growth and development and provide examples to support the level identified.

2. Have the students discuss the different approaches used to support the nutritional status of patients at each level of development.

3. Discuss with the students the order in which the following patient needs should be met, according to Maslow's hierarchy of needs.

   Bleeding

   Requesting water

   Needing to have hearing aid batteries changed

   Asking for help filling out the daily menu

   Concern that the front door at home is not locked

   Missing having family come visit every day

   Upset because has not had hair done for two weeks

   Asking if there are any library books available to read

   Requesting assistance getting to the chapel for weekly services

© 2022 Cengage Learning. All Rights Reserved. May not be scanned, copied or duplicated, or posted to a publicly accessible website, in whole or in part.

Comfort, Pain, Rest, and Sleep

OBJECTIVES

After completing this chapter, you will be able to:

10-1 Spell and define terms.

10-2 Explain how noise affects patients and hospital staff.

10-3 Explain why nursing comfort measures are important to patients' well-being.

10-4 List six observations to make and report for patients having pain.

10-5 State the purpose of the pain rating scale.

10-6 Briefly describe how a pain scale is used.

10-7 Describe nursing assistant measures to increase comfort, relieve pain, and promote rest and sleep.

10-8 Name the phases of the sleep cycle.

10-9 Describe the importance of each phase of the sleep cycle.

VOCABULARY BUILDER

Matching

Match each definition with the correct term.

1. _____ bedwetting
2. _____ sleepwalking
3. _____ grinding teeth
4. _____ the part of the sleep cycle in which dreams occur
5. _____ prolonged sleep loss, or inadequate quality or quantity of sleep
6. _____ a state of mental and physical comfort, calmness, and relaxation

a. bruxism
b. sleep
c. apnea
d. narcolepsy
e. somnambulism
f. insomnia

© 2022 Cengage Learning. All Rights Reserved. May not be scanned, copied or duplicated, or posted to a publicly accessible website, in whole or in part.

7. _____ the part of the sleep cycle that begins when the patient first falls asleep

8. _____ a disorder characterized by sleeping very late in the morning and napping during the day

9. _____ a potentially serious condition in which breathing stops for periods of 10 seconds or more during sleep

10. _____ a chronic deprivation of quality or quantity of sleep because sleep is ended or interrupted prematurely

11. _____ a state of physical and emotional well-being in which the patient is calm and relaxed, and is not in pain or upset

12. _____ a condition in which the patient has sudden, uncontrollable, unpredictable urges to fall asleep during the daytime hours

13. _____ a basic human need that consists of a period of continuous or intermittent unconsciousness in which physical movements are decreased

g. REM

h. deprivation

i. rest

j. enuresis

k. hypersomnia

l. NREM

m. comfort

CHAPTER REVIEW

Short Answer

Complete the assessment in the space provided.

1. List eight factors that may interfere with a patient's ability to sleep.

   a. _____

   b. _____

   c. _____

   d. _____

   e. _____

   f. _____

   g. _____

   h. _____

2. List eight observations that you may see, hear, feel, or smell that should be reported to the nurse regarding a patient's pain.

   a. _____

   b. _____

   c. _____

   d. _____

   e. _____

   f. _____

   g. _____

   h. _____

© 2022 Cengage Learning. All Rights Reserved. May not be scanned, copied or duplicated, or posted to a publicly accessible website, in whole or in part.

3. How is the patient's outward expression of pain affected by culture?

   _____

4. List at least eight factors that affect patients' comfort, rest, and sleep.

   a. _____

   b. _____

   c. _____

   d. _____

   e. _____

   f. _____

   g. _____

   h. _____

5. What is the purpose of the pain rating scale?

   _____

6. Why is using the pain rating scale a key to consistent pain evaluation?

   _____

7. Why is uninterrupted REM sleep important?

   _____

8. Define the following.

   a. acute pain _____

   b. radiating pain _____

   c. chronic pain _____

   d. phantom pain _____

True/False

Mark the following true or false by circling T or F.

1. T F The nurse's assessment is always more accurate than a patient's self-report of pain intensity.

2. T F A patient must be lying in bed to rest properly.

3. T F Comfort is a state of well-being.

4. T F A patient with somnambulism is at high risk of injury during sleep.

5. T F Full-color dreams occur during the NREM phase of the sleep cycle.

6. T F Elderly adults require about 5–7 hours of sleep per day.

7. T F Toddlers require 12–14 hours of sleep a day.

8. T F Phantom pain is psychological pain.

9. T F The body repairs itself during sleep.

10. T F A patient who is resting may pray or say the rosary.

11. T F Hunger and thirst do not interfere with the ability to rest when a person is sick.

© 2022 Cengage Learning. All Rights Reserved. May not be scanned, copied or duplicated, or posted to a publicly accessible website, in whole or in part.

12. T   F   Lack of privacy may affect the patient's comfort and ability to rest.

13. T   F   There are two phases of the NREM sleep cycle.

14. T   F   The patient passes into REM sleep within approximately 60–90 minutes after falling asleep.

15. T   F   Hypersomnia is a chronic deprivation of quality or quantity of sleep because sleep is ended or interrupted prematurely.

16. T   F   According to the EPA, hospital noises should not exceed 138 decibels during the day.

17. T   F   Some patients regard excessive noise as an invasion of their privacy.

18. T   F   Excessive noise has no effect on the stress level of staff.

19. T   F   Hospital workers must be active listeners for good communication.

20. T   F   Body language is not affected by pain.

21. T   F   A confused patient with garbled speech may be able to describe their pain accurately.

22. T   F   Because nurses assess pain, the nursing assistant need not bother learning about the pain scales the facility uses.

23. T   F   Unrelieved pain affects the patient's health.

24. T   F   Unrelieved pain may cause feelings of anxiety.

CERTIFICATION REVIEW

Complete the following multiple-choice assessments.

1. Which is an uncontrollable factor that contributes to discomfort?

    a. Age

    b. Odor

    c. Noise

    d. Lack of privacy

2. Which causes the highest decibel level?

    a. Hair dryer

    b. Whispering

    c. Ringing telephone

    d. Normal conversation

3. Which patient problem that is preventable slows recovery and increases health care costs?

    a. Pain

    b. Hunger

    c. Sadness

    d. Arthritis

4. Which type of pain occurs as a result of an amputation?

    a. Acute

    b. Phantom

    c. Persistent

    d. Radiating

© 2022 Cengage Learning. All Rights Reserved. May not be scanned, copied or duplicated, or posted to a publicly accessible website, in whole or in part.

5. Which action should the nursing assistant take if a patient reports pain as a level 8 an hour after receiving pain medication?

   a. Report it to the nurse

   b. Reposition the patient

   c. Ask the patient again in an hour

   d. Measure the patient's blood pressure

6. When would it be appropriate to provide care to a patient who received pain medication?

   a. Immediately afterward

   b. Several hours afterward

   c. Before the end of the shift

   d. At least 30 minutes afterward

7. Which activity helps promote a patient's rest?

   a. Backrub

   b. Mouth care

   c. Offering a cup of tea

   d. Assisting to the bathroom

8. Which patient needs the most sleep?

   a. Adolescent

   b. Young adult

   c. School-age child

   d. Preschool-age child

9. Which is a characteristic of stage 4 NREM sleep?

   a. Eyes move

   b. Full-color dreaming

   c. Incontinence may occur

   d. Feels like daydreaming

10. Which term describes grinding of the teeth?

    a. Bruxism

    b. Enuresis

    c. Narcolepsy

    d. Sleep apnea

© 2022 Cengage Learning. All Rights Reserved. May not be scanned, copied or duplicated, or posted to a publicly accessible website, in whole or in part.

CHAPTER APPLICATION

Fill-in-the-Blank

Your patient uses the horizontal numeric pain scale. The nurse gave her pain medication an hour ago. The patient tells you that her pain has increased from number 4 to number 6. You should _____

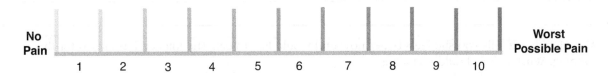

No Pain · 1 · 2 · 3 · 4 · 5 · 6 · 7 · 8 · 9 · 10 · Worst Possible Pain

Relating to the Nursing Process

1. List 10 things the nursing assistant can do to enhance comfort, rest, and sleep and relieve pain.

a. _____

b. _____

c. _____

d. _____

e. _____

f. _____

g. _____

h. _____

i. _____

j. _____

DEVELOPING GREATER INSIGHT

1. Your patient, Mrs. Hernandez, has spinal stenosis and frequently complains of pain. The nurse alternates an injection for pain with an oral medication every two hours.

a. Mrs. Hernandez is laughing and visiting with her family. When you enter the room with fresh ice water, she tells you she is in pain. Can a patient who is laughing and visiting be having pain? Explain your answer.

_____

_____

_____

_____

_____

© 2022 Cengage Learning. All Rights Reserved. May not be scanned, copied or duplicated, or posted to a publicly accessible website, in whole or in part.

b. Mrs. Hernandez refuses her supper tray. She tells you she is in too much pain to eat. What action should you take?

_____

_____

_____

_____

c. Mrs. Hernandez tells you she feels better now and would like to eat. The kitchen has closed for the evening. What action should you take?

_____

_____

_____

_____

d. Why do you think that hunger, thirst, pain, and need to use the bathroom affect patients' comfort and ability to rest or sleep?

_____

_____

_____

_____

e. Mrs. Hernandez cannot sleep. She tells you that her lower back really hurts. What nursing assistant measures can you take to help her be more comfortable?

_____

_____

_____

_____

© 2022 Cengage Learning. All Rights Reserved. May not be scanned, copied or duplicated, or posted to a publicly accessible website, in whole or in part.

CHAPTER **11**

Developing Cultural Sensitivity

OBJECTIVES

After completing this chapter, you will be able to:

11-1 Spell and define terms.

11-2 Name six major cultural groups in the United States.

11-3 Describe ways nursing assistants can develop sensitivity about cultures other than their own.

11-4 List ways the nursing assistant can help patients in practicing rituals appropriate to their cultures.

11-5 State ways the nursing assistant can demonstrate appreciation of and sensitivity to other cultures.

VOCABULARY BUILDER

Fill-in-the-Blank

Write the term for each definition.

1. customs _____

2. object used to ward off evil _____

3. rigid beliefs based on generalizations _____

4. special group within a race as defined by national origin and/or culture _____

5. ability to be aware of and to appreciate the personal characteristics of others _____

6. classification of people according to shared physical characteristics such as skin color, bone structure, facial features, hair texture, and blood type _____

© 2022 Cengage Learning. All Rights Reserved. May not be scanned, copied or duplicated, or posted to a publicly accessible website, in whole or in part.

Matching

Match each definition with correct term.

1. _____ rules
2. _____ placement of metal needles in the body
3. _____ solemn ceremonial act that reinforces faith
4. _____ parents and children living in the same household
5. _____ traditional spiritual leader, healer, or medicine man
6. _____ different terminology and usage of a common language
7. _____ father and/or mother and their children, uncles, aunts, cousins, and grandparents
8. _____ process of removing sins, diseases, and negative energy through ritual washing
9. _____ mental acceptance of and conviction in the truth, actuality, or validity of something
10. _____ the customary beliefs, social forms, and material traits of a racial, religious, or social group
11. _____ actual physical closeness that one person is comfortable with during social interaction with others
12. _____ customs and practices followed by members of a culture and passed from generation to generation
13. _____ part of a person that gives a sense of wholeness by fulfilling the need to feel connected to the world and to a higher power

a. ablutions
b. acupuncture
c. belief
d. culture
e. dialect
f. extended family
g. nuclear family
h. personal space
i. ritual
j. shaman
j. spirituality
l. standards
m. tradition

CHAPTER REVIEW

Short Answer

Briefly answer the following questions.

1. What are the six major ethnic groups in the United States?

   a. _____
   b. _____
   c. _____
   d. _____
   e. _____
   f. _____

© 2022 Cengage Learning. All Rights Reserved. May not be scanned, copied or duplicated, or posted to a publicly accessible website, in whole or in part.

2. What is meant by cross-cultural nursing?

_____

_____

3. People are classified as a race according to which shared physical characteristics?

_____

_____

_____

4. What features do members of ethnic groups have in common?

_____

_____

_____

_____

5. What are five cultural differences between ethnic groups?

a. _____

b. _____

c. _____

d. _____

e. _____

6. What are the five major religions in the United States?

a. _____

b. _____

c. _____

d. _____

e. _____

True/False

Mark the following true or false by circling T or F.

1. T   F   Family organization determines who is responsible for making health care decisions.

2. T   F   Dialects may vary between different groups that share a common culture.

3. T   F   Amish women must be covered from neck to ankles.

4. T   F   Members of Native American tribes wear short-legged underwear at all times.

5. T   F   A language learned in school is the same language that a patient will speak.

© 2022 Cengage Learning. All Rights Reserved. May not be scanned, copied or duplicated, or posted to a publicly accessible website, in whole or in part.

CERTIFICATION REVIEW

Complete the following multiple-choice assessments.

1. Which term is used to describe the way a patient follows traditions learned as a child?

   a. Mores

   b. Culture

   c. Ethnicity

   d. Stereotype

2. Which action violates a patient's personal space?

   a. Emptying a water pitcher

   b. Removing a meal tray from the room

   c. Bringing fresh linens to change the bed

   d. Touching the patient without permission

3. Which action should be done if a female patient does not want to receive care from a male nursing assistant?

   a. Document that the patient refuses care.

   b. Reassign the patient to a female nursing assistant.

   c. Ask the nurse manager to discuss the patient's lack of cooperation with care.

   d. Explain to the patient that the gender of the nursing assistant does not matter.

4. In which religion are long underwear–type garments to be worn at all times?

   a. Muslim

   b. Mormon

   c. Protestant

   d. Roman Catholic

5. Which action would the nursing assistant take to learn how to care for a patient from a different culture?

   a. Ask the health care provider the actions to take.

   b. Wait for the patient to explain what they wants done.

   c. Research the patient's cultural group on the Internet.

   d. Watch the interactions of the patient with family and other staff.

6. In which way would a nursing assistant communicate with a patient who does not understand English?

   a. Speak in a loud voice.

   b. Use common hand gestures.

   c. Explain what is to be done in English.

   d. Provide the care silently while smiling.

7. Which action should be taken if a patient's amulet is in the way of providing care?

   a. Remove the amulet.

   b. Work around the amulet.

   c. Pin the amulet to the patient's gown.

   d. Move the amulet to another body area.

© 2022 Cengage Learning. All Rights Reserved. May not be scanned, copied or duplicated, or posted to a publicly accessible website, in whole or in part.

8. Which item is considered a hot medical remedy?

   a. Milk

   b. Sage

   c. Honey

   d. Aspirin

9. Which action should be taken if a patient's clergy member arrives to visit with the patient?

   a. Provide privacy.

   b. Escort the patient and clergy to the patient lounge.

   c. Stay in the room while the clergy member is visiting.

   d. Ask the clergy member to have a seat in the waiting room.

10. Which religion uses a prayer rug as part of a religious practice?.

   a. Islam

   b. Hinduism

   c. Protestant

   d. Roman Catholic

CHAPTER APPLICATION

Relating to the Nursing Process

Write the step of the nursing process that is related to each nursing assistant action.

Nursing Assistant Action	Nursing Process Step
1. The nursing assistant reports their observations that the patient cannot speak and understand English easily.	_____
2. The nursing assistant stands at a distance that is comfortable for the patient when giving care.	_____
3. The nursing assistant asks politely about practices that are unfamiliar.	_____
4. The nursing assistant provides privacy when a spiritual advisor visits.	_____

Clinical situations

1. Your patient, Mr. Topolov, is 82 and has lived in this country for several years. He was born in China, is an Orthodox Christian, and is bilingual.

   a. Of what major ethnic group is Mr. Topolov a member?

   _____

   b. What should you do if Mr. Topolov will not take off his cross for an X-ray?

   _____

   c. What will you do when Mr. Topolov's clergy arrives for a visit?

   _____

© 2022 Cengage Learning. All Rights Reserved. May not be scanned, copied or duplicated, or posted to a publicly accessible website, in whole or in part.

2. Your patient, Ms. Ruiz, is 76. Her leg was fractured in several places when she was hit by a car. She is in balanced traction on your unit. She is originally from Costa Rica and speaks Spanish with limited English.

a. How might you improve your ability to communicate with her?

_____

_____

b. What three religious articles might be important to her?

_____

_____

c. In what religious ceremony might she wish to participate?

_____

_____

DEVELOPING GREATER INSIGHT

1. List some family practices, events, or celebrations related to your ethnicity.

2. List as many countries as you can related to the origin of people that you know. Provide as much information about each person as possible.

3. Make a list of food, music, or attire that are associated with a specific ethnicity. Discuss the items on the list with other members of the class.

© 2022 Cengage Learning. All Rights Reserved. May not be scanned, copied or duplicated, or posted to a publicly accessible website, in whole or in part.

Infection and Infection Control

C H A P T E R **12**

Infection

OBJECTIVES

After completing this chapter, you will be able to:

12-1 Spell and define terms.

12-2 Identify the most common microbes and describe some of their characteristics.

12-3 List the links in the chain of infection.

12-4 List the ways in which infectious diseases are spread.

12-5 Name and briefly describe five serious infectious diseases.

12-6 Identify the causes of several important infectious diseases.

12-7 Define spores and explain how spores differ from other pathogens.

12-8 Define biofilms and explain how they are different from other microbes.

12-9 Describe common treatments for infectious disease.

12-10 List natural body defenses against infections.

12-11 Explain why patients are at risk for infections.

© 2022 Cengage Learning. All Rights Reserved. May not be scanned, copied or duplicated, or posted to a publicly accessible website, in whole or in part.

VOCABULARY BUILDER

Matching

Match each term with its description.

1. _____ round bacterium growing in chains
2. _____ simple one-celled organisms that cause malaria
3. _____ pathogenic microbe that stimulates the production of antibodies
4. _____ systemic bacterial infection spread through the bloodstream
5. _____ capable of passing an infection to others
6. _____ visible human biofilm
7. _____ organism that grows best on living matter
8. _____ rod-shaped microbes
9. _____ microbes that grow in pairs
10. _____ microbes that grow in clusters

a. antigen
b. bacilli
c. contagious
d. streptococci
e. vector
f. parasite
g. protozoa
h. dental plaque
i. staphylococci
j. bacteremia
k. diplococci

Match each causative organism with the correct disease. Answers may be used more than once.

Disease	Organism
11. _____ diarrhea	a. bacterium
12. _____ abscess	b. virus
13. _____ gonorrhea	c. protozoan
14. _____ destroys brain tissue	d. yeast
15. _____ herpes	e. mold
16. _____ hepatitis	f. prion
17. _____ boil	
18. _____ common cold	
19. _____ toxic shock	
20. _____ athlete's foot	

CHAPTER REVIEW

Short Answer

Complete the assessment in the space provided.

1. List four external defense mechanisms against disease.

   a. _____

   b. _____

   c. _____

© 2022 Cengage Learning. All Rights Reserved. May not be scanned, copied or duplicated, or posted to a publicly accessible website, in whole or in part.

2. List four internal defense mechanisms against disease.

   a. _____

   b. _____

   c. _____

   d. _____

3. A human carrier is a person who _____

   _____

4. List the five major portals of entry.

   a. _____

   b. _____

   c. _____

   d. _____

   e. _____

5. List seven portals of exit.

   a. _____

   b. _____

   c. _____

   d. _____

   e. _____

   f. _____

   g. _____

6. The causative agent of infectious disease means the _____

   _____

7. In the health care setting, three potential reservoirs of infection must be considered and controlled. They are as follows:

   a. _____

   b. _____

   c. _____

8. List three ways microbes may be spread.

   a. _____

   b. _____

   c. _____

9. Name the six components of the chain of infection.

   a. _____

   b. _____

   c. _____

   d. _____

   e. _____

   f. _____

© 2022 Cengage Learning. All Rights Reserved. May not be scanned, copied or duplicated, or posted to a publicly accessible website, in whole or in part.

10. Three common viruses that cause hepatitis are as follows:

    a. _____

    b. _____

    c. _____

11. Why is hepatitis a major public health concern? _____

    _____

12. What organ is most commonly damaged as a result of hepatitis? _____

    _____

13. Why is proper functioning of the organ in question 10 so important to overall body function and health? _____

    _____

14. Two groups of organisms that have become resistant to methicillin and vancomycin are as follows:

    a. methicillin-resistant _____

    b. vancomycin-resistant _____

15. Explain the difference between tuberculosis infection and tuberculosis disease. _____

True/False

Mark the following true or false by circling T or F.

1. T F People who are HIV-positive are less resistant to tuberculosis.
2. T F The barrier that forms around the tuberculosis infection is called an abscess.
3. T F Weight gain is a sign associated with tuberculosis infection.
4. T F A positive Mantoux test indicates the presence of antibodies to tuberculosis.
5. T F HIV is much more infectious than hepatitis B.
6. T F Renal failure is a possible complication of infection with *E. coli* 0157:H7.
7. T F *C. difficile* is not commonly contracted in health care facilities.
8. T F Infection with *C. difficile* causes severe diarrhea.
9. T F Pseudomembranous colitis is a very serious condition.
10. T F Hantavirus is transmitted from person to person in respiratory secretions.
11. T F Bioterrorism involves the use of biological agents for terrorist purposes.
12. T F Cutaneous anthrax can be passed from one person to another by skin contact.
13. T F *Klebsiella* normally resides in the colon, where it takes part in normal bowel function.
14. T F Listeria cannot contaminate cooked hot dogs.
15. T F *Acinetobacter baumannii* is a common cause of pneumonia.
16. T F *Aspergillosis* is a serious bacterial infection.
17. T F *Streptococcus* B can cause necrotizing fasciitis.

© 2022 Cengage Learning. All Rights Reserved. May not be scanned, copied or duplicated, or posted to a publicly accessible website, in whole or in part.

18. T F Necrotizing fasciitis causes tissue death.
19. T F Necrotizing fasciitis is not painful.
20. T F Necrotizing fasciitis can cause organ failure.
21. T F Prompt diagnosis and treatment are essential for a positive outcome with strep A infection.
22. T F Spores cannot spread disease.
23. T F Spores cannot live long in a dormant form.
24. T F Spores are readily eliminated with alcohol and many disinfectants.
25. T F Rotavirus and norovirus cause infectious diarrhea.
26. T F Rotavirus and norovirus remain active on the hands for at least four hours and on wet surfaces for weeks.
27. T F Shingles are not contagious.
28. T F A patient who is jaundiced will have a gray tinge to the skin.
29. T F Scientists believe that prion disease is spread by very close person-to-person contact.
30. T F Biofilms are readily eliminated by hospital-grade disinfectants.
31. T F Nits are easily removed by brushing them off the hair and scalp.
32. T F The scabies mite is a parasite.
33. T F Scabies is rarely contagious.
34. T F Bedbugs are imaginary pests from a nursery rhyme.
35. T F Dark spots in the bed are a strong indication that bedbugs are present.
36. T F Bedbugs can live on bats, chickens, pigeons, other birds, laboratory animals, and some domestic pets.
37. T F Bedbugs can live for up to a year without food.

CERTIFICATION REVIEW

Complete the following multiple choice assessments.

1. Which microbe is named according to shape and arrangement?

   a. Virus

   b. Fungus

   c. Bacteria

   d. Protozoa

2. What causes drug-resistant organisms to develop?

   a. Poor handwashing

   b. Overuse of antibiotics

   c. Insufficient oral hygiene

   d. Inconsistent body hygiene

© 2022 Cengage Learning. All Rights Reserved. May not be scanned, copied or duplicated, or posted to a publicly accessible website, in whole or in part.

3. What is an example of a biofilm?

   a. Scab

   b. Peritoneum

   c. Dental plaque

   d. Granulation tissue

4. In which way is an infection stopped from spreading?

   a. Provide prophylactic antibiotics.

   b. Ingest adequate vitamins everyday.

   c. Ensure adequate moisture for the skin.

   d. Break one link in the chain of infection.

5. In which way are droplets transmitted?

   a. Singing

   b. Clothing

   c. Touching

   d. Dressings

6. Which infection is the most expensive condition treated in U.S. hospitals each year?

   a. Boil

   b. Sepsis

   c. Abscess

   d. Pneumonia

7. Which response occurs when a pathogen enters the body?

   a. Sequestration of antigens

   b. Development of antibodies

   c. Activation of inflammation

   d. Elevation of body temperature

8. At which time is a Mantoux test evaluated for results?

   a. After 1 day

   b. In 1 week

   c. Immediately

   d. Between 48 and 72 hours

9. In which way are spores removed from the hands?

   a. Rinsing with hot water

   b. Cleansing with waterless cleanser

   c. Washing with soap, water, and friction

   d. Pouring rubbing alcohol over the hands

© 2022 Cengage Learning. All Rights Reserved. May not be scanned, copied or duplicated, or posted to a publicly accessible website, in whole or in part.

10. What should be done if a patient develops a rash?

    a. Apply lotion over the area.

    b. Notify the nurse immediately.

    c. Wrap the area with clean gauze.

    d. Cleanse the area with soap and water.

CHAPTER APPLICATION

Clinical Situations

1. Your patient, Alan Corbin, is 19 years old and is in end-stage AIDS. Mark the following statements true or false to demonstrate your understanding of the disease.

    a. T F The disease is caused by a bacterium.

    b. T F Everyone who comes in contact with the patient's blood will contract AIDS.

    c. T F An asymptomatic period may last from months to years following infection.

    d. T F Progression of the disease is determined by the effect of the viruses on the red blood cells.

    e. T F AIDS suppresses the immune system.

    f. T F Drug resistance is not a problem with HIV disease and AIDS.

    g. T F Drug therapy is used to cure the disease.

    h. T F There is no evidence that touching or hugging a patient with AIDS will transmit the disease.

    i. T F HIV can be transmitted by unsterile instruments used in medical procedures and tattooing.

2. Amy Lee, age 87, was admitted to your unit. Her admission diagnosis was lobar pneumonia. Her initial vital signs were: T 104.4°F; P 112; R 24 (labored). She is 5 feet 6 inches tall and weighs 89 pounds. She is in generally poor health, presenting with a history of emphysema and congestive heart failure. Identify three types of pathogens that can cause pneumonia.

    a. _____

    b. _____

    c. _____

3. Mrs. Bustemonte is 67 years of age and a patient on your unit. She has been diagnosed with carbapenem-resistant *Enterobacteriaceae* (CRE). In the following list, circle four actions you should take to prevent the spread of this infection to other patients.

respiratory precautions	standard precautions	good hand hygiene	strict isolation
medical asepsis	wear a mask	standard precautions	bathe the patient twice a day

© 2022 Cengage Learning. All Rights Reserved. May not be scanned, copied or duplicated, or posted to a publicly accessible website, in whole or in part.

4. Complete the chain of infection.

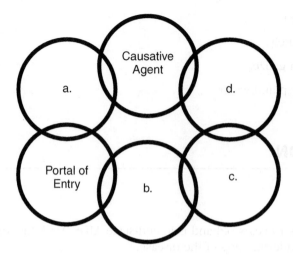

a. _____

b. _____

c. _____

d. _____

5. If one link in the chain of infection is broken, _____

_____

6. Give four examples of fomites found in the health care facility.

a. _____

b. _____

c. _____

d. _____

RELATING TO THE NURSING PROCESS

Write the nursing process step defined by the action in the space provided.

Nursing Assistant Action	**Nursing Process Step**
1. The nursing assistant reports an elevation of Mr. Bergen's temperature and redness near his infusion site.	_____
2. The nursing assistant makes sure that Mr. Popejoy, who has pneumonia, has plenty of tissues and a place to dispose of them.	_____
3. The nursing assistant reports that Mr. Menendez is coughing frequently as he is admitted.	_____

© 2022 Cengage Learning. All Rights Reserved. May not be scanned, copied or duplicated, or posted to a publicly accessible website, in whole or in part.

DEVELOPING GREATER INSIGHT

Match each action with the related portion of breaking the chain of infection.

1. _____ receiving antibiotics when infected
2. _____ disinfecting bedpans
3. _____ covering a draining pressure ulcer
4. _____ not coming to work when you have a cold
5. _____ putting a Band-Aid over a cut in your skin

a. protecting the portal of entry
b. protecting the portal of exit
c. protecting a susceptible host
d. controlling the causative agents
e. eliminating the reservoir

6. Discuss with the class the value of immunization procedures. Try to answer the following:

a. Which vaccines are commonly given?

b. When should vaccines be given?

c. How do vaccines offer protection?

d. Are there some infections for which there are no immunizations?

© 2022 Cengage Learning. All Rights Reserved. May not be scanned, copied or duplicated, or posted to a publicly accessible website, in whole or in part.

Infection Control

OBJECTIVES

After completing this chapter, you will be able to:

13-1 Spell and define terms.

13-2 Explain the principles of medical asepsis.

13-3 State the purpose of standard precautions.

13-4 List the types of personal protective equipment.

13-5 State the purpose of each type of personal protective equipment.

13-6 Describe nursing assistant actions related to standard precautions.

13-7 Describe airborne, droplet, and contact precautions.

13-8 Demonstrate the following procedures:

- Procedure 1: Handwashing
- Procedure 2: Putting on a Mask
- Procedure 3: Putting on a Gown
- Procedure 4: Putting on Gloves
- Procedure 5: Removing Contaminated Gloves
- Procedure 6: Removing Contaminated Gloves, Eye Protection, Gown, and Mask
- Procedure 7: Serving a Meal in an Isolation Unit
- Procedure 8: Measuring Vital Signs in an Isolation Unit
- Procedure 9: Transferring Nondisposable Equipment Outside of the Isolation Unit
- Procedure 10: Specimen Collection from a Patient in an Isolation Unit (Expand Your Skills)
- Procedure 11: Caring for Linens in an Isolation Unit
- Procedure 12: Transporting a Patient to and from the Isolation Unit
- Procedure 13: Opening a Sterile Package

© 2022 Cengage Learning. All Rights Reserved. May not be scanned, copied or duplicated, or posted to a publicly accessible website, in whole or in part.

VOCABULARY BUILDER

Matching

Match each term with its definition.

1. _____ spreads long distances in the air on dust and moisture

2. _____ Centers for Disease Control and Prevention

3. _____ an infectious disease easily transmitted to others

4. _____ protective hand coverings

5. _____ expendable

6. _____ separate ill patients from others

7. _____ entryway to AIIR room

8. _____ eye protection that is always worn with a mask

9. _____ one type of mask used for airborne precautions

10. _____ human immunodeficiency virus

11. _____ pressure air flow that is used in an airborne precautions room

12. _____ contaminated

13. _____ precautions that are used any time contact with blood, body fluid, secretions, excretions, mucous membranes, or nonintact skin is likely

14. _____ PPE that covers the uniform

a. anteroom

b. disposable

c. HIV

d. CDC

e. standard

f. HEPA

g. dirty

h. droplet

i. communicable

j. gloves

k. gown

l. isolate

m. goggles

CHAPTER REVIEW

True/False

Mark the following true or false by circling T or F.

1. T   F   Linens found on a linen cart are considered clean.

2. T   F   Linens that have touched the floor are clean as long as the floor is not wet.

3. T   F   Medical aseptic techniques destroy all organisms on an item.

4. T   F   One patient's items may be used by another as long as the first patient does not have a communicable disease.

5. T   F   Handwashing is not necessary if gloves were worn during patient care.

6. T   F   You can safely touch environmental surfaces with used gloves as long as the gloves are not contaminated with blood.

7. T   F   The nursing assistant is responsible for understanding the principles of standard precautions and selecting personal protective equipment appropriate to the procedure.

8. T   F   Wash your gloves promptly if they become soiled.

© 2022 Cengage Learning. All Rights Reserved. May not be scanned, copied or duplicated, or posted to a publicly accessible website, in whole or in part.

9. T   F   Artificial nails are usually acceptable for health care workers as long as they have been professionally applied.

10. T   F   The housekeeping cart and the clean linens cart should be positioned close to each other in the hallway.

11. T   F   Personal medical asepsis includes a daily bath.

12. T   F   Complete personal protective equipment is required when working with all patients.

When washing hands correctly:

13. T   F   Always use cool water.

14. T   F   Lean against the sink so no water will get on the floor.

15. T   F   A soap dispenser is preferable to a bar of soap.

16. T   F   Always rinse the bar of soap (if used) after use.

17. T   F   Turn faucets on and off with gloves.

18. T   F   Always point fingertips up when washing.

19. T   F   It is the use of soap that actually removes microbes from hands.

20. T   F   Hands can be washed effectively in 5 to 10 seconds.

21. T   F   Alcohol-based gel may be used instead of handwashing, unless the hands are visibly soiled.

22. T   F   When using an alcohol-based hand cleaner, rub the product into all surfaces for at least 15 seconds.

Short Answer

Complete the statements in the spaces provided.

1. The purpose of transmission-based precautions is _____

_____.

2. Apply a _____when you enter a droplet precautions room.

3. Isolation is the responsibility of _____

4. The purpose of wearing a mask and gown in the isolation unit is to _____

_____.

5. Gloves should be used whenever there may be contact with _____

_____.

6. To be effective, a mask must cover both _____ and _____.

7. To be effective, a gown should _____ correctly.

8. The contaminated gown should be folded _____ before you dispose of it in the proper receptacle.

9. Disposable equipment is used only _____.

10. List seven secretions or excretions that are potentially infectious.

  a. _____

  b. _____

© 2022 Cengage Learning. All Rights Reserved. May not be scanned, copied or duplicated, or posted to a publicly accessible website, in whole or in part.

c. _____

d. _____

e. _____

f. _____

g. _____

11. Breaks in the skin of a health care worker should be immediately treated by _____ and applying
_____.

12. What must be done before these items are used?

    stethoscope   bathtub

    shower chair   wheelchair

    _____.

Short Answer

Complete the assessment in the space provided.

1. State the type of infection control that is used in all situations in which care providers may contact body fluids. _____

2. List the three types of transmission-based precautions.

    a. _____

    b. _____

    c. _____

3. List three ways communicable diseases may be spread.

    a. _____

    b. _____

    c. _____

4. List six articles to be placed on a cart outside an isolation room.

    a. _____

    b. _____

    c. _____

    d. _____

    e. _____

    f. _____

5. State the sequence for applying personal protective equipment.

    a. _____

    b. _____

    c. _____

    d. _____

© 2022 Cengage Learning. All Rights Reserved. May not be scanned, copied or duplicated, or posted to a publicly accessible website, in whole or in part.

6. List seven precautions to keep in mind when handling soiled linens.

   a. _____

   b. _____

   c. _____

   d. _____

   e. _____

   f. _____

   g. _____

7. State the measures that are to be taken to care for vital sign equipment used with a patient in isolation.

   a. _____

   b. _____

8. Explain what to do with food not eaten by a patient in isolation. _____

   _____

9. Name the type of bag that is used for the transport of specimens. _____

   _____

10. Name two ways of sterilizing an item.

    a. _____

    b. _____

11. List three respiratory hygiene/cough etiquette practices that patients should be instructed to follow to prevent the spread of infection.

    a. _____

    b. _____

    c. _____

12. UVGI:

    a. Uses _____ light in the _____ or _____.

    b. The purpose of UVGI is to _____.

    c. Does the UVGI light remain on 24 hours a day? _____

    d. Does the radiation emitted from the bright UVGI harm patients' or staff members' eyes? _____

13. When entering the room of a patient who is in isolation for chickenpox, what PPE should you apply?

    _____

    _____

    _____

14. List at least three reasons for wearing gloves. _____

    _____

    _____

© 2022 Cengage Learning. All Rights Reserved. May not be scanned, copied or duplicated, or posted to a publicly accessible website, in whole or in part.

15. List at least five situations when gloves should be worn.

_____

_____

_____

_____

_____

16. Where is PPE removed when leaving a contact precautions room?

_____

_____

17. Where should the respirator be removed when you have finished working in an airborne precautions room?

_____

_____

18. What should be done with the face mask when leaving the room of a patient who is on droplet precautions?

_____

_____

CERTIFICATION REVIEW

Complete the following multiple-choice assessments.

1. Which is the most important method of preventing the spread of infection?

    a. Handwashing

    b. Receiving vaccinations

    c. Discarding used tissues

    d. Changing bed linens every day

2. Which action needs to be taken when using an alcohol-based hand rub?

    a. Wash afterward with soap and water.

    b. Dry excess product with paper towels.

    c. Rinse the hands with hot water after rubbing the hands.

    d. Rub the product for 20 to 30 seconds and allow to air dry.

3. Which action should be taken first if an exposure incident occurs on nonintact skin?

    a. Report it to the nurse.

    b. Complete an incident report.

    c. Wash the area with soap and water.

    d. Blot the area with disposable towels.

© 2022 Cengage Learning. All Rights Reserved. May not be scanned, copied or duplicated, or posted to a publicly accessible website, in whole or in part.

4. Which action should be taken if goggles are required and the staff member wears glasses?

   a. Remove the glasses.

   b. Use the glasses as the goggles.

   c. Tape the goggle over the glasses.

   d. Place the goggles over the glasses.

5. Which type of transmission-based precaution is used for influenza?

   a. Airborne

   b. Contact

   c. Droplet

   d. Reverse

6. Which is a characteristic of a high-efficiency particulate air (HEPA) filter mask?

   a. Disposed after each use

   b. Can be shared between users

   c. Must be professionally fitted

   d. Cleansed with alcohol after use

7. Which should be done for a patient who needs contact precautions?

   a. Apply gloves before providing care.

   b. Place a mask on the patient when leaving the room.

   c. Place in a room with a patient with the same type of infection.

   d. Wear a mask, gown, gloves, and goggles when providing care.

8. Which personal protective equipment should be applied first?

   a. Mask

   b. Gown

   c. Gloves

   d. Goggles

9. Which personal protective equipment should be removed first?

   a. Mask

   b. Gown

   c. Gloves

   d. Goggles

10. Which action is done before using equipment for surgical asepsis?

   a. Cleansing

   b. Protection

   c. Disinfection

   d. Sterilization

© 2022 Cengage Learning. All Rights Reserved. May not be scanned, copied or duplicated, or posted to a publicly accessible website, in whole or in part.

CHAPTER APPLICATION

Clinical Situations

Briefly describe how a nursing assistant should react to the following situations.

1. You saw an airborne precautions sign on Mr. Keene's door. You are assigned to serve his breakfast tray.

   _____

   _____

   _____

2. You are responsible for caring for nondisposable equipment from a contact precautions unit.

   _____

   _____

Identification

1. Identify each sign and indicate the type of precaution to be used.

   a.

   _____

   _____

   b.

   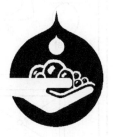

   _____

   _____

© 2022 Cengage Learning. All Rights Reserved. May not be scanned, copied or duplicated, or posted to a publicly accessible website, in whole or in part.

c.

_____

_____

d.

_____

_____

e.

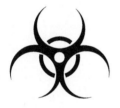

_____

_____

2. Label the diagram of the isolation room.

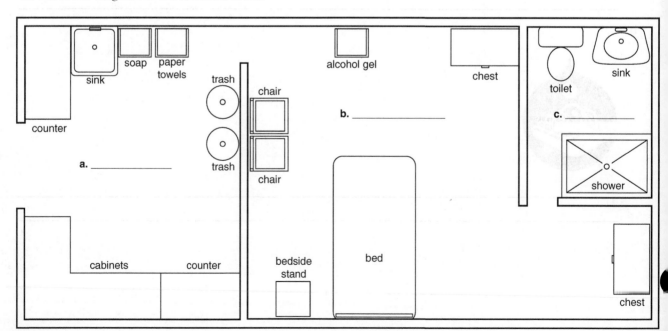

© 2022 Cengage Learning. All Rights Reserved. May not be scanned, copied or duplicated, or posted to a publicly accessible website, in whole or in part.

a. _____

b. _____

c. _____

3. Identify what is wrong with each picture. What should be done to correct it?

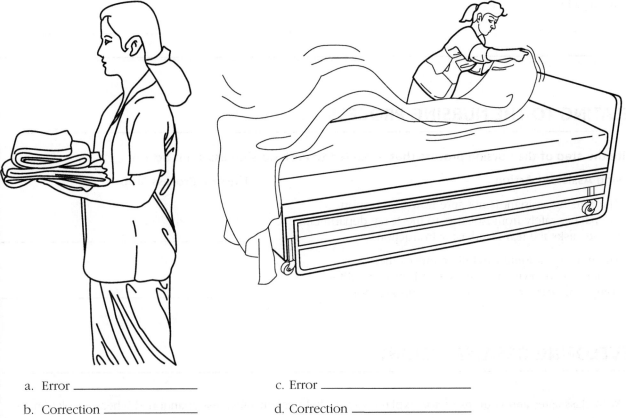

a. Error _____   c. Error _____

b. Correction _____   d. Correction _____

4. What is wrong with the figure on the left? Correct it in the figure on the right. Use the empty bedside table to demonstrate the correction by locating the articles properly or writing in the words.

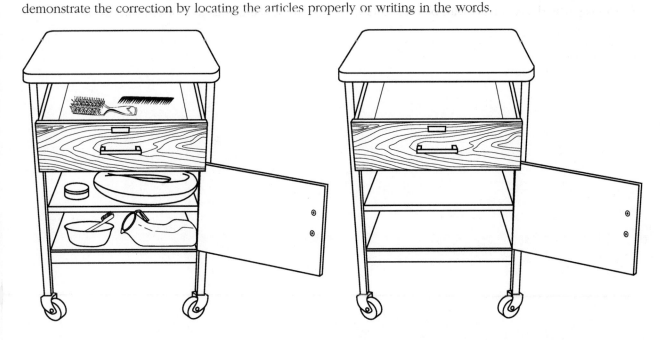

© 2022 Cengage Learning. All Rights Reserved. May not be scanned, copied or duplicated, or posted to a publicly accessible website, in whole or in part.

a. Error: _____

b. Correction: _____

5. Briefly explain how the nursing assistant should react to the following. You are assisting the nurse in setting up a sterile field to change a surgical dressing. You open some 4 × 4 gauze pads and reach across the field and place them on the towel. The nurse tells you the setup cannot be used and must be discarded and set up again. Why?

_____

_____

RELATING TO THE NURSING PROCESS

Write the step of the nursing process that is related to each nursing assistant action.

Nursing Assistant Action	Nursing Process Step
1. The nursing assistant is not sure how to transport the patient safely from isolation to the X-ray department, so they asks the team leader for instructions.	_____
2. The nursing assistant carefully removes their contaminatedgown and disposes of it properly after completing care in the contact precautions room.	_____

DEVELOPING GREATER INSIGHT

1. With classmates and your instructor, explain ways to help patients feel less abandoned when in isolation.

2. Investigate the transmission-based isolation precautions in your facility and report back to the class.

3. Discuss why direct contact with blood and body fluids can be dangerous to a health care worker.

© 2022 Cengage Learning. All Rights Reserved. May not be scanned, copied or duplicated, or posted to a publicly accessible website, in whole or in part.

Safety and Mobility

C H A P T E R **14**

Environmental and Nursing Assistant Safety

OBJECTIVES

After completing this chapter, you will be able to:

14-1 Spell and define terms.

14-2 Describe the health care facility environment.

14-3 Identify measures to promote environmental safety.

14-4 List situations when equipment must be repaired.

14-5 Describe the elements required for fire.

14-6 List five measures to prevent a fire.

14-7 Describe the procedure to follow if a fire occurs.

14-8 Demonstrate the use of a fire extinguisher.

14-9 List techniques for using ergonomics on the job.

14-10 Demonstrate appropriate body mechanics.

14-11 Describe the types of information contained in Safety Data Sheets (SDS).

© 2022 Cengage Learning. All Rights Reserved. May not be scanned, copied or duplicated, or posted to a publicly accessible website, in whole or in part.

VOCABULARY BUILDER

Spelling

Each line has four different spellings of a word from this unit. Circle the correctly spelled word.

1. incident	incedent	incidant	incydent
2. ralys	rails	riles	rhales
3. warde	werd	ward	whard
4. privite	privat	pryvate	private
5. ergonomecs	ergonomics	erkonomics	ergonomicks
6. concurent	concurrent	concurrant	concarrent
7. seme private	semiprivote	semepryvate	semiprivate
8. envyromental	environmantyl	environmental	enviromental

Matching

Match each term with the correct definition.

1. _____ room with one bed
2. _____ daily care of equipment
3. _____ condition of an entire facility
4. _____ what to do when a fire occurs
5. _____ what to do to use a fire extinguisher
6. _____ lists what to do for a hazardous exposure
7. _____ form that explains an unexpected occurrence

a. concurrent cleaning
b. environmental safety
c. incident report
d. PASS
e. private room
f. RACE
g. Safety Data Sheet (SDS)

CHAPTER REVIEW

Fill-in-the-Blank

Complete the statements related to safety practices by selecting the correct term from the list provided.

alcohol	all health care	available to the patient	calm
checked	concern	electrical	fuel
grounded	hazard	heat	incident
indirect	locked	SDS	nail polish remover
never	oils	OSHA	oxygen
patients	right away	screens, curtains	shut off
supervisor	tagged	upright	work
work-related	71	ungloved hands	importance

© 2022 Cengage Learning. All Rights Reserved. May not be scanned, copied or duplicated, or posted to a publicly accessible website, in whole or in part.

1. Keeping the environment safe and clean is the responsibility of _____ workers.

2. Prevention of injuries to patients and others is of primary _____.

3. Wheels should always be _____ unless a bed is being moved.

4. The best temperature for the patient's room is about _____ degrees.

5. The best way to shield patients from drafts is by _____ or _____.

6. The best kind of light is _____.

7. When leaving a patient's room, be sure that the ceiling lights are _____.

8. Report frayed _____ cords at once.

9. For safety, never pick up broken glass with _____.

10. An unexpected, undesirable event that occurs in a health care facility is called an _____.

11. Broken electrical equipment must be _____.

12. Mechanical lifts should be _____ before use.

13. Plugs that are not properly _____ are a fire hazard.

14. Smoking in bed should _____ be permitted.

15. Make sure the call signal (call light) is always _____.

16. The three elements that form the fire triangle are _____, _____, and _____.

17. Possible fire hazards should be reported _____ to the _____.

18. When oxygen is in use, flammable liquids such as _____, _____, or _____ should not be used.

19. A fire extinguisher should be carried in the _____ position.

20. When there is an emergency, it is very important for you to keep _____.

21. When there is a fire, always move _____ to safety first.

22. The term *ergonomic* refers to _____ musculoskeletal conditions.

23. The federal agency that is responsible for employee safety is called _____.

24. By law, hazards communication information called _____ must be supplied by manufacturers.

Short Answer

Complete the assessment in the space provided.

1. Briefly list seven items you would expect to find in a patient's environment.

    a. _____

    b. _____

    c. _____

    d. _____

    e. _____

    f. _____

    g. _____

© 2022 Cengage Learning. All Rights Reserved. May not be scanned, copied or duplicated, or posted to a publicly accessible website, in whole or in part.

2. Name two pieces of fire control equipment.

   a. _____

   b. _____

3. The acronym PASS is important for fire control. The:

   a. P stands for _____.

   b. A stands for _____.

   c. S stands for _____.

   d. S stands for _____.

4. List six ergonomic techniques you can use to decrease the risk of injury.

   a. _____

   b. _____

   c. _____

   d. _____

   e. _____

   f. _____

5. State five types of information you expect to learn from the SDS of a product.

   a. _____

   b. _____

   c. _____

   d. _____

   e. _____

6. List four potential benefits of using side rails.

   a. _____

   b. _____

   c. _____

   d. _____

7. List six potential risks of using side rails.

   a. _____

   b. _____

   c. _____

   d. _____

   e. _____

   f. _____

© 2022 Cengage Learning. All Rights Reserved. May not be scanned, copied or duplicated, or posted to a publicly accessible website, in whole or in part.

8. List five areas that are usually equipped with emergency lighting in the event of a power failure.

a. _____

b. _____

c. _____

d. _____

e. _____

9. List six methods of preventing a fire.

a. _____

b. _____

c. _____

d. _____

e. _____

f. _____

10. Draw the fire triangle, showing its elements.

CERTIFICATION REVIEW

Complete the following multiple-choice assessments.

1. Which is a part of the patient unit?

a. Chair

b. Toilet

c. Room door

d. Bathroom sink

2. For which reason is a gatch handle used?

a. Signal for help.

b. Lower the bedside table.

c. Adjust the oxygen concentrator.

d. Change the position on a nonelectric bed.

3. Which type of light may be used for catheterization?

a. Flashlight

b. Night light

c. Ceiling light

d. Over bed light

4. What should be done with a patient's personal care items?

a. Placed in the bathroom

b. Placed in a community area

c. Stored under the patient's bed

d. Labeled with the patient's name

© 2022 Cengage Learning. All Rights Reserved. May not be scanned, copied or duplicated, or posted to a publicly accessible website, in whole or in part.

5. Which should be the priority when providing patient care?

    a. Safety

    b. Comfort

    c. Hygiene

    d. Communication

6. What should be done to ensure proper functioning of the sprinkler system?

    a. Run water in the bathroom sink.

    b. Keep items 18 inches from the ceiling.

    c. Limit the use of showers to the morning.

    d. Make sure the lights are properly working.

7. In addition to heat and fuel, what else is needed for a fire to occur?

    a. Oil

    b. Paper

    c. Plastic

    d. Oxygen

8. Which type of fire extinguisher is used for an electrical fire?

    a. A

    b. B

    c. C

    d. K

9. Which is the first action when a fire occurs?

    a. Alarm.

    b. Contain the fire.

    c. Remove patients.

    d. Extinguish the fire.

10. Which is the first action when using a fire extinguisher?

    a. Pull the pin.

    b. Aim the nozzle.

    c. Squeeze the handle.

    d. Sweep over the fire.

© 2022 Cengage Learning. All Rights Reserved. May not be scanned, copied or duplicated, or posted to a publicly accessible website, in whole or in part.

CHAPTER APPLICTION

Hidden Picture

Look carefully at the picture and list each violation of a safety measure in the space provided.

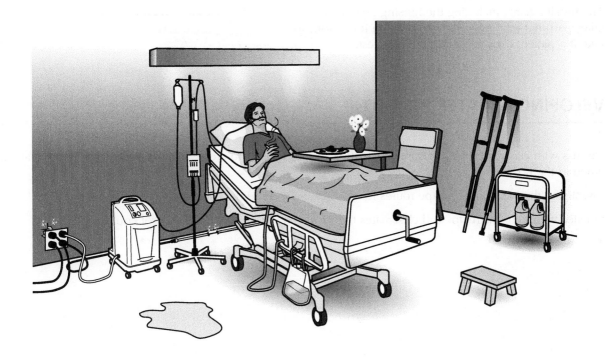

1. _____
2. _____
3. _____
4. _____
5. _____
6. _____
7. _____
8. _____
9. _____
10. _____
11. _____
12. _____
13. _____
14. _____
15. _____

© 2022 Cengage Learning. All Rights Reserved. May not be scanned, copied or duplicated, or posted to a publicly accessible website, in whole or in part.

RELATING TO THE NURSING PROCESS

Write the step of the nursing process that is related to each nursing assistant action.

Nursing Assistant Action   **Nursing Process Step**

1. The nursing assistant participates in a conference   _____
   regarding patient evacuation in case of an emergency.

2. The nursing team, including the nursing assistants,   _____
   takes part in a training session to prepare for actions to
   take if a patient experiences a cardiac arrest.

DEVELOPING GREATER INSIGHT

1. Discuss with classmates why consistent attention to safety helps to create feelings of security for the patient when in the hospital.

2. Investigate the location of escape routes for your facility. Locate the escape plan on your unit.

3. Practice with your instructor and classmates the proper way to operate fire control equipment.

© 2022 Cengage Learning. All Rights Reserved. May not be scanned, copied or duplicated, or posted to a publicly accessible website, in whole or in part.

CHAPTER 15

Patient Safety and Positioning

OBJECTIVES

After completing this chapter, you will be able to:

15-1 Spell and define terms.

15-2 Identify patients who are at risk for having incidents.

15-3 List alternatives to the use of physical restraints.

15-4 Describe the guidelines for the use of restraints.

15-5 Demonstrate the correct application of restraints.

15-6 Describe two measures for preventing accidental poisoning, thermal injuries, skin injuries, and choking.

15-7 List the elements that are common to all procedures.

15-8 Describe correct body alignment for the patient.

15-9 List the purposes of repositioning patients.

15-10 State the purpose of assistive moving devices.

15-11 Demonstrate these positions using the correct supportive devices: supine, semisupine, prone, semiprone, lateral, Fowler's, and orthopneic.

15-12 Demonstrate the following procedures:

- Procedure 14: Turning the Patient Toward You
- Procedure 15: Turning the Patient Away from You
- Procedure 16: Moving a Patient to the Head of the Bed (Expand Your Skills)
- Procedure 17: Logrolling the Patient (Expand Your Skills)

© 2022 Cengage Learning. All Rights Reserved. May not be scanned, copied or duplicated, or posted to a publicly accessible website, in whole or in part.

VOCABULARY BUILDER

Matching

Match each term to its definition.

1. _____ on the back

2. _____ ability to move

3. _____ another term for orthosis

4. _____ involving muscle contractions

5. _____ device that inhibits movement

6. _____ steps to follow to carry out a task

7. _____ devices for maintaining the position of extremities

8. _____ occurs when muscles become fixed in one position

a. spasms

b. orthoses

c. restraint

d. mobility

e. contracture

f. supine

g. procedure

h. splint

Matching

Match each term with the correct definition.

1. _____ flat slippery sheet

2. _____ side-lying position

3. _____ sitting position in bed

4. _____ lying on the abdomen

5. _____ folded large sheet or half-sheet

6. _____ capable of burning living tissue

7. _____ involuntary muscle contraction

8. _____ move from one position to another

9. _____ bath blanket rolled into 12-inch-long shape

10. _____ item to maintain body position and alignment

11. _____ position to use when a patient is in a wheelchair

12. _____ accidental entry of food or a foreign object into the trachea

a. 90-90-90 position

b. aspiration

c. caustic

d. draw sheet

e. Fowler's position

f. lateral

g. postural support

h. prone

i. slider

j. spasticity

k. transfer

l. trochanter roll

© 2022 Cengage Learning. All Rights Reserved. May not be scanned, copied or duplicated, or posted to a publicly accessible website, in whole or in part.

CHAPTER REVIEW

Fill-in-the-Blank

Complete the statements in the spaces provided.

1. Before beginning any patient contact, you must _____ and _____.

2. A good principle to follow is never to attempt to move a patient who weighs more than you do if you are
_____

3. A heavy or helpless patient can be more easily positioned in bed if a _____ is used.

4. A good way to help a patient maintain a side-lying position is to form a pillow roll and place it _____
_____
_____

5. Before rolling a patient away from you, be sure the _____.

6. When moving the patient to the head of the bed, the nursing assistant should _____
the head of the bed.

7. The patient's position must be changed at least every_____.

8. When a patient is in the prone position, the bed is in the _____ position and the
patient is placed on their _____.

9. Two forms of restraint are _____ and _____.

10. When restraints are released, the patient must be _____.

11. Three incidents that may occur are _____, _____, and
_____ injury.

True/False

Mark the following true or false by circling T or F.

1. T   F   Restraints should be used only as a last resort.

2. T   F   Side rails may safely be left down when restraints are in use.

3. T   F   Restraints should be secured to the immovable part of the bed frame.

4. T   F   To prevent accidental poisoning, store a patient's personal food items in the bedside table.

5. T   F   When preparing bath water, always turn the hot water on last.

6. T   F   Using a microwave oven to reheat foods is safe and economical because food is evenly heated.

7. T   F   Always knock before entering a room.

8. T   F   Special boots or shoes may be worn in bed to maintain feet in the proper alignment.

9. T   F   A patient positioned on their left side should be moved to the left side of the bed.

10. T   F   A trochanter roll should extend from under the arm, along the trunk, to the top of the hip.

© 2022 Cengage Learning. All Rights Reserved. May not be scanned, copied or duplicated, or posted to a publicly accessible website, in whole or in part.

Short Answer

Briefly explain the reasoning behind each of the following statements.

1. To lift, the nursing assistant should use leg muscles and shoulder muscles—not the muscles of the back. Why?

   _____

   _____

   _____

2. Proper positioning of the patient's body must be conscientiously done because

   _____

   _____

   _____

3. The staff must take specific steps before applying restraints. What are these steps, and why must they be done?

   _____

   _____

   _____

CERTIFICATION REVIEW

Complete the following multiple-choice assessments.

1. What must be done before applying a restraint on a patient?

   a. Obtain a physician's order.

   b. Ask the patient for permission.

   c. Take the patient to the bathroom.

   d. Measure the patient's current weight.

2. Which device helps to prevent falls when ambulating a patient?

   a. Cane

   b. Walker

   c. Gait belt

   d. Crutches

3. Which item can be used to prevent a patient from pulling on tubes?

   a. Hand mitt

   b. Vest restraint

   c. Wrist restraint

   d. Wheelchair belt

© 2022 Cengage Learning. All Rights Reserved. May not be scanned, copied or duplicated, or posted to a publicly accessible website, in whole or in part.

4. Which approach is used to ensure the safety of a patient with a seizure disorder?

   a. Pad the side rails.

   b. Apply a vest restraint.

   c. Remove wrist restraints.

   d. Keep all side rails raised at all times.

5. Which action is done for a patient who is being restrained?

   a. Unlock the wheels on the bed.

   b. Provide sedation before restraining.

   c. Pull the draw curtains around the bed.

   d. Release the restraint every 2 hours for 10 minutes.

6. In which way can a patient's fragile skin be protected?

   a. Cover with clothing.

   b. Apply petroleum jelly.

   c. Keep the skin open to air.

   d. Cleanse daily with soap and water.

7. Which action should be taken before performing any procedure?

   a. Wash hands.

   b. Set up supplies.

   c. Identify yourself.

   d. Provide for privacy.

8. Which action should be taken first after completing a procedure?

   a. Wash hands.

   b. Remove gloves.

   c. Remove used equipment.

   d. Provide for patient privacy.

9. What should be done before moving a patient from one surface to another?

   a. Position the patient for comfort.

   b. Place a draw sheet under the patient.

   c. Ensure the surfaces are of the same height.

   d. Have the patient cross the arms over the chest.

10. Which position is used to administer an enema?

   a. Sims'

   b. Prone

   c. Supine

   d. Fowler's

© 2022 Cengage Learning. All Rights Reserved. May not be scanned, copied or duplicated, or posted to a publicly accessible website, in whole or in part.

CHAPTER APPLICATION

Name the Position

In the space provided, name each position pictured.

1. _____

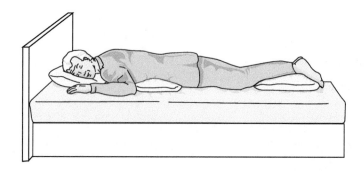

2. _____

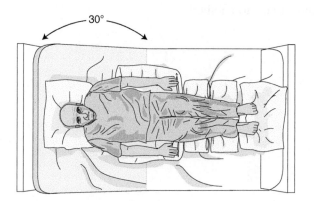

3. _____

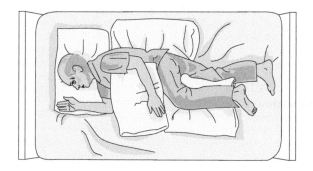

© 2022 Cengage Learning. All Rights Reserved. May not be scanned, copied or duplicated, or posted to a publicly accessible website, in whole or in part.

Clinical Situations

Complete the assessment in the space provided.

1. Mrs. Grover wears a hearing aid and glasses. She has difficulty ambulating and is unsteady on her feet. She is sometimes disoriented and tends to wander in search of food when she becomes hungry. List ways a nursing assistant might protect this patient and avoid the need for protective restraints.

   a. _____

   b. _____

   c. _____

   d. _____

   e. _____

   f. _____

2. What might be done if physical restraint alternatives fail and the protocol for restraints has been followed?

   a. _____

   b. _____

3. Mr. Kinsey is 82 years of age, weighs 215 pounds, and has a respiratory problem (emphysema). He tends to slide to the foot of the bed and often complains of feeling uncomfortable. What action should you take when you find him in this position?

   a. _____

   b. _____

   c. _____

4. Mr. Milhouse is 91 years old and has had difficulty swallowing since suffering from stroke. His left side is paralyzed, and he needs assistance feeding himself. What might the nursing assistant do to help avoid aspiration?

   a. _____

   b. _____

   c. _____

DEVELOPING GREATER INSIGHT

1. Divide the class into groups of two or three. With one person acting as the patient, have classmates practice positioning the patient using proper supportive devices.

2. With classmates, practice applying restraints on one another, leaving them in place for 15 minutes. Think how you would feel if you wanted a drink of water or had to use the bathroom and no one was nearby to help you.

3. With classmates, practice positioning each other in the four basic patient positions.

© 2022 Cengage Learning. All Rights Reserved. May not be scanned, copied or duplicated, or posted to a publicly accessible website, in whole or in part.

CHAPTER 16

The Patient's Mobility: Transfer Skills

OBJECTIVES

After completing this chapter, you will be able to:

16-1 Spell and define terms.

16-2 List at least seven factors to consider before lifting or moving a patient to determine whether additional equipment or assistance is necessary.

16-3 Demonstrate the principles of good body mechanics and ergonomics to moving and transferring patients.

16-4 List the guidelines for safe transfers.

16-5 Describe the difference between a standing transfer and a sitting transfer.

16-6 List the guidelines for using the manual handling sling.

16-7 List the guidelines for using the pivot disk.

16-8 Demonstrate correct application and use of a transfer belt.

16-9 Demonstrate the following procedures:

- Procedure 18: Applying a Transfer Belt
- Procedure 19: Transferring the Patient from Bed to Chair—One Assistant
- Procedure 20: Transferring the Patient from Bed to Chair—Two Assistants (Expand Your Skills)
- Procedure 21: Sliding-Board Transfer from Bed to Wheelchair (Expand Your Skills)
- Procedure 22: Transferring the Patient from Chair to Bed—One Assistant
- Procedure 23: Transferring the Patient from Chair to Bed—Two Assistants (Expand Your Skills)
- Procedure 24: Transferring the Patient from Bed to Stretcher (Expand Your Skills)
- Procedure 25: Transferring the Patient from Stretcher to Bed (Expand Your Skills)
- Procedure 26: Transferring the Patient with a Mechanical Lift (Expand Your Skills)
- Procedure 27: Transferring the Patient onto and off of the Toilet (Expand Your Skills)

© 2022 Cengage Learning. All Rights Reserved. May not be scanned, copied or duplicated, or posted to a publicly accessible website, in whole or in part.

VOCABULARY BUILDER

Fill-in-the-Blank

Complete each sentence using the best term. Select terms from the list provided.

dependent	full weight-	gait	paralyzed
partial weight-	pivot	self	sitting

1. A mechanical lift may be used to transfer a _____ patient.
2. Having the ability to stand on both legs is called _____ bearing.
3. The ability to stand on one leg is called _____ bearing.
4. A _____ patient does not have the ability to move.
5. A transfer belt is also called a _____ belt.
6. To _____ means to turn the entire body to one side.

Matching

Match each term with its definition.

1. _____ weakness of an extremity
2. _____ inability to move extremities
3. _____ manually operated hydraulic lift
4. _____ ability to stand on one or both legs
5. _____ webbed belt used as a safety device
6. _____ unable to place full weight on the legs
7. _____ moving a patient by hand or bodily force
8. _____ situation in which something is not indicated
9. _____ moving to another surface in a seated position
10. _____ plastic or wooden board with a slippery surface
11. _____ moving from one surface to another while standing

a. contraindication
b. manual patient handling
c. mechanical lift
d. nonweight-bearing (NWB)
e. paralysis
f. paresis
g. sitting (lateral) transfer
h. sliding board
i. standing transfer
j. transfer belt
k. weight-bearing (WB)

CHAPTER REVIEW

Short Answer

Complete each statement in the space provided.

1. Before attempting to move a patient, always determine if _____ is needed.
2. Before transferring a patient from bed to chair, you should know whether the patient is _____-bearing.

© 2022 Cengage Learning. All Rights Reserved. May not be scanned, copied or duplicated, or posted to a publicly accessible website, in whole or in part.

3. When assisting the patient from bed to wheelchair, make sure that the footrests are _____.

4. When moving a patient with a mechanical lift, make sure the sling is positioned from _____ to _____.

5. Four people should be positioned to move an unconscious person from a stretcher to bed, as follows:

_____

_____

_____

_____

Corrections

Correct the statements that are wrong by crossing out the incorrect word or words. Write the correct words under them. Do not make any changes to the correct statements.

1. Know a patient's capabilities before attempting a transfer.

_____

2. Allow patients to place their hands around your neck.

_____

3. Use a lift sheet for standing transfers.

_____

4. Always explain the transfer plan to the patient.

_____

5. Transfer patients toward their weakest side.

_____

6. Patient shoes should have smooth soles and heels.

_____

7. Placing your hands under the patient's arms is acceptable during transfers.

_____

8. IVs, drainage bags, and other items must be considered during a transfer.

_____

9. Give patients who are transferring only the assistance they needs.

_____

10. Before making a transfer, the bed should be in the high horizontal position.

_____

11. Always use correct body mechanics when making transfers.

_____

12. During transfer, encourage patients to focus their eyes on your hands.

_____

13. Stand close to the patient during a transfer.

_____

© 2022 Cengage Learning. All Rights Reserved. May not be scanned, copied or duplicated, or posted to a publicly accessible website, in whole or in part.

True/False

Mark the following true or false by circling T or F.

1. T F A transfer belt is used to assist patients to transfer.
2. T F A transfer belt can be used to lift a patient who has no ability to bear weight.
3. T F A transfer belt should be applied under the patient's clothing.
4. T F Always apply a transfer belt with the patient lying on their side.
5. T F The buckle of the transfer belt should be positioned in the front.
6. T F The transfer belt should be positioned around a female patient's breasts.
7. T F The transfer belt should be held using an underhand grasp.
8. T F The use of a transfer belt is contraindicated for a patient with an abdominal aneurysm.
9. T F The transfer belt can be removed after the transfer is complete.
10. T F The transfer belt should be very tight.
11. T F Two 16-year-old nursing assistants may not operate the mechanical lift in the skills lab for the nursing assistant class.
12. T F The maximum weight capacity for the pivot disk is about 250 to 300 pounds.
13. T F Close the leg spreader before moving a patient in the mechanical lift.
14. T F Transferring patients into and out of vehicles is a high-risk task.
15. T F A manual handling sling helps make you stronger.
16. T F Position the small part of the front caster wheels facing forward and lock the brakes during transfers and when a wheelchair is parked.

CERTIFICATION REVIEW

Complete the following multiple-choice assessments.

1. What does a "zero-lift" policy mean?

    a. Never lift a box

    b. Never lift a patient

    c. Never lift equipment

    d. Never do manual lifting

2. For which patient situation would a transfer belt be avoided?

    a. Obesity

    b. Weakness

    c. Colostomy

    d. Joint replacement

© 2022 Cengage Learning. All Rights Reserved. May not be scanned, copied or duplicated, or posted to a publicly accessible website, in whole or in part.

3. Which type of device is a walker with a seat for the patient to rest if needed?

   a. Rollator

   b. Standing lifter

   c. Merry motivator

   d. Merry stand by me

4. Which device is used to pivot a patient for seated or standing transfers?

   a. Rollator

   b. Swivel disk

   c. Transfer belt

   d. Handling sling

5. Which is an advantage of using a manual handling sling?

   a. Prevents falls.

   b. Stabilizes the patient.

   c. Provides better control.

   d. Ensures ease of moving between surfaces.

6. Which patient characteristic is required when performing a sliding-board transfer?

   a. Sitting balance

   b. Ability to stand

   c. Strong thigh muscles

   d. Maximum foot control

7. What should be done when using a mechanical lift?

   a. Place shoes on the patient's feet.

   b. Place padding on the sling surface.

   c. Ask someone to assist with the lift.

   d. Prepare the seated surface with a bath blanket.

8. Which item is needed to transfer a patient to use the toilet?

   a. Sink

   b. Wall rail

   c. Towel rack

   d. Elevated commode seat

9. What should be done after transferring a patient to the bathtub?

   a. Cover the back with a bath blanket.

   b. Turn on the cold water before the hot.

   c. Hand the patient a handheld shower head.

   d. Place a slip-proof mat on the floor of the tub.

© 2022 Cengage Learning. All Rights Reserved. May not be scanned, copied or duplicated, or posted to a publicly accessible website, in whole or in part.

10. What should be done when transferring a patient into a car?

    a. Use the front seat

    b. Use the back seat

    c. Loosen the seat belt

    d. Recline the back of the seat

CHAPTER APPLICATION

Clinical Situations

Briefly describe how a nursing assistant should react in the following situations.

1. There is no one available in the radiology department when you arrive. You need help to move a patient.

2. Your heavy patient is unable to help himself. He has returned from physical therapy and is sitting in a wheelchair waiting to be returned to bed.

3. You must assist one other person to transfer a conscious patient from a stretcher to bed following an X-ray.

4. You are assigned to use a mechanical lift to transfer a patient to a chair. The sling is frayed where it hooks onto the lift frame.

5. Mr. Dunn is able to be up but is unstable when standing. He needs to empty his bladder.

© 2022 Cengage Learning. All Rights Reserved. May not be scanned, copied or duplicated, or posted to a publicly accessible website, in whole or in part.

Identification

Look carefully at each picture. List the corrections that should be made in each.

1.

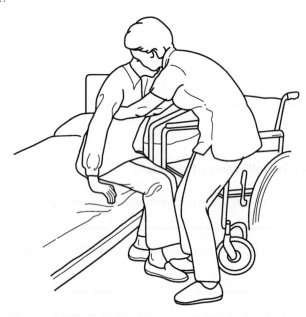

Corrections

a. _____
b. _____
c. _____

2.

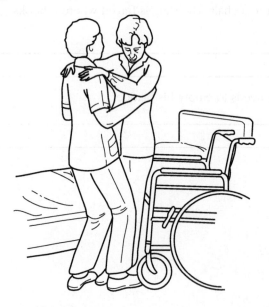

Corrections

a. _____
b. _____
c. _____

© 2022 Cengage Learning. All Rights Reserved. May not be scanned, copied or duplicated, or posted to a publicly accessible website, in whole or in part.

3.

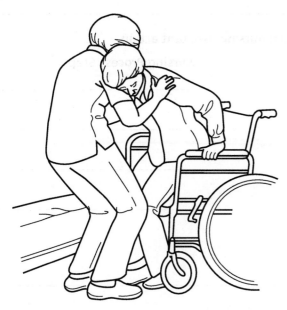

Corrections

a. _____

b. _____

c. _____

4.

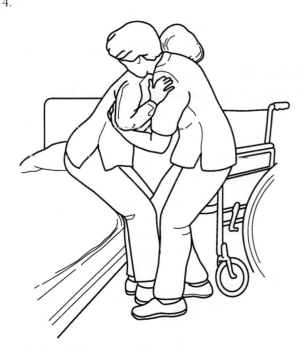

Corrections

a. _____

b. _____

c. _____

© 2022 Cengage Learning. All Rights Reserved. May not be scanned, copied or duplicated, or posted to a publicly accessible website, in whole or in part.

RELATING TO THE NURSING PROCESS

Write the step of the nursing process that is related to each nursing assistant action.

Nursing Assistant Action	Nursing Process Step
1. The nursing assistant carefully applies the transfer belt.	_____
2. The nursing assistant reports that the patient weighs 216 pounds and is paralyzed on the right side.	_____
3. The nursing assistant assembles all needed equipment at the bedside before attempting a transfer.	_____
4. The nursing assistant carefully checks the mechanical lift before using it.	_____

DEVELOPING GREATER INSIGHT

1. With classmates, practice transferring one another from bed to chair using one and then two assistants. Follow these special directions.

   a. Patient: put one arm in a sling and do not use it in the transfer.

   b. Patient: stand on right foot but bear no weight on the left.

2. Apply a transfer belt that is:

   a. too loose.

   b. too tight.

3. Practice using a mechanical lift. Select a student to act as the patient.

4. Discuss why, when assisting a patient to get up or down, the patient should not place their hands on the body of the nursing assistant.

© 2022 Cengage Learning. All Rights Reserved. May not be scanned, copied or duplicated, or posted to a publicly accessible website, in whole or in part.

CHAPTER 17

The Patient's Mobility: Ambulation

OBJECTIVES

After completing this chapter, you will be able to:

17-1 Spell and define terms.
17-2 Describe the purpose of assistive devices used in ambulation.
17-3 List safety measures for using assistive ambulation devices.
17-4 Describe safety measures for using a wheelchair.
17-5 Describe nursing assistant actions for:
  • Ambulating a patient using a gait belt.
  • Propelling a patient in a wheelchair.
  • Positioning a patient in a wheelchair.
  • Transporting a patient on a stretcher.
17-6 Demonstrate the following procedures:
  • Procedure 28: Assisting the Patient to Walk with a Cane and Three-Point Gait
  • Procedure 29: Assisting the Patient to Walk with a Walker and Three-Point Gait
  • Procedure 30: Assisting the Falling Patient (Expand Your Skills)

VOCABULARY BUILDER

Matching

Match each term with the correct definition.

1. _____ to walk
2. _____ artificial body part
3. _____ the way a person walks
4. _____ related to bones and muscles
5. _____ item that makes walking easier and safer

a. ambulate
b. assistive device
c. orthopedic
d. prosthesis
e. gait

© 2022 Cengage Learning. All Rights Reserved. May not be scanned, copied or duplicated, or posted to a publicly accessible website, in whole or in part.

Fill-in-the-Blank

Complete the following statements in the spaces provided. Select terms from the list provided.

affected	ambulation	arms	ball	four	heel
joint	need	ninety	rails	right	shoes
spills	strong	swinging	unsafe		

1. Walking is also known as _____.

2. In normal walking, the _____ strikes the floor before the _____ of the foot.

3. During walking, the arms normally have a slight _____ movement.

4. To walk safely, the patient must have adequate _____ motion.

5. The type of assistive device selected depends upon a particular patient's _____.

6. Patients should be encouraged to use hand _____ when walking.

7. When walking with a patient, the nursing assistant should stand on the patient's _____ side.

8. The nursing assistant should always check floors for clutter or _____.

9. No assistive device should be used if it is _____.

10. When forearm crutches with platforms are used, the elbows are constantly at a _____-degree angle to the shoulder.

11. When patients ambulate, clothes should not hang down over the _____.

12. A patient needs strength in both _____ to safely use a walker.

13. When ambulating with a walker, the patient shifts weight to the _____ leg as the walker is lifted and moved forward.

14. A wheelchair that fits properly will have about _____ inches between the top of the back and the patient's axillae.

15. When the feet are on the footrests of a wheelchair, the feet should be at _____ degrees to the legs.

CHAPTER REVIEW

True/False

Mark the following true or false by circling T or F.

1. T F   The arthritic patient has involuntary movements that disturb balance.

2. T F   Protheses are used by patients who have had amputations, to aid mobility.

3. T F   Before initiating an ambulation program, a physical therapist evaluates the patient.

4. T F   If a patient requires assistance but is using a cane, a gait belt need not be used.

5. T F   Quad canes provide a narrow base of support.

6. T F   Canes are recommended for aiding balance rather than providing support.

7. T F   A walker should be narrow so the patient can walk behind it.

© 2022 Cengage Learning. All Rights Reserved. May not be scanned, copied or duplicated, or posted to a publicly accessible website, in whole or in part.

8. T   F   The walker can safely be used as a transfer device.

9. T   F   Patients who are ambulating with a walker may use a two-point or three-point gait.

10. T   F   A wheelchair that fits the patient properly will have a two- to three-inch clearance between the front edge of the seat and the back of the patient's knees.

Short Answer

Complete the assessment in the space provided.

1. List six disorders that may affect a person's gait.

    a. _____

    b. _____

    c. _____

    d. _____

    e. _____

    f. _____

2. Identify eight abilities that must be evaluated by a therapist before an ambulation program may be started.

    a. _____

    b. _____

    c. _____

    d. _____

    e. _____

    f. _____

    g. _____

    h. _____

3. Name three commonly used assistive devices.

    a. _____

    b. _____

    c. _____

4. Explain why standard crutches are seldom recommended for older adults.

5. Explain the value of encouraging patients to do wheelchair push-ups.

6. List six guidelines for safely transporting a patient on a stretcher.

    a. _____

    b. _____

    c. _____

    d. _____

    e. _____

    f. _____

© 2022 Cengage Learning. All Rights Reserved. May not be scanned, copied or duplicated, or posted to a publicly accessible website, in whole or in part.

7. List six observations to make and report about a patient's ability to ambulate and the amount of assistance required.

a. _____

b. _____

c. _____

d. _____

e. _____

f. _____

CHAPTER REVIEW

Complete the following multiple-choice assessments.

1. Which term describes moving about in a wheelchair?

   a. Self-propel

   b. Locomotion

   c. Range of motion

   d. Assistive ambulation

2. In which position does walking begin?

   a. Having ankle in dorsiflexion.

   b. Heel striking the floor.

   c. Bring the other leg forward.

   d. Rolling onto the ball of the foot.

3. Which action will be taken when ambulating a patient?

   a. Limit the use of a gait belt.

   b. Encourage use of the handrail.

   c. Stand on the patient's strong side.

   d. Remind the patient to take off shoes.

4. For which reason will a patient use a cane?

   a. Uneven gait

   b. Leg weakness

   c. Support balance

   d. Partial weight bearing

5. Which instruction will a patient be provided when using a cane?

   a. Hold the cane on the stronger side.

   b. Move the weak leg forward ahead of the cane.

   c. Shift weight to the weak leg and advance the cane half a foot.

   d. Place the tip of the cane 1 inch on the side of the weaker foot.

© 2022 Cengage Learning. All Rights Reserved. May not be scanned, copied or duplicated, or posted to a publicly accessible website, in whole or in part.

6. Which action will be taken when ambulating a patient with a walker?

   a. Apply slippers or socks

   b. Stand on the person's weak side

   c. Remove the gait belt before ambulating

   d. Instruct to advance the walker while standing on the weak leg

7. Which action will be taken if a patient begins to fall?

   a. Search for help.

   b. Grasp the transfer belt.

   c. Attempt to break the patient's fall.

   d. Bend as the patient falls to the floor.

8. Which action ensures safety when using a wheelchair?

   a. Remove pillows and props.

   b. Replace the armrest if removed.

   c. Lower footrests when getting into the chair.

   d. Position with the knees higher than the hips.

9. Which action relieves pressure on the buttocks when in a wheelchair?

   a. Lean backward.

   b. Wheelchair push-ups.

   c. Elevate the legs on the footrests.

   d. Place the knees higher than the hips.

10. Which action will be taken when transporting a patient on a stretcher?

    a. Apply the safety belt.

    b. Enter the elevator feet first.

    c. Raise one side of the side rails.

    d. Stand at the foot of the stretcher.

CHAPTER APPLICATION

Clinical Situations

Briefly describe how a nursing assistant should react to the following situations.

1. Mrs. Keane is poststroke and weak on her left side. She uses a walker when walking. You note that the hand grip is cracked and one of the bolt nuts is missing.

   _____

   _____

   _____

© 2022 Cengage Learning. All Rights Reserved. May not be scanned, copied or duplicated, or posted to a publicly accessible website, in whole or in part.

2. Mr. Jacks is using a walker for stability because he is still weak following abdominal surgery for colon cancer. You notice that he seems fatigued after walking the length of the corridor away from his room.

_____

_____

_____

3. Mrs. De Koniger is ambulating with her walker. As she moves across the room, she moves her walker 15 inches in front of her, putting her weight on her weak leg as she brings her strong foot forward.

_____

_____

_____

4. You enter Ebony Norman's room and find her on the floor. She is bleeding from somewhere on her scalp and is more confused than usual. She points at the corner and says, "He pushed me." There is no one else in the room.

_____

_____

_____

Identification

1. Circle the letter of the figure below that shows the proper way to approach a closed door with a wheelchair.

A.   B.

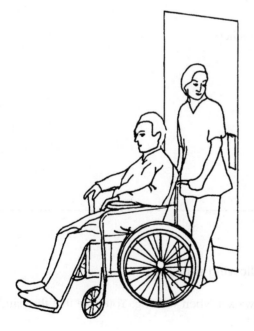   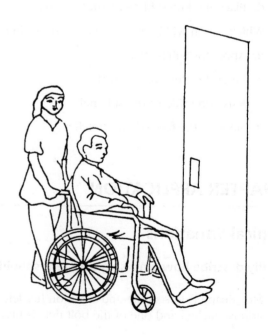

© 2022 Cengage Learning. All Rights Reserved. May not be scanned, copied or duplicated, or posted to a publicly accessible website, in whole or in part.

RELATING TO THE NURSING PROCESS

Write the step of the nursing process that is related to each nursing assistant action.

Nursing Assistant Action   **Nursing Process Step**

1. Two nursing assistants use a small sheet under the patient's
   buttocks to move the patient up in his wheelchair.   _____

2. The nursing assistant reports to the nurse that the patient wishes to
   ambulate but has only poorly fitting slippers at the bedside.   _____

3. The nursing assistant uses alcohol and cotton swabs to clean
   debris out of the ridges of a cane tip.   _____

4. The nursing assistant picks up old newspapers from the floor
   and disposes of them.   _____

DEVELOPING GREATER INSIGHT

1. Try sitting in a wheelchair for one hour without moving anything other than your arms. Discuss your reaction and concerns with your classmates.

2. Gather different types of assistive devices. Practice using them yourself. Discuss any problems with your instructor.

3. Select one student to be the patient and others to be nursing assistants. Practice assisting the patient who has slipped down in the wheelchair to regain proper alignment.

© 2022 Cengage Learning. All Rights Reserved. May not be scanned, copied or duplicated, or posted to a publicly accessible website, in whole or in part.

Measuring and Recording Vital Signs, Height, and Weight

CHAPTER **18**

Body Temperature

OBJECTIVES

After completing this chapter, you will be able to:

18-1 Spell and define terms.

18-2 Explain the uses of the three types of clinical thermometers.

18-3 Read a thermometer.

18-4 Identify the range of normal temperature values.

18-5 Demonstrate the following procedures:

- Procedure 31: Measuring an Oral Temperature (Electronic Thermometer)
- Procedure 32: Measuring a Rectal Temperature (Electronic Thermometer)
- Procedure 33: Measuring an Axillary Temperature (Electronic Thermometer)
- Procedure 34: Measuring a Tympanic Temperature
- Procedure 35: Measuring a Temporal Artery Temperature

© 2022 Cengage Learning. All Rights Reserved. May not be scanned, copied or duplicated, or posted to a publicly accessible website, in whole or in part.

VOCABULARY BUILDER

Definitions

Define the terms in the spaces provided.

1. body core

_____

2. body shell

_____

3. probe

_____

4. tympanic

_____

5. vital signs

_____

Matching

Match each term with the correct definition.

1. _____ notation to follow up
2. _____ exposure to high temperatures
3. _____ lowering of core body temperature
4. _____ device used to measure temperature
5. _____ chemical reaction that produces heat
6. _____ device that displays a measurement with numbers
7. _____ condition caused by inability to regulate temperature
8. _____ scale used in countries that follow the metric system
9. _____ device most commonly used to measure temperature
10. _____ scale used in the United States to measure temperature
11. _____ measures temperature using skin on the side of the head

a. Celsius scale
b. clinical thermometer
c. digital thermometer
d. electronic thermometer
e. Fahrenheit scale
f. flagged
g. heat exhaustion
h. heat stroke
i. hypothermia
j. metabolism
k. temporal artery thermometer (TAT)

CHAPTER REVIEW

Short Answer

Complete the assessment in the space provided.

1. The measurement of body heat is called _____.

© 2022 Cengage Learning. All Rights Reserved. May not be scanned, copied or duplicated, or posted to a publicly accessible website, in whole or in part.

2. Measurement of body heat is one of the vital signs. Name three others.

   a. _____

   b. _____

   c. _____

3. List eight factors that can influence body temperature.

   a. _____

   b. _____

   c. _____

   d. _____

   e. _____

   f. _____

   g. _____

   h. _____

4. In healthy adults, what is the usual daily variation in temperature?

   _____

5. When compared to adult body temperature, the temperature of children is _____ stable.

6. When using an electronic thermometer, the _____ is inserted into the patient.

7. How is the part named in question 6 protected?

   _____

8. What happens to the protector after use? _____

   _____

9. Glass thermometers are long cylindrical tubes that contain a column of _____.

10. Write the names of the two scales used to measure temperature.

    a. _____

    b. _____

11. You enter Odelia Michaud's room to take vital signs and learn that she just returned from outside, where she was drinking gourmet coffee, eating doughnuts, and smoking with her friends. What action should you take?

    _____

12. List three advantages of the tympanic thermometer.

    a. _____

    b. _____

    c. _____

13. Indicate which method of temperature determination (oral or rectal) is best in each of the following circumstances if only glass thermometers are available.

© 2022 Cengage Learning. All Rights Reserved. May not be scanned, copied or duplicated, or posted to a publicly accessible website, in whole or in part.

a. patient has diarrhea   _____

b. patient is confused   _____

c. patient cannot breathe through his nose   _____

d. patient has rectal bleeding   _____

e. patient is comatose   _____

f. patient has hemorrhoids   _____

g. patient is restless   _____

h. patient is a child   _____

i. patient has fecal impaction   _____

j. patient is coughing   _____

14. Name three areas other than the mouth or rectum that can be used to determine body temperature.

a. _____

b. _____

c. _____

15. Write the names of the thermometers pictured.

a. _____

b. _____

© 2022 Cengage Learning. All Rights Reserved. May not be scanned, copied or duplicated, or posted to a publicly accessible website, in whole or in part.

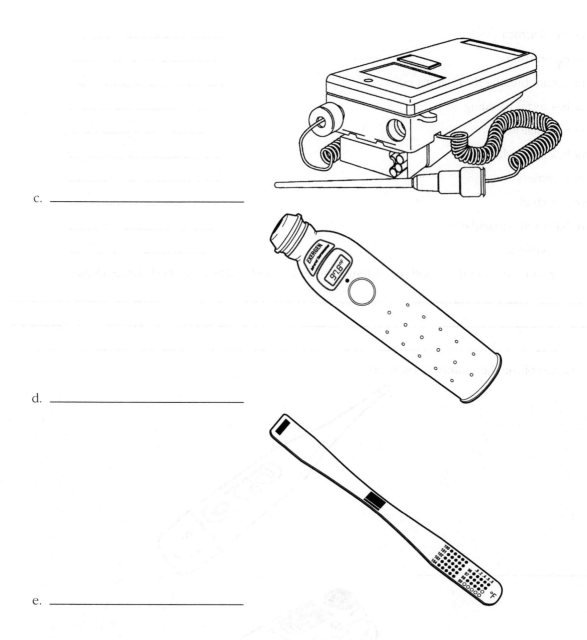

c. _____

d. _____

e. _____

True/False

Mark the following true or false by circling T or F.

1. T   F   Body temperature is lower the closer to the body surface it is measured.

2. T   F   The tympanic thermometer is the most accurate.

3. T   F   The same person may have different temperatures when the value is determined at different parts of the body.

4. T   F   Hydration levels have no effect on body temperature.

5. T   F   Body heat is managed by special cells in the liver.

6. T   F   The tip of a rectal thermometer should always be lubricated before insertion.

7. T   F   Oxygen use will alter the temperature value of a temporal artery thermometer.

© 2022 Cengage Learning. All Rights Reserved. May not be scanned, copied or duplicated, or posted to a publicly accessible website, in whole or in part.

8. T   F   A new disposable cover should be used to protect the electronic thermometer for each patient.

9. T   F   The probe of the tympanic thermometer should be placed directly under the patient's tongue.

10. T   F   A patient's temperature should be recorded as soon as it is taken.

11. T   F   When taking a tympanic temperature on an adult, gently pull the ear pinna back and up.

12. T   F   There is no need to cover the tip of the tympanic thermometer if you wipe it with alcohol before each use.

13. T   F   Always wear gloves when taking a temporal artery temperature.

14. T   F   The temporal artery thermometer measures centigrade values only.

CERTIFICATION REVIEW

Complete the following multiple-choice assessments.

1. Which statement is correct about temperature control?

    a. Sweating raises body temperature.

    b. Shivering increases body heat when the patient is cold.

    c. Heat loss is regulated through breathing.

    d. Body temperature is regulated by the heart.

2. Which is a symptom of heat exhaustion?

    a. Dizziness

    b. Dilated pupils

    c. Slurred speech

    d. Poor coordination

3. Which is a symptom of hypothermia?

    a. Cyanosis

    b. Confusion

    c. Low blood pressure

    d. Nausea and vomiting

4. Which type of thermometer should *not* be used?

    a. Glass

    b. Digital

    c. Electronic

    d. Tympanic

5. Which type of thermometer is associated with the most errors?

    a. Digital

    b. Electronic

    c. Tympanic

    d. Temporal

© 2022 Cengage Learning. All Rights Reserved. May not be scanned, copied or duplicated, or posted to a publicly accessible website, in whole or in part.

6. Which type of thermometer has a reading similar to that of the temporal artery thermometer?

    a. Oral

    b. Rectal

    c. Digital

    d. Electronic

7. For which reason would a rectal temperature be contraindicated?

    a. Coughing

    b. Hemorrhoids

    c. Unconscious

    d. Has dentures

8. When should an oral temperature be taken after a patient smoked a cigarette?

    a. 5 minutes

    b. 10 minutes

    c. 15 minutes

    d. 30 minutes

9. Which equipment is used for measuring an axillary temperature?

    a. Oral

    b. Rectal

    c. Tympanic

    d. Temporal artery

10. On which area is a temporal artery thermometer placed before moving to the location to measure the temperature?

    a. Neck

    b. Cheek

    c. Shoulder

    d. Forehead

CHAPTER APPLICATION

Clinical Situations

Answer the following questions in the space provided.

1. Mrs. Morgan's oral temp was 98.4°F at 9:00 a.m. When you see her at 10:30 a.m., she is flushed and her skin is dry. What action should you take? _____

_____

© 2022 Cengage Learning. All Rights Reserved. May not be scanned, copied or duplicated, or posted to a publicly accessible website, in whole or in part.

2. You are assigned to use the electronic thermometer to recheck the temperatures of two patients. The probe cover package is empty. You only have two temperatures to take and new covers are at the far end of the hall. What do you do? _____

_____

_____

RELATING TO THE NURSING PROCESS

Write the step of the nursing process that is related to each nursing assistant action.

Nursing Assistant Action   **Nursing Process Step**

1. The nursing assistant covers the digital thermometer   _____
   with a disposable sheath before placing it under the
   patient's tongue.

2. The nursing assistant accurately reports that the patient's _____
   temperature is 102°F orally.

3. Before inserting a rectal thermometer, the nursing assistant _____
   lubricates the tip with water-soluble lubricant.

4. The nursing assistant checks the nursing care plan   _____
   before measuring an oral temperature when she notices
   that the patient is receiving oxygen by face mask.

5. The nursing assistant reports that the patient feels faint   _____
   and has hot, flushed skin.

DEVELOPING GREATER INSIGHT

1. Practice taking temperatures using different types of thermometers.

2. Discuss with your instructor and classmates why proper placement of the tympanic thermometer is important.

3. Think about the times and reasons for using disposable gloves for temperature-taking procedures.

4. Explain to classmates why the forehead is a useful site for taking a patient's temperature and explain why this value is accurate even though the temperature value is obtained on the outside of the body.

© 2022 Cengage Learning. All Rights Reserved. May not be scanned, copied or duplicated, or posted to a publicly accessible website, in whole or in part.

Pulse and Respiration

OBJECTIVES

After completing this chapter, you will be able to:

19-1 Spell and define terms.
19-2 Define pulse.
19-3 Explain the importance of monitoring a pulse rate.
19-4 Locate the pulse sites.
19-5 Identify the range of normal pulse rates.
19-6 Identify the range of normal respiratory rates.
19-7 Measure the pulse at different locations.
19-8 List the characteristics of the pulse.
19-9 List the characteristics of respiration.
19-10 List eight guidelines for using a stethoscope.
19-11 Demonstrate the following procedures:

- Procedure 36: Counting the Radial Pulse
- Procedure 37: Counting the Apical–Radial Pulse
- Procedure 38: Counting Respirations
- Procedure 39: Using a Pulse Oximeter

VOCABULARY BUILDER

Spelling

Each line has four different spellings of a word. Circle the correctly spelled word.

1. appical	apical	apecal	apicale
2. cyanosis	sianosis	syanosis	cyanoses
3. poulse	pullse	polse	pulse
4. despnea	dypnea	disnea	dyspnea
5. apnea	epnea	apnia	appnea

© 2022 Cengage Learning. All Rights Reserved. May not be scanned, copied or duplicated, or posted to a publicly accessible website, in whole or in part.

6. tachipnea   tachypnea   takipnea   tachipnia

7. rhythm   rhythem   rhethem   rytham

8. bradekardia   bradicardea   bradycardia   bradykardya

Matching

Match each term with the correct definition.

1. _____ inhalation
2. _____ exhalation
3. _____ moist respirations
4. _____ pulse that feels weak
5. _____ depth of respirations
6. _____ snoring-like respirations
7. _____ most commonly measured pulse
8. _____ whistling sound when breathing
9. _____ supply the body cells with oxygen
10. _____ number of respirations per minute
11. _____ ability of the chest to expand equally
12. _____ respiratory rate more than 25 per minute
13. _____ pulse of more than 100 beats per minute
14. _____ instrument to listen to sounds inside the body
15. _____ a period of dyspnea followed by periods of apnea
16. _____ difference between the apical pulse and the radial pulse
17. _____ test used to determine how well the body uses oxygen

a. accelerated
b. Cheyne–Stokes respirations
c. expiration
d. inspiration
e. pulse deficit
f. pulse oximetry
g. radial pulse
h. rales
i. rate
j. respiration
k. stertorous
l. stethoscope
m. symmetry
n. tachycardia
o. thready pulse
p. volume
q. wheezing

CHAPTER REVIEW

Short Answer

Complete the assessment in the space provided.

1. The pulse is the _____ of blood felt against the wall of a(n) _____.
2. The pulse can be felt best in _____ that come close to the _____ and can be gently pressed against a(n) _____.
3. You should measure the _____ pulse when the patient is unconscious.
4. Pulse measurement includes determining the pulse character, which means the _____ and _____.

© 2022 Cengage Learning. All Rights Reserved. May not be scanned, copied or duplicated, or posted to a publicly accessible website, in whole or in part.

5. To check circulation to the toes of your patient with diabetes, you should palpate the _____ artery.

6. Seven major arteries used to measure pulse rates are:

   a. _____

   b. _____

   c. _____

   d. _____

   e. _____

   f. _____

   g. _____

7. In an adult, the normal pulse rate is between _____ bpm and _____ bpm.

8. Ten factors that can alter the pulse rate are:

   a. _____

   b. _____

   c. _____

   d. _____

   e. _____

   f. _____

   g. _____

   h. _____

   i. _____

   j. _____

9. Your patient is eight years old and has a pulse rate of 120 bpm. You know this is _____ for a child of this age.

10. To accurately measure a pulse rate, your watch must have a _____.

11. You should locate the pulse with your _____.

12. The pulse should be counted for _____.

© 2022 Cengage Learning. All Rights Reserved. May not be scanned, copied or duplicated, or posted to a publicly accessible website, in whole or in part.

True/False

Mark the following true or false by circling T or F.

1. T   F   Normally the apical pulse is 4 bpm higher than the radial pulse in the same person.

2. T   F   Three health care providers are needed to accurately measure an apical pulse.

3. T   F   When determining an apical pulse, you will need a stethoscope.

4. T   F   The earpieces of the stethoscope must be cleaned before use.

5. T   F   Moist respirations are best documented as stertorous.

6. T   F   Each respiration consists of one inspiration and one expiration.

7. T   F   *Symmetry* of respirations refers to the depth of respiration.

8. T   F   The regularity of respirations is referred to as the *rhythm*.

9. T   F   The normal adult rate is 25 respirations per minute.

10. T   F   Always count the respiratory rate after you tell the patient what you intend to do.

CERTIFICATION REVIEW

Complete the following multiple-choice assessments.

1. Which of these describes the purpose of the pulse?

    a. Determines if the patient has an illness.

    b. Estimates the volume of blood in the body.

    c. Measures the amount of oxygen in the blood.

    d. Indicates functioning of the cardiovascular system.

2. Which pulse rate will the nursing assistance report to the nurse immediately?

    a. 64 bpm

    B. 72 bpm

    c. 92 bpm

    d. 112 bpm

3. In which way will the nursing assistant count the pulse of a patient with an irregular heartbeat?

    a. 10 seconds × 6

    b. 15 seconds × 4

    c. 30 seconds × 2

    d. 1 full minute

4. In which area will the nursing assistant place the stethoscope when counting the number of a patient's heartbeats?

    a. Below the left nipple.

    b. Just above the left nipple.

    c. Right side of the sternum.

    d. Between the third and fourth ribs.

© 2022 Cengage Learning. All Rights Reserved. May not be scanned, copied or duplicated, or posted to a publicly accessible website, in whole or in part.

5. Which action will the nursing assistant take when using a stethoscope?

   a. Position the diaphragm at an angle.

   b. Place the diaphragm over the gown.

   c. Wrap tape around cracks in the tubing.

   d. Hold the diaphragm flat against the skin.

6. In which way will a patient's apical–radial pulse be measured?

   a. Count the heart rate first and then count the radial pulse.

   b. Ask another assistant to count the heart rate while counting the radial pulse.

   c. Count the heartbeat for a minute then count the radial pulse after 2 minutes.

   d. Count the heart rate for 15 minutes and then count the radial pulse for a minute.

7. Which factor will increase a patient's heart rate?

   a. Smoking

   b. Sleeping

   c. Resting in bed

   d. Looking out the window

8. Which finding will the nursing assistant report to the nurse?

   a. Heart rate of 74 beats per minute.

   b. Heart rate of 118 beats per minute.

   c. Respiratory rate of 16 breaths per minute.

   d. Respiratory rate of 20 breaths per minute.

9. When should the nursing assistant measure a patient's pulse oximetry?

   a. Before lunch

   b. After breakfast

   c. At hour of sleep

   d. When measuring vital signs

10. Which action will the nurse take when a patient's pulse oximeter measurement is 70 percent?

    a. Notify the nurse.

    b. Provide the patient with oxygen.

    c. Check the location of the sensor.

    d. Raise the head of the bed.

© 2022 Cengage Learning. All Rights Reserved. May not be scanned, copied or duplicated, or posted to a publicly accessible website, in whole or in part.

CHAPTER APPLICATION

Clinical Situations

Briefly describe how a nursing assistant should react to the following situations.

1. You are measuring vital signs and notice that the patient in 112B, whose pulse rate has been 84 to 88 bpm, now has a pulse rate of 112 and the pulse is weak.

   _____

2. Mr. Murray has a medical diagnosis of congestive heart failure. When you measure his pulse, you find it irregular and weak. The nurse says she suspects a pulse deficit.

   _____

3. You report that Mr. Rossi has a pulse deficit of 24 and a pulse rate of 84. What was the patient's apical pulse, and how would you document the reading? Show your work.

   _____

   _____

   _____

4. Find the pulse deficit in each of the following readings and show proper documentation.

   a. apical pulse 120, radial pulse 104 _____

   b. apical pulse 118, radial pulse 88 _____

   c. apical pulse 92, radial pulse 50 _____

   d. apical pulse 102, radial pulse 68 _____

   e. apical pulse 98, radial pulse 76 _____

Label the diagrams.

5. This piece of medical equipment is a _____ .

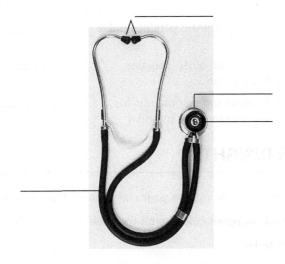

© 2022 Cengage Learning. All Rights Reserved. May not be scanned, copied or duplicated, or posted to a publicly accessible website, in whole or in part.

6. Each dot on this diagram represents the location of a _____.

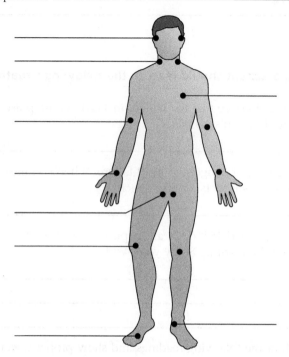

RELATING TO THE NURSING PROCESS

Write the step of the nursing process that is related to each nursing assistant action.

Nursing Assistant Action	Nursing Process Step
1. The nursing assistant tells the nurse that the patient's respirations have become labored.	_____
2. The nursing assistant has an order to measure the apical pulse. She seeks help because she is not sure how to perform this procedure.	_____
3. The nursing assistant notifies the nurse that the patient's pulse rate is 60.	_____
4. The nursing assistant listens closely as the nurse explains the new, revised care plans for her patients.	_____
5. The nursing assistant listens and counts the respirations for a full minute when the patient's respirations are irregular.	_____

DEVELOPING GREATER INSIGHT

1. Practice taking pulse and respiration readings on your classmates. Have your instructor check your findings.

2. Discuss ways of handling the following situations with the class.

   a. Mr. Volaire has an irregular pulse.

   b. Mrs. Benton has an IV on the thumb side of one wrist.

   c. Mrs. Zeldane seems to stop breathing shortly after you start counting the pulse, making it impossible for you to count her respirations.

   d. Mr. Capione's pulse and respiratory rates have increased markedly since your last measurement.

© 2022 Cengage Learning. All Rights Reserved. May not be scanned, copied or duplicated, or posted to a publicly accessible website, in whole or in part.

Blood Pressure

OBJECTIVES

After completing this chapter, you will be able to:

20-1 Spell and define terms.

20-2 Describe the factors that influence blood pressure.

20-3 Identify the range of normal blood pressure values.

20-4 Identify the causes of inaccurate blood pressure readings.

20-5 Describe how to select the proper size blood pressure cuff.

20-6 List precautions associated with use of the sphygmomanometer.

20-7 Demonstrate the following procedures:

• Procedure 40: Taking Blood Pressure

• Procedure 41: Taking Blood Pressure with an Electronic Blood Pressure
   Apparatus

VOCABULARY BUILDER

Matching

Match each term with the correct definition.

1. _____ unit of measurement of blood pressure

2. _____ low blood pressure

3. _____ drugs that slow down body function

4. _____ felt

5. _____ artery most often used to determine blood pressure

6. _____ stretchability

a. aneroid

b. brachial

c. depressants

d. diastolic

e. elasticity

f. fasting

© 2022 Cengage Learning. All Rights Reserved. May not be scanned, copied or duplicated, or posted to a publicly accessible website, in whole or in part.

7. _____ type of gauge

8. _____ blood pressure cuff and gauge

9. _____ not eating

10. _____ lowest blood pressure reading

11. _____ an instrument used to hear body sounds

12. _____ drugs that speed up body functions

g. hypotension

h. mm Hg

i. palpated

j. stethoscope

k. stimulants

l. sphygmomanometer

CHAPTER REVIEW

Short Answer

Complete the assessment in the space provided.

1. Blood pressure depends on four specific factors. They are:

   a. _____

   b. _____

   c. _____

   d. _____

2. List five factors other than heredity that can cause elevated blood pressure.

   a. _____

   b. _____

   c. _____

   d. _____

   e. _____

3. List five factors other than grief that can lower blood pressure.

   a. _____

   b. _____

   c. _____

   d. _____

   e. _____

4. A properly sized blood pressure cuff should measure approximately _____ of the patient's arm.

5. Three types of sphygmomanometers in common use are:

   a. _____

   b. _____

   c. _____

© 2022 Cengage Learning. All Rights Reserved. May not be scanned, copied or duplicated, or posted to a publicly accessible website, in whole or in part.

6. The patient has a blood pressure reading of 148/98. You recognize this as _____.

7. The difference between the systolic and diastolic pressure is called the _____.

8. Three reasons for not using an arm to measure blood pressure are: the arm is _____, the arm is the site of an _____, or the arm is _____.

9. Sound that fades out for 10 to 15 mm Hg and then resumes as you deflate the cuff is known as _____.

10. The large lines on the blood pressure gauge are at increments of _____ mm Hg.

11. Each small line on the blood pressure gauge indicates _____ intervals.

12. The cuff should be applied _____ above the elbow.

13. The center of the rubber bladder should be placed directly over the _____.

14. Three situations that you should immediately report regarding blood pressure measurement are:

    a. _____

    b. _____

    c. _____

15. Unusual blood pressure readings ought to be checked after _____.

16. Identify the equipment and the specific parts.

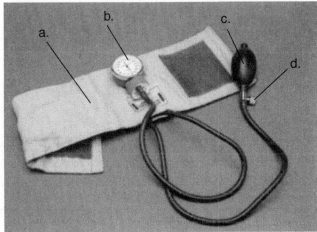

    a. _____

    b. _____

    c. _____

    d. _____

© 2022 Cengage Learning. All Rights Reserved. May not be scanned, copied or duplicated, or posted to a publicly accessible website, in whole or in part.

17. Determine the systolic and diastolic readings.

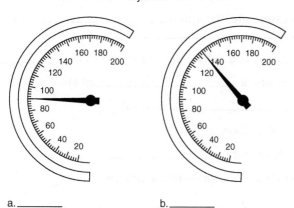

Systolic

a. _____   b. _____

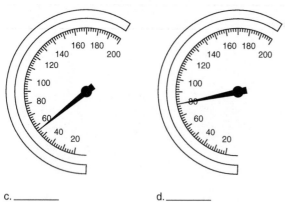

Diastolic

c. _____   d. _____

a. _____

b. _____

c. _____

d. _____

© 2022 Cengage Learning. All Rights Reserved. May not be scanned, copied or duplicated, or posted to a publicly accessible website, in whole or in part.

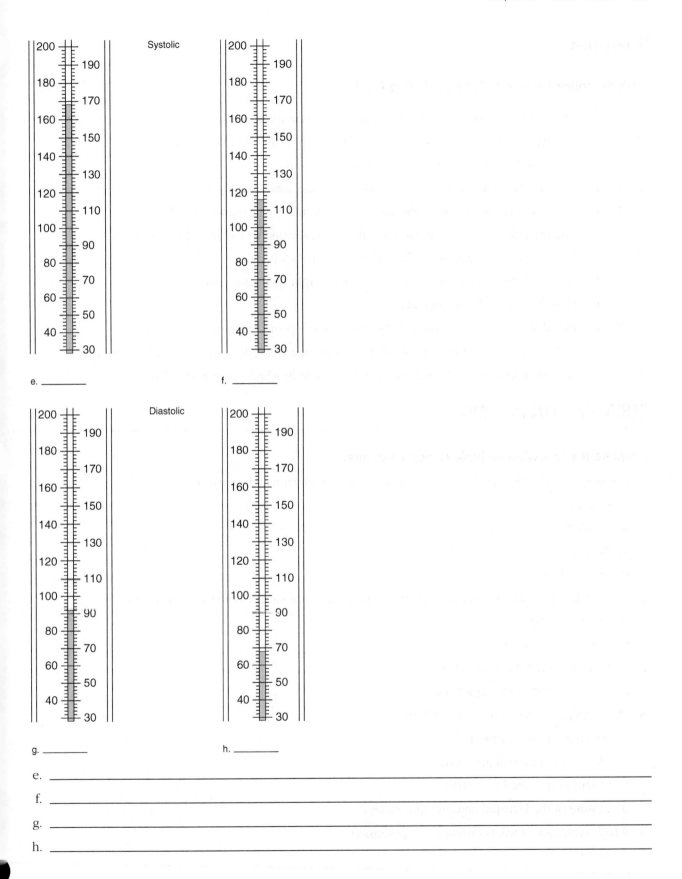

Systolic

Diastolic

e. _____   f. _____

g. _____   h. _____

e. _____

f. _____

g. _____

h. _____

© 2022 Cengage Learning. All Rights Reserved. May not be scanned, copied or duplicated, or posted to a publicly accessible website, in whole or in part.

True/False

Mark the following true or false by circling T or F.

1.   T   F   The same size blood pressure cuff may be used for all patients.

2.   T   F   The highest point of blood pressure measurement is the diastolic reading.

3.   T   F   Hereditary factors can cause elevated blood pressure.

4.   T   F   Deflating the cuff too slowly can result in an inaccurate reading.

5.   T   F   All blood pressure readings should be made with the gauge above eye level.

6.   T   F   The diastolic pressure is measured at the change sound or last sound that is heard.

7.   T   F   The blood pressure is most often taken over the brachial artery.

8.   T   F   Always clean the stethoscope earpieces and diaphragm before and after use.

9.   T   F   Grief lowers the blood pressure.

10.   T   F   Blood pressure readings are always recorded as a proper fraction such as 40/110.

11.   T   F   It is very important to use a cuff of the proper size when determining the blood pressure.

12.   T   F   A blood pressure may be measured using an arm in which an IV is inserted.

CERTFICATION REVIEW

Complete the following multiple-choice assessments.

1. Controlling high blood pressure can delay the onset of which health problem?

   a. Obesity

   b. Cataracts

   c. Renal failure

   d. Osteoarthritis

2. For which reason do some facilities prefer to measure the blood pressure on the left arm?

   a. Easier to obtain

   b. Closest to the heart

   c. Usually the nondominant hand

   d. IVs are placed in the right hand

3. The systolic pressure reflects which heart action?

   a. Initiation of the heartbeat.

   b. Closure of the semilunar valve.

   c. Contraction of the left ventricle.

   d. Closure of the bicuspid and tricuspid valves.

4. Which symptom indicates orthostatic hypotension?

   a. Nausea

   b. Sneezing

   c. Dizziness

   d. Muscle cramps

© 2022 Cengage Learning. All Rights Reserved. May not be scanned, copied or duplicated, or posted to a publicly accessible website, in whole or in part.

5. Which blood pressure measurement indicates prehypertension?

    a. 98/54 mm Hg

    b. 136/88 mm Hg

    c. 142/92 mm Hg

    d. 168/102 mm Hg

6. Which action will the nursing assistant take if a patient's blood pressure cannot be heard?

    a. Notify the nurse.

    b. Remove and reapply the cuff.

    c. Place the cuff on the other arm.

    d. Ensure the stethoscope is placed correctly.

7. At which speed will the nursing assistant release the bulb valve when measuring the blood pressure?

    a. 1 mm Hg per second

    b. 2 to 3 mm Hg per second

    c. 5 mm Hg per second

    d. 10 mm Hg per second

8. At which level will the nursing assistance roll the sleeve of a patient's shirt above the elbow to measure the blood pressure?

    a. 2 inches

    b. 3 inches

    c. 5 inches

    d. 10 inches

9. Which technique is the most reliable for measuring the blood pressure?

    a. Using a disposable cuff.

    b. Measuring on both arms.

    c. Following the two-step method.

    d. Using an electronic monitoring device.

10. Which action will the nursing assistant take after hearing the last sound when measuring the blood pressure?

    a. Remove the cuff

    b. Reinflate the cuff

    c. Release the bulb valve

    d. Listen for 10 to 20 mm Hg longer

© 2022 Cengage Learning. All Rights Reserved. May not be scanned, copied or duplicated, or posted to a publicly accessible website, in whole or in part.

CHAPTER APPLICATION

Yes or No

Determine if the following actions are to be taken when measuring a blood pressure with an electronic blood pressure apparatus by identifying Y for Yes or N for No.

1. Y N   Plug into a source of electricity.
2. Y N   Turn the machine on.
3. Y N   Apply cuff over clothing.
4. Y N   Make sure the artery arrow on the cuff is over the elbow.
5. Y N   Press the start button.
6. Y N   Ensure two fingers can fit between the cuff and the patient's arm.

RELATING TO THE NURSING PROCESS

Write the step of the nursing process that is related to each nursing assistant action.

Nursing Assistant Action	Nursing Process Step
1. The nursing assistant finds that the patient's blood pressure is higher than the previous reading and reports this information.	_____
2. The patient is very heavy, and the nursing assistant seeks guidance as to which size blood pressure cuff to use.	_____
3. The nursing assistant informs the team leader of the patient's vital signs before leaving for a break.	_____

DEVELOPING GREATER INSIGHT

1. Practice taking blood pressure readings on patients whose arms are different sizes.
2. Explain why narrowing of the blood vessels raises blood pressure.
3. Explain why a blood pressure cuff should not be placed on the same side as a recent mastectomy.

© 2022 Cengage Learning. All Rights Reserved. May not be scanned, copied or duplicated, or posted to a publicly accessible website, in whole or in part.

CHAPTER 21

Measuring Height and Weight

OBJECTIVES

After completing this chapter, you will be able to:

21-1 Spell and define terms.

21-2 Understand why accurate weight measurements are important.

21-3 Describe the proper use of an overbed scale.

21-4 Demonstrate the following procedures:

- Procedure 42: Weighing and Measuring the Patient Using an Upright Scale (Expand Your Skills)
- Procedure 43: Weighing the Patient on a Chair Scale
- Procedure 44: Measuring Weight with an Electronic Wheelchair Scale
- Procedure 45: Measuring and Weighing the Patient in Bed

VOCABULARY BUILDER

Matching

Match each term with the correct definition.

1. _____ amount
2. _____ structure on the upright scale
3. _____ original measurement of height and weight
4. _____ weight measurement using the metric system
5. _____ weight measurement using the imperial system

a. balance bar

b. baseline

c. increment

d. kilogram (kg)

e. pound (lb)

© 2022 Cengage Learning. All Rights Reserved. May not be scanned, copied or duplicated, or posted to a publicly accessible website, in whole or in part.

CHAPTER REVIEW

Short Answer

Complete each statement in the spaces provided. Select terms from the list provided.

bed	chair	clothing	empty	kilograms
metric	paper towel	same	scale	
sling	tape measure	upright	wheelchair	

1. Choose the correct scale for each patient.

   a. Mr. Graham is in a wheelchair and cannot stand. He should be weighed with a(n) _____ scale.

   b. Mrs. Almos is recovering from pneumonia and is up and about as desired. She should be weighed with a(n) _____ scale.

   c. Mrs. DerHagopian is elderly. Her condition requires constant bedrest. She should be weighed with a(n) _____ scale.

2. Patients should be weighed at the _____ time each day.

3. Patients should wear the same type of _____ each time they are weighed.

4. The same method and _____ should be used each time a patient is weighed.

5. Patients should _____ their bladders before weighing.

6. When a patient cannot get out of bed, height measurement may be made with a _____.

7. Before weighing a patient, the platform of an upright scale should be covered with a _____.

8. Some facilities use the _____ system, which records weights in _____.

True/False

Mark the following true or false by circling T or F.

1. T   F   Weights should be moved to the extreme left before weighing.

2. T   F   Patients may hold the bar while being weighed as long as they do not lean on the scale.

3. T   F   Before weighing a patient on a wheelchair scale, be sure to weigh the wheelchair only.

4. T   F   The wheels of a wheelchair need not be locked when weighing the patient on a wheelchair scale.

5. T   F   When using a bed scale, the patient's body must be suspended freely above the bed before a reading is taken.

CERTIFICATION REVIEW

Complete the following multiple-choice assessments.

1. Where are a patient's original height and weight documented?

   a. On the Kardex

   b. On a flow sheet

   c. In the nurse's notes

   d. On the demographic form

© 2022 Cengage Learning. All Rights Reserved. May not be scanned, copied or duplicated, or posted to a publicly accessible website, in whole or in part.

2. For which reason will a patient be prescribed a daily weight?

    a. On bedrest

    b. Taking a diuretic

    c. Receiving antibiotics

    d. Receiving physical therapy

3. What does a patient's weight indicate?

    a. Nutritional status

    b. Response to medications

    c. Recovery from an illness

    d. Condition to have surgery

4. Which action should be taken when a built-in bed scale is being used to weigh a patient?

    a. Lower the head of the bed.

    b. Raise the bed to waist height.

    c. Ask the patient to bed the knees.

    d. Remove all extraneous items from the bed.

5. Which amount of fluid is equivalent to a 2-lb weight gain?

    a. One liter

    b. Two liters

    c. Half a liter

    d. Three liters

6. Which incremental amount of weight is measured by the lower bar on a standing scale?

    a. 5 lb

    b. 10 lb

    c. 25 lb

    d. 50 lb

7. Which direction will the patient face when their height is being measured using a standing scale?

    a. Face the left.

    b. Face the right.

    c. Face the balance bar.

    d. Face away from the balance bar.

8. Which information will the nursing assistant report to the nurse?

    a. Patient consumed an entire meal.

    b. Patient is losing weight every day.

    c. Patient wants the television on during a meal.

    d. Patient requested assistance opening containers.

© 2022 Cengage Learning. All Rights Reserved. May not be scanned, copied or duplicated, or posted to a publicly accessible website, in whole or in part.

9. How will a patient in a wheelchair be weighed on a chair scale?

   a. Weigh the wheelchair empty.

   b. Open the metal ramp sides on the scale.

   c. Roll the wheelchair onto the scale platform.

   d. Transfer the patient from the wheelchair to the chair on the scale.

10. Which action will the nursing assistant take first when using a sling scale to weigh a patient?

   a. Raise the head of the bed.

   b. Raise the bed to waist height.

   c. Guide the lift to the foot of the bed.

   d. Cover the canvas sling with a sheet.

CHAPTER APPLICATION

Reading Weights and Heights

Read each weight measurement and record it in pounds.

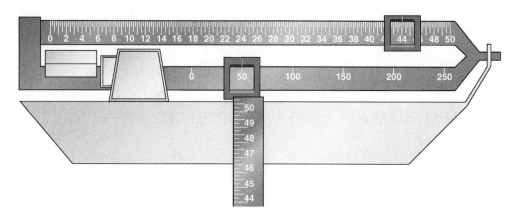

1. _____

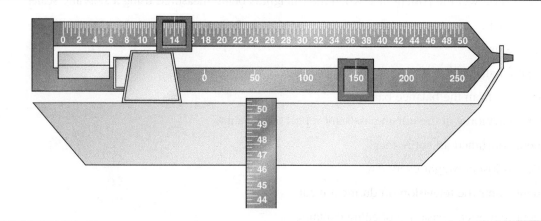

2. _____

© 2022 Cengage Learning. All Rights Reserved. May not be scanned, copied or duplicated, or posted to a publicly accessible website, in whole or in part.

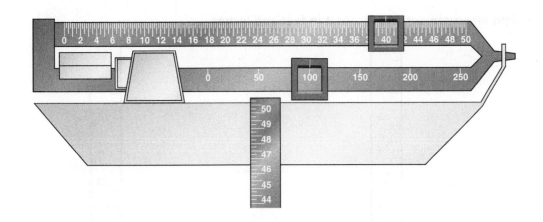

3. _____

4. _____

© 2022 Cengage Learning. All Rights Reserved. May not be scanned, copied or duplicated, or posted to a publicly accessible website, in whole or in part.

Read each height measurement and record it in feet and inches.

1. _____

67
66
65
64
63
62
→ 61
60
59
58
57
56
55

2. _____

→ 67
66
65
64
63
62
61
60
59
58
57
56
55

3. _____

67
66
65
64
63
62
61
→ 60
59
58
57
56
55

4. _____

67
66
65
→ 64
63
62
61
60
59
58
57
56
55

© 2022 Cengage Learning. All Rights Reserved. May not be scanned, copied or duplicated, or posted to a publicly accessible website, in whole or in part.

RELATING TO THE NURSING PROCESS

Write the step of the nursing process that is related to each nursing assistant action.

Nursing Assistant Action	Nursing Process Step
1. The nursing assistant measures and weighs the new patient as instructed.	_____
2. The nursing assistant reports information about the patient's height and weight to the nurse and records it on the patient's record.	_____

DEVELOPING GREATER INSIGHT

1. With classmates, practice the safe use of different types of scales.

2. Explain why a patient whose height is 64 inches is recorded as being 5 feet 4 inches.

3. Mrs. Menitt is a new admission. She cannot get out of bed. Think through the steps you will take to obtain an accurate height measurement.

© 2022 Cengage Learning. All Rights Reserved. May not be scanned, copied or duplicated, or posted to a publicly accessible website, in whole or in part.

Patient Care and Comfort Measures

CHAPTER **22**

Admission, Transfer, and Discharge

OBJECTIVES

After completing this chapter, you will be able to:

22-1 Spell and define terms.

22-2 List the ways the nursing assistant can help in the processes of admission, transfer, and discharge.

22-3 Describe family dynamics and emotions that occur when a loved one is admitted to the hospital.

22-4 List ways in which the nursing assistant can develop positive relationships with a patient's family members.

22-5 Demonstrate the following procedures:

- Procedure 46: Admitting the Patient (Expand Your Skills)
- Procedure 47: Transferring the Patient
- Procedure 48: Discharging the Patient (Expand Your Skills)

© 2022 Cengage Learning. All Rights Reserved. May not be scanned, copied or duplicated, or posted to a publicly accessible website, in whole or in part.

VOCABULARY BUILDER

Matching

Match each term with the correct definition.

1. _____ initial evaluation of a patient's condition
2. _____ movement of a patient to another unit or facility
3. _____ authorized release of a patient from a health care facility
4. _____ evaluation of a problem that has the potential to harm a patient
5. _____ entry to a health care facility for treatment of an illness or injury

a. admission

b. baseline assessment

c. discharge

d. risk assessment

e. transfer

CHAPTER REVIEW

Short Answer

Complete the statements in the spaces provided.

1. Admission to a care facility is a cause of great concern for both _____ and _____.

2. The nursing assistant should identify the patient by speaking the patient's name and _____.

3. _____ helps identify issues that could become problematic for the patient.

4. The nursing assistant can help orient the patient to the unit by explaining how to use the telephone or television and the times _____ are served.

5. Never leave the patient, their records, or medications _____ during the transfer procedure.

6. After a transfer is completed, you should be sure the patient is _____ and _____.

7. Before preparing the patient for discharge, make sure the _____ has been written.

8. The nursing assistant's _____ are very valuable in the nurse's baseline assessment.

9. The patient is the facility's _____ until they have left the building.

10. After discharge, a final _____ is made on the patient's chart.

11. Before the patient is discharged, make sure the _____ have been given to him.

12. DRGs were introduced for the purpose of _____.

© 2022 Cengage Learning. All Rights Reserved. May not be scanned, copied or duplicated, or posted to a publicly accessible website, in whole or in part.

Short Answer

Briefly provide the requested information in the spaces provided.

1. List six items you can expect to find in the admission kit.

   a. _____

   b. _____

   c. _____

   d. _____

   e. _____

   f. _____

2. The nursing assistant can facilitate the admission procedure if seven points are kept in mind and carried out. List them.

   a. _____

   b. _____

   c. _____

   d. _____

   e. _____

   f. _____

   g. _____

3. Before admitting a patient, you will need specific information. What three questions should you ask the nurse?

   a. _____

   b. _____

   c. _____

CERTIFICATION REVIEW

Complete the following multiple-choice assessments.

1. Which observation will the nursing assistant report to the nurse when admitting a patient?

   a. Has dentures

   b. Wears cotton socks

   c. Requested some water

   d. Ulcer on the left buttock

2. For which reason would family members be angry during an admission process?

   a. Feel a loss of control

   b. Feeling of uncertainty

   c. Difficulty coping with separation

   d. Concern the patient's condition has worsened

© 2022 Cengage Learning. All Rights Reserved. May not be scanned, copied or duplicated, or posted to a publicly accessible website, in whole or in part.

3. In which area will the nursing assistant place the completed personal belongings inventory?

    a. Kardex

    b. Medical record

    c. Nurse manager's office

    d. Top drawer of the bedside table

4. For which reason might a patient need to wear a hospital gown instead of their own nightwear?

    a. Eating a meal

    b. After a shower

    c. Having surgery

    d. Before seeing the physician

5. Which response will the nursing assistant make when a family member asks about a patient's condition?

    a. "She's doing very well today."

    b. "What did the patient tell you?"

    c. "Let me read you the last nurse's note."

    d. "I will ask the nurse to come and talk with you."

6. Which action will the nursing assistant take if a patient is arguing with visiting family members?

    a. Leave the room.

    b. Ask the family to leave.

    c. Encourage the patient to calm down.

    d. Give an opinion about the argument.

7. What is the primary goal when admitting a pediatric patient to the hospital?

    a. Limiting contact with the child

    b. Beginning treatment as soon as possible

    c. Making the child and parents comfortable

    d. Asking the parents to leave while the child is being admitted

8. Which action will the nursing assistant take if an ambulance service is transporting a patient to the unit?

    a. Stay with the patient until the service leaves.

    b. Leave the room until the transfer is complete.

    c. Obtain paperwork for the ambulance service.

    d. Close the doors of all the other patient rooms.

9. Which action will the nursing assistant take when admitting an ambulatory patient to the care area?

    a. Ask the patient to be seated.

    b. Tell the patient to put on a hospital gown.

    c. Provide the patient with a water pitcher and cup.

    d. Ask family members to explain the reason for the hospitalization.

© 2022 Cengage Learning. All Rights Reserved. May not be scanned, copied or duplicated, or posted to a publicly accessible website, in whole or in part.

10. What will the nursing assistant do with medications, the care plan, and the medical record when transferring a patient?

    a. Hand them to the nurse in charge.

    b. Ask the patient to hold them until the nurse arrives.

    c. Place them in the nurse's station of the new care area.

    d. Place them on the bedside table of the patient's new bed space.

CHAPTER APPLICATION

Clinical Situations

Briefly describe how a nursing assistant should react to the following situations.

1. Your patient tells you they intends to leave the health care facility without their physician's permission.

   _____

   _____

   _____

   _____

2. Your patient has just been discharged.

   _____

   _____

   _____

   _____

3. The family accompanies your patient to the unit and must wait as you carry out the admission procedure. How can you show courtesy to them?

   _____

   _____

   _____

   _____

   _____

4. Your assignment is to admit the patient. List the equipment you will gather.

   _____

   _____

   _____

   _____

   _____

© 2022 Cengage Learning. All Rights Reserved. May not be scanned, copied or duplicated, or posted to a publicly accessible website, in whole or in part.

RELATING TO THE NURSING PROCESS

Write the step of the nursing process that is related to each nursing assistant action.

Nursing Assistant Action   **Nursing Process Step**

1. The nursing assistant carefully prepares the patient's unit before   _____
   admission.

2. The nursing assistant measures the vital signs during the admis-   _____
   sion procedure.

3. During admission, the nursing assistant carefully observes the   _____
   patient and listens to the patient's statements.

4. The nursing assistant makes sure that all the patient's personal   _____
   articles are transported to the new unit when the patient is
   transferred.

5. The nursing assistant documents the correct time and method   _____
   of patient discharge on the proper record.

DEVELOPING GREATER INSIGHT

1. With classmates, role-play the following situations (consider equipment, psychological, and physical needs).

   a. Mrs. Coe is being admitted. She is in a wheelchair and very frail.

   b. Mr. Fletcher is ambulatory and is being discharged to the care of his son and daughter-in-law. The daughter-in-law seems very nervous and is pacing back and forth.

   c. Mrs. Barkley spends most of the day in a wheelchair. She is to be transferred to another floor.

© 2022 Cengage Learning. All Rights Reserved. May not be scanned, copied or duplicated, or posted to a publicly accessible website, in whole or in part.

Bedmaking

OBJECTIVES

After completing this chapter, you will be able to:

23-1 Spell and define terms.

23-2 List the different types of beds and their uses.

23-3 Describe how to operate each type of bed.

23-4 Explain how to properly handle clean and soiled linens.

23-5 Demonstrate the following procedures:

- Procedure 49: Making a Closed Bed (Expand Your Skills)
- Procedure 50: Making an Occupied Bed

VOCABULARY BUILDER

Definitions

Define the following terms.

1. gatch bed _____

_____

2. toe pleat _____

_____

3. mitered corner _____

_____

4. box (square) corner _____

_____

© 2022 Cengage Learning. All Rights Reserved. May not be scanned, copied or duplicated, or posted to a publicly accessible website, in whole or in part.

5. closed bed _____

_____

6. electric bed _____

_____

7. low bed

_____

_____

8. open bed

_____

_____

CHAPTER REVIEW

True/False

Mark the following true or false by circling T or F.

1.	T	F	Gatch beds are most commonly used in home health care.
2.	T	F	After the bottom of the bed has been made, pull the mattress to the head of the bed.
3.	T	F	Before making a bed, lower it to its lowest horizontal height.
4.	T	F	When completing an open bed, position the top bedding under the pillow.
5.	T	F	The top linen of a surgical bed is left untucked and fan-folded to one side.
6.	T	F	Position the lift sheet from the patient's waist to their knees.
7.	T	F	CPR is not effective on a low air loss bed.
8.	T	F	The risk of side rail entrapment increases in low air loss beds.
9.	T	F	A mattress pad is applied to the mattress before the bottom sheet is put on.
10.	T	F	Fitted sheets are used in some facilities in place of top sheets.
11.	T	F	Before making an unoccupied bed, arrange the linens in the order they are to be used.
12.	T	F	Always position a patient comfortably before leaving the room.
13.	T	F	The flat bottom sheet should be placed so the bottom edge is even with the end of the mattress at the foot of the bed.
14.	T	F	Place the clean bed linens on the overbed table.

© 2022 Cengage Learning. All Rights Reserved. May not be scanned, copied or duplicated, or posted to a publicly accessible website, in whole or in part.

15. T   F   Never shake the linens when making a bed because this may spread germs.

16. T   F   When making the bottom of an occupied bed, the linens should be rolled against the patient's back and then tucked under the patient's body.

17. T   F   Loosen the top linens when a bed is occupied.

18. T   F   Side rails should be up and secure before you leave an occupied bed.

Short Answer

Briefly answer the following questions.

1. Why should one side of the bed be made at a time?

    _____

2. Why are the sheets unfolded rather than shaken out?

    _____

3. How should the pillow be placed on the bed?

    _____

4. What is the purpose of the open bed?

    _____

5. What is the purpose of the surgical bed?

    _____

6. Why is it necessary to turn patients who are in low air loss beds that reduce pressure on the skin?

    _____

7. What is the proper position for the overbed table when the bed is closed or unoccupied?

    _____

8. When is the closed bed made in the hospital?

    _____

9. Why would the wheels of the bed be locked before the nursing assistant starts to make the bed?

    _____

© 2022 Cengage Learning. All Rights Reserved. May not be scanned, copied or duplicated, or posted to a publicly accessible website, in whole or in part.

'0. COMPLETE THE CHART

Method of Bedmaking	Procedure Variations	Rationale
Unoccupied bed	a. Most _____ type of bedmaking procedure. • Used for making all types of beds	b. Making the unoccupied bed is _____ and faster for the nursing assistant. It is more comfortable for the patient.
Occupied bed	c. Used when the patient is _____ to bed.	Changes wet or soiled linen for patient comfort and prevention of skin breakdown. Provides fresh, clean linen for feeling of comfort and security.
d. _____ bed	• The bed is made with the top sheet, blanket, and spread pulled all the way to the top. • The pillow may be covered or placed on top of the spread, depending on facility policy. • The open end of the pillowcase faces away from the door.	e. Used when the patient is expected to be _____ all day or when making a bed after the patient has been discharged. Presents a neat, tidy appearance.
Open bed	• The bed is made in the normal manner. f. The top sheet and spread are _____ to the foot of the bed.	This procedure is used when the patient is temporarily out of bed. The patient or nursing assistant can easily and quickly cover the patient upon return to bed.

CERTIFICATION REVIEW

Complete the following multiple-choice assessments.

1. Which action will the nursing assistant take to make it easier to make a low bed?

    a. Stand on the mat.

    b. Push the mat under the bed.

    c. Cover the mat and kneel on it.

    d. Move the mat away from the bed.

2. What is the purpose of the ribbon on a low air loss bed?

    a. Increases air inflation

    b. Deflates the air pillows

    c. Raises the head of the bed

    d. Lowers the height of the bed

3. In which location can the nursing assistant place soiled linens until they can be taken to the laundry hamper?

    a. On a chair

    b. On the floor

    c. Near the door

    d. Pillowcase on the back of the chair

© 2022 Cengage Learning. All Rights Reserved. May not be scanned, copied or duplicated, or posted to a publicly accessible website, in whole or in part.

4. Which item should the nursing assistant use when changing the linens on a low air loss bed?

    a. Bath blanket

    b. Regular sheets

    c. Cloth soaker pads

    d. Paper bed protectors

5. Which bedmaking item is used to ensure the patient's modesty and warmth?

    a. Bedspread

    b. Bath blanket

    c. Mattress pad

    d. Regular blanket

6. What needs to be done before a closed bed is made?

    a. Remove used linens.

    b. Clean the entire unit.

    c. Collect necessary linens.

    d. Place new linens on a chair.

7. Where should the draw sheet be placed when making the bed?

    a. On the mattress

    b. Over the top sheet

    c. Under the bottom sheet

    d. On top of the bottom sheet

8. Which action will the nursing assistant take when removing wet or soiled linens?

    a. Apply gloves.

    b. Apply a gown.

    c. Place the linens in a plastic bag.

    d. Place the linens in the bathroom sink.

9. Which action will the nursing assistant take if they needs to obtain an item when making an occupied bed?

    a. Lower the bed.

    b. Raise the side rails.

    c. Ensure the patient is supine.

    d. Direct the patient to hold the position.

10. Which action will the nursing assistant take when making a surgical bed?

    a. Make a toe pleat.

    b. Remove the pillow.

    c. Tighten the bottom sheet.

    d. Keep the top sheet pulled to the pillow.

© 2022 Cengage Learning. All Rights Reserved. May not be scanned, copied or duplicated, or posted to a publicly accessible website, in whole or in part.

CHAPTER APPLICATION

Identification

Identify the following items.

1. Name the type of corner that has been made in the linen.

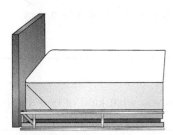

2. Identify the items pictured here.

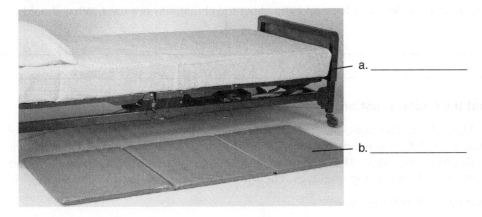

a. _____

b. _____

3. a. Name the fold the nursing assistant is making in the linen.

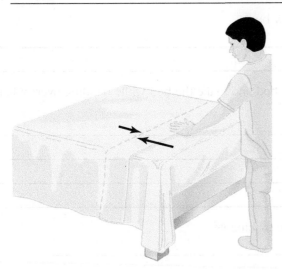

   b. State the purpose of folding the linen in this manner.

© 2022 Cengage Learning. All Rights Reserved. May not be scanned, copied or duplicated, or posted to a publicly accessible website, in whole or in part.

Clinical Situations

Briefly describe how a nursing assistant should react to the following situations.

1. You finish making an occupied bed and you notice that the bed is at the working horizontal height.

   _____

   _____

2. Your patient asks you to raise the side rails before leaving the room so they can pull on them when they moves.

   _____

   _____

3. A visitor tells you that her father is to be placed on a low air loss bed and asks you what kind of bed that is.

   _____

   _____

4. You finish giving a patient a bath and find you have an extra clean towel that was not used. What should be done with the towel?

   _____

   _____

Answer the questions about the clinical situation. Briefly explain your answers.

It is career day for your local high school. The nurse manager of your unit has asked you to allow a high school student to "shadow" you during your shift. You know that only the best nursing assistants are asked to work with these students, and you feel honored to be asked. The student, who is close to your age, is glad to be there and very excited to be working with you. She has many questions. The student asks you the following:

5. What is the purpose of the low bed in Room 321?

   _____

   _____

6. What is the purpose of the mat on the floor next to the low bed?

   _____

   _____

7. Doesn't it hurt your back to care for the patient in the low bed and make the bed while bending over? What can you do to prevent a backache?

   _____

   _____

   _____

   _____

8. Why do you elevate the electric hospital bed when you are making it?

   _____

   _____

© 2022 Cengage Learning. All Rights Reserved. May not be scanned, copied or duplicated, or posted to a publicly accessible website, in whole or in part.

9. Why do you lower the bed when you have finished making it?

_____

_____

10. Why did you leave the room to put the soiled bed linens in the hamper in the hallway? Wouldn't it be easier to put them on the floor and take them to the hamper when you have finished?

_____

_____

_____

11. What is the purpose of the half-sheet in the center of the bed?

_____

_____

12. After you finished making the bed, you pulled the top linen down and folded it at the foot of the bed. That seems like undoing what you just finished. Why did you do this?

_____

_____

_____

_____

13. Why do you make one side of a bed at a time?

_____

_____

RELATING TO THE NURSING PROCESS

Write the step of the nursing process that is related to each nursing assistant action.

Nursing Assistant Action	Nursing Process Step
1. The nursing assistant makes sure the bottom bed linen is free of wrinkles.	_____
2. The nursing assistant applies gloves before removing wet and soiled bed linens.	_____
3. The nursing assistant makes sure the patient is not exposed when the bed linens are changed.	_____
4. The nursing assistant is assigned to prepare a bed for a post-operative patient. She has not done this before and asks the nurse for clarification.	_____

© 2022 Cengage Learning. All Rights Reserved. May not be scanned, copied or duplicated, or posted to a publicly accessible website, in whole or in part.

DEVELOPING GREATER INSIGHT

1. Wrinkle the bottom linen on a bed. Make sure there are wrinkles. Put on your nightwear and spend 30 minutes on the wrinkles.

2. Make the top linen very tight. Be sure to tuck in the top sheet and spread tightly. Spend 30 minutes in this bed.

3. Discuss with classmates the reasons making beds would be very fatiguing if proper procedures were not followed.

4. Discuss with classmates the importance of turning and repositioning patients who are in low air loss beds.

© 2022 Cengage Learning. All Rights Reserved. May not be scanned, copied or duplicated, or posted to a publicly accessible website, in whole or in part.

CHAPTER 24

Patient Bathing

OBJECTIVES

After completing this chapter, you will be able to:

24-1 Spell and define terms.

24-2 Describe the safety precautions for patient bathing.

24-3 List the purposes of bathing patients.

24-4 State the value of whirlpool baths.

24-5 Demonstrate the following procedures:
- Procedure 51: Assisting with the Tub Bath or Shower
- Procedure 52: Bed Bath
- Procedure 53: Changing the Patient's Gown
- Procedure 54: Waterless Bed Bath
- Procedure 55: Partial Bath (Expand Your Skills)
- Procedure 56: Female Perineal Care
- Procedure 57: Male Perineal Care
- Procedure 58: Hand and Fingernail Care
- Procedure 59: Foot and Toenail Care
- Procedure 60: Bed Shampoo (Expand Your Skills)
- Procedure 61: Dressing and Undressing the Patient

VOCABULARY REVIEW

Spelling

Each line has four different spellings of a word. Circle the correctly spelled word.

1. axilla   axiller   axella   arxilla
2. genetala   genitalia   genetalea   ginetalia
3. parineal   pirineal   paraneal   perineal
4. perineum   parineum   pirineum   perinaum

© 2022 Cengage Learning. All Rights Reserved. May not be scanned, copied or duplicated, or posted to a publicly accessible website, in whole or in part.

CHAPTER REVIEW

Fill-in-the-Blank

Complete the statements in the spaces provided.

1. A partial bath ensures cleansing of the hands, face, _____, buttocks, and _____.

2. The best temperature for bath water is about _____°F.

3. A _____ should be in the bath area in case of an emergency.

4. After the tub bath is completed and the patient has returned to the unit, return to the tub room and _____ the tub.

5. To provide privacy during a tub bath or shower, the patient may use a _____ to wrap around their _____.

6. Hold a(n) _____ around the patient to provide privacy as they steps out of the tub.

7. Privacy can be provided during a bed bath by _____.

8. Offer the patient a(n) _____ before giving a bath.

9. When preparing the patient for a bed bath, remove the top bedding and replace it with a(n) _____.

10. Do not use soap near the _____.

11. Clean and wipe the eyes from _____ to _____ corner.

12. Pay special attention to the folds under a female patient's _____ as you wash her.

13. A bag bath may be used instead of using _____.

14. Apply _____ to the feet of a patient with dry skin.

15. Clip the fingernails _____ and do not clip below the _____.

16. When finishing the bath for a male patient, carefully wash and dry the _____, _____, and groin area.

17. The whirlpool tub provides the beneficial action of a _____ in addition to cleaning.

18. Allow the patient to soak the feet for _____ minutes.

19. Two abnormalities you might note during foot care are _____ and calluses.

20. When giving a bed shampoo, _____ the scalp with your _____.

21. Protect the patient's eyes with a(n) _____ during a shampoo.

22. Dry the hair following a shampoo with a(n) _____ or portable hair dryer.

Short Answer

Complete the assessment in the space provided.

1. Three values patients derive from a bath include the following:

   a. _____

   b. _____

   c. _____

© 2022 Cengage Learning. All Rights Reserved. May not be scanned, copied or duplicated, or posted to a publicly accessible website, in whole or in part.

2. Three precautions.you should take when the patient is able to bathe himself or herself in a tub include the following:

a. _____

b. _____

c. _____

3. Special care must be given during the bath to the patient who:

a. _____

b. _____

c. _____

4. There are 13 ending procedure (procedure completion) actions. They are as follows:

a. _____

b. _____

c. _____

d. _____

e. _____

f. _____

g. _____

h. _____

i. _____

j. _____

k. _____

l. _____

m. _____

5. List at least five situations in which gloves must be worn when bathing a patient.

a. _____

b. _____

c. _____

d. _____

e. _____

6. Describe how a bath mitt is made.

_____

_____

_____

7. List three advantages to using the waterless bathing system compared with a regular bed bath.

a. _____

b. _____

c. _____

© 2022 Cengage Learning. All Rights Reserved. May not be scanned, copied or duplicated, or posted to a publicly accessible website, in whole or in part.

8. Why should the patient help you with the bed bath as much as their condition permits?

_____

_____

9. What is the nursing assistant's responsibility when the patient is unable to complete their bath?

_____

_____

10. What other procedures may be carried out in conjunction with the bath procedure?

_____

11. What are four advantages of the whirlpool bath?

a. _____

b. _____

c. _____

d. _____

12. What seven measures can be taken to help avoid patient falls during tub bathing?

a. _____

b. _____

c. _____

d. _____

e. _____

f. _____

g. _____

CERTIFICATION REVIEW

Complete the following multiple-choice assessments.

1. For which reason will the nursing assistant apply powder in a patient's skin folds?

   a. Reduce odor

   b. Prevent itching

   c. Reduce moisture

   d. Prevent sweating

2. Which action will the nursing assistant take if all the cloths are not used for a bag bath?

   a. Place them in the bathroom.

   b. Use them on another patient.

   c. Throw the unused ones away.

   d. Reseal the package and date it.

© 2022 Cengage Learning. All Rights Reserved. May not be scanned, copied or duplicated, or posted to a publicly accessible website, in whole or in part.

3. Which gloving technique will the nursing assistant practice when bathing a patient?

    a. Do not apply gloves.

    b. Apply sterile gloves.

    c. Wear clean gloves at all times.

    d. Wear a glove on the dominant hand.

4. Which action will be taken when assisting a patient with a tub bath?

    a. Undress the patient in the tub room.

    b. Place a nonskid surface on the bottom of the tub.

    c. Leave the patient once safely positioned in the tub.

    d. Position the patient in the tub before filling it with water.

5. Which action should be taken if a patient with Alzheimer disease becomes agitated during a bath?

    a. Skip the bath.

    b. Continue with the bath.

    c. Change the type of bath.

    d. Tell the patient to calm down.

6. Which item will be used to make a bath mitt?

    a. Towel

    b. Washcloth

    c. Draw sheet

    d. Bath blanket

7. Which action should be taken if assisting a patient wash the genitalia?

    a. Apply gloves.

    b. Assist to a seated position.

    c. Hold a bath blanket over the area.

    d. Change the basin water afterward.

8. What is an advantage of a towel bath?

    a. Can be done quickly

    b. Can be done by the patient

    c. Focuses on specific body areas

    d. Does not require rinsing with water

9. What should be done before combing a patient's hair?

    a. Apply gloves.

    b. Wash the comb.

    c. Apply water to the hair.

    d. Place a towel over the pillowcase.

© 2022 Cengage Learning. All Rights Reserved. May not be scanned, copied or duplicated, or posted to a publicly accessible website, in whole or in part.

10. What should be done when providing perineal care after a patient is incontinent of stool?

    a. Apply sterile gloves

    b. Cleanse from clean to dirty

    c. Scrub the area back and forth

    d. Use the same cloth to save time

CHAPTER APPLICATION

Clinical Situations

Briefly describe how a nursing assistant should react to the following situations.

1. Your patient feels weak or faint during a tub bath.

    _____

    _____

2. You have not yet finished bathing the legs of a bed patient and the water feels cool.

    _____

    _____

3. Your patient has diabetes and their toenails need cutting.

    _____

    _____

4. Describe the technique to be used when washing the penis and the scrotum.

    _____

    _____

© 2022 Cengage Learning. All Rights Reserved. May not be scanned, copied or duplicated, or posted to a publicly accessible website, in whole or in part.

RELATING TO THE NURSING PROCESS

Write the step of the nursing process that is related to each nursing assistant action.

Nursing Assistant Action	Nursing Process Step

1. The nursing assistant carefully cleans the tub before and after each patient use.   _____

2. The nursing assistant has to bathe a patient who has an IV line and is not sure how to remove the patient's gown. They asks a nurse for help.   _____

3. The nursing assistant offers a bedpan to the patient before giving a bed bath.   _____

4. The nursing assistant finds that the patient cannot separate their legs sufficiently to allow good perineal care, so the assistant asks the nurse for directions on how to give care.   _____

5. The nursing assistant is giving foot care to a patient with long, thick toenails. He asks the nurse if the nails should be cut.   _____

6. The nursing assistant listens carefully as the nurse explains that the care plan for a bed bath will be modified the next day to allow the patient to shower if they feels well enough.   _____

DEVELOPING GREATER INSIGHT

1. Discuss why frequent perineal care is important for the patient's hygiene.

2. Discuss why nursing assistants are not permitted to cut the toenails of a patient with diabetes.

3. Discuss ways to give perineal care if the patient cannot separate their legs.

4. Working with another student, demonstrate the proper way to assist a person to put on a shirt that slips over the head when the patient cannot use one side of their body.

5. Think through the reasons you should be ready to assist patients to put on shoes and socks.

© 2022 Cengage Learning. All Rights Reserved. May not be scanned, copied or duplicated, or posted to a publicly accessible website, in whole or in part.

General Comfort Measures

OBJECTIVES

After completing this chapter, you will be able to:

25-1 Spell and define terms.

25-2 Discuss the reasons for early morning and bedtime care.

25-3 Identify patients who require frequent oral hygiene.

25-4 List the purposes of oral hygiene.

25-5 Explain nursing assistant responsibilities related to a patient's dentures.

25-6 State the purpose of backrubs.

25-7 Describe safety precautions when shaving a patient.

25-8 Describe the importance of hair care.

25-9 Explain the use of comfort devices.

25-10 State the purpose of bed boards and list guidelines for their use.

25-11 Explain why regular elimination is essential to good health.

25-12 Demonstrate the following procedures:

- Procedure 62: Assisting with Routine Oral Hygiene
- Procedure 63: Assisting with Special Oral Hygiene—Dependent and Unconscious Patients
- Procedure 64: Assisting the Patient to Floss and Brush Teeth
- Procedure 65: Caring for Dentures
- Procedure 66: Providing Backrubs
- Procedure 67: Shaving a Male Patient (Expand Your Skills)
- Procedure 68: Providing Daily Hair Care
- Procedure 69: Giving and Receiving the Bedpan
- Procedure 70: Giving and Receiving the Urinal (Expand Your Skills)
- Procedure 71: Assisting with Use of the Bedside Commode (Expand Your Skills)

© 2022 Cengage Learning. All Rights Reserved. May not be scanned, copied or duplicated, or posted to a publicly accessible website, in whole or in part.

VOCABULARY BUILDER

Matching

1. _____ stool
2. _____ bad breath
3. _____ tooth decay
4. _____ contracture of the foot
5. _____ removable artificial teeth
6. _____ care of the mouth and teeth
7. _____ medication that thins the blood
8. _____ care provided early in the morning
9. _____ prepare the patient for a night of rest
10. _____ device to keep the feet at right angles
11. _____ elevate the body off the surface of the bed
12. _____ condition that affects the tissue and bone that supports the teeth

a. a.m. care
b. anticoagulant
c. bridging
d. caries
e. dentures
f. feces
g. footboard
h. foot drop
i. halitosis
j. oral hygiene
k. periodontal disease
l. p.m. care

CHAPTER REVIEW

Fill-in-the-Blank

Complete the following statements in the spaces provided.

1. When out of the mouth, dentures should be stored in a _____

_____.

2. The purpose of applying lubricant to the lips is _____

_____.

3. Handle dentures _____ to prevent damage.

4. Label each patient's denture cup with _____

_____.

5. Proper mouth cleaning helps prevent halitosis and dental _____.

6. Insert the toothbrush into the mouth with the bristles in a _____ position.

7. Special oral hygiene is given by using _____ or _____.

8. Apply lubricant to the lips with _____.

9. Position the patient in a(n) _____ position during toothbrushing, if possible.

10. Always _____ to protect dentures during cleaning.

11. _____ lotion in _____ before giving a backrub.

12. A special order may be needed to shave the face of a patient who is taking _____.

© 2022 Cengage Learning. All Rights Reserved. May not be scanned, copied or duplicated, or posted to a publicly accessible website, in whole or in part.

13. Hold the skin _____ when shaving a patient's face.

14. Brushing the hair makes the patient feel better and _____ the scalp.

15. Give the patient the opportunity to go to the bathroom or to use the _____ before breakfast.

16. Give evening care in a _____, _____ manner.

17. Clear the _____ table and adjust the _____ of the bed during evening care.

18. Tightening the _____ and straightening the _____ linen is part of a.m. and p.m. care.

19. Position the bed in the _____ horizontal position after p.m. care if the patient's condition permits.

20. Remove all used _____ from the patient's room at bedtime.

Short Answer

Complete the assessment in the space provided.

1. Why is oral hygiene important?

   _____.

2. How are dentures stored when the patient is not wearing them?

   _____.

3. Why are backrubs important to the patient who is not permitted out of bed?

   _____.

4. Why should nursing assistants keep their fingernails short?

   _____.

5. Why should the skin be held taut while using the razor?

   _____.

6. What would you do if you accidentally nicked a patient during the shaving procedure?

   _____.

7. What action would you take if a patient's hair were tangled?

   _____.

8. Why must gloves be worn when shaving a patient's intact face with a disposable razor?

   _____.

9. Six patients requiring special oral hygiene are those who are

   a. _____

   b. _____

   c. _____

   d. _____

   e. _____

   f. _____

© 2022 Cengage Learning. All Rights Reserved. May not be scanned, copied or duplicated, or posted to a publicly accessible website, in whole or in part.

'0. Five times when backrubs are usually given are as follows:

a. _____

b. _____

c. _____

d. _____

e. _____

11. List four pieces of equipment you would need to give a backrub.

a. _____

b. _____

c. _____

d. _____

12. Why is mouth care given before the patient has breakfast?

_____.

13. Why is a backrub given to the patient at bedtime?

_____.

14. How do you wake the patient?

_____.

15. Two instances when you would not waken the patient before breakfast are if they is

a. _____

b. _____

16. Four activities you will carry out as part of bedtime care include the following:

a. _____

b. _____

c. _____

d. _____

True/False

Mark the following true or false by circling T or F.

1. T F Never place a bedpan on the overbed table.

2. T F Place the bedpan cover on the bedside stand.

3. T F A bariatric bedpan must be used for patients who have had orthopedic surgery.

4. T F You do not need to cover a used bedpan if the bathroom is close to the patient's room.

5. T F A small folded towel can be used to pad a bedpan if the patient is very thin.

6. T F If the patient is very heavy, you may need assistance placing him or her on a bedpan.

7. T F The patient's buttocks should rest on the narrow end of the fracture bedpan.

© 2022 Cengage Learning. All Rights Reserved. May not be scanned, copied or duplicated, or posted to a publicly accessible website, in whole or in part.

8. T   F   Draw the cubicle curtains around a patient who is using a bedpan.

9. T   F   Make sure the signal cord is close at hand when the patient is on a bedpan.

10. T   F   Note and document bedpan contents.

CERTIFICATION REVIEW

Complete the following multiple-choice assessments.

1. Which is the minimal personal protective equipment that should be worn when providing mouth care?

    a. Mask

    b. Gown

    c. Gloves

    d. Face shield

2. Which length of dental floss should be used to floss a patient's teeth?

    a. 6 inches

    b. 8 inches

    c. 10 inches

    d. 12 inches

3. Which item is needed when assisting a patient to self-brush teeth while in bed?

    a. Gloves

    b. Plastic bag

    c. Emesis basin

    d. Cotton-tipped applicators

4. What should be done with the dentures of a patient who is comatose?

    a. Kept in the mouth

    b. Cleansed every day

    c. Soaked in hot water

    d. Removed and stored

5. Which action should be taken when a reddened area does not blanch when providing a back rub?

    a. Massage the area.

    b. Report it to the nurse.

    c. Apply gentle pressure.

    d. Apply a warm compress.

6. Which action should be avoided when providing a backrub to a patient?

    a. Bend from the waist.

    b. Rock back and forth.

    c. Use strong leg muscles.

    d. Use arm and shoulder muscles.

© 2022 Cengage Learning. All Rights Reserved. May not be scanned, copied or duplicated, or posted to a publicly accessible website, in whole or in part.

7. Which guideline will the nursing assistant follow when applying lotion to a patient's skin?

   a. Pat on the legs.

   b. Rub reddened areas.

   c. Use the patient's lotion.

   d. Apply between the toes.

8. What needs to be done when applying a bed board on a patient's bed?

   a. Remove the mattress linens.

   b. Wrap the board with a bath blanket.

   c. Place the board under the draw sheet.

   d. Ensure a physician's order has been written.

9. What should be done if a footboard is not available for a patient?

   a. Have the patient wear shoes while in bed.

   b. Wait until a footboard becomes available.

   c. Place a firm board at the end of the mattress.

   d. Fold a pillow lengthwise and place it at the foot of the bed.

10. Which action should be taken after placing a patient on a bedpan?

    a. Apply gloves.

    b. Turn down the top sheet.

    c. Raise the head of the bed.

    d. Lower the head of the bed.

© 2022 Cengage Learning. All Rights Reserved. May not be scanned, copied or duplicated, or posted to a publicly accessible website, in whole or in part.

CHAPTER APPLICATION

Identify Strokes

Using a colored pencil or crayon, draw in the indicated strokes.

1. Soothing

2. Passive

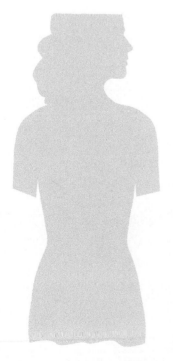

© 2022 Cengage Learning. All Rights Reserved. May not be scanned, copied or duplicated, or posted to a publicly accessible website, in whole or in part.

3. Circular

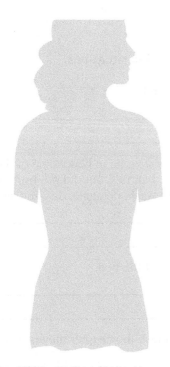

Name the Equipment

Write the name of the equipment pictured in the space provided.

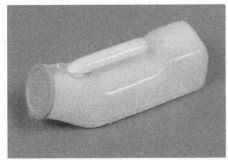

1. _____.

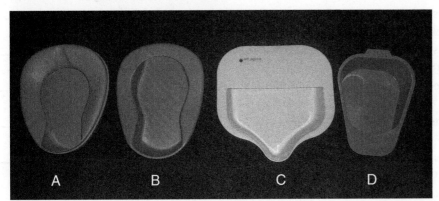

2. A. _____.

   B. _____

   C. _____

   D. _____

© 2022 Cengage Learning. All Rights Reserved. May not be scanned, copied or duplicated, or posted to a publicly accessible website, in whole or in part.

Clinical Situations

Briefly describe how a nursing assistant should react to the following situations.

1. You note a pressure area on your patient's hip while giving a backrub.

   _____

   _____

2. You must wash the hair of an African American patient who vomited while in bed. Some of the vomitus accidentally got in her hair. The patient has a comb, brush, and elastic hair ties, but did not bring any hair care products to the hospital. What hair care products will you need to wash, detangle, dry, and style her hair?

   _____

   _____

3. Your patient needs to use the bedpan but cannot lift her buttocks off the bed.

   _____

   _____

4. You are giving p.m. care and the patient says they would like to finish the chapter they is reading.

   _____

   _____

5. Your patient is settled for the night and you are ready to leave the room.

   _____

   _____

RELATING TO THE NURSING PROCESS

Write the step of the nursing process that is related to each nursing assistant action.

Nursing Assistant Action	Nursing Process Step
1. The nursing assistant allows the patient to sleep and omits early a.m. care because the patient is going to surgery.	_____
2. The nursing assistant makes sure that bedtime care has been given before the nurse administers sleep medications.	_____
3. The nursing assistant uses cool water when brushing the dentures for the patient.	_____
4. The nursing assistant reports that the patient's lips are very dry and cracked.	_____
5. The nursing assistant listens carefully when the patient says that they does not want to put their dentures in because they hurt.	_____
6. The nursing assistant reports and documents the condition of the patient's skin each time they gives back care.	_____

© 2022 Cengage Learning. All Rights Reserved. May not be scanned, copied or duplicated, or posted to a publicly accessible website, in whole or in part.

DEVELOPING GREATER INSIGHT

1. In the learning lab, divide the class into pairs. Have the students simulate completing the following:

   a. Assisting with toothbrushing

   b. Providing hair care

   c. Providing a bedpan (or urinal)

2. Have the students practice giving backrubs to each other while sitting in a chair.

3. Ask the students to brainstorm approaches for the following situations:

   a. Patient does not want mouth care.

   b. Patient refuses p.m. care.

   c. Patient does want hair care but is obviously dirty.

© 2022 Cengage Learning. All Rights Reserved. May not be scanned, copied or duplicated, or posted to a publicly accessible website, in whole or in part.

Principles of Nutrition and Fluid Balance

C H A P T E R **26**

Nutritional Needs and Diet Modifications

OBJECTIVES

After completing this chapter, you will be able to:

26-1 Spell and define terms.

26-2 Define normal nutrition.

26-3 List the essential nutrients.

26-4 Name the food groups and list the foods included in each group.

26-5 Identify the basic facility diets and describe each.

26-6 State the purposes of the following diets:
- Clear liquid
- Full liquid
- Soft
- Mechanically altered

26-7 State the purpose of calorie counts and food intake studies.

26-8 Define dysphagia and explain the risks of this condition.

26-9 Describe general care for the patient with dysphagia and swallowing problems.

26-10 State the purposes of therapeutic diets.

26-11 List types of alternative nutrition.

26-12 Describe the nursing assistant actions when patients are unable to drink fluids independently.

26-13 Demonstrate the following procedures:
- Procedure 72: Assisting the Patient Who Can Feed Self
- Procedure 73: Feeding the Dependent Patient
- Procedure 74: Abdominal Thrusts—Heimlich Maneuver

© 2022 Cengage Learning. All Rights Reserved. May not be scanned, copied or duplicated, or posted to a publicly accessible website, in whole or in part.

VOCABULARY BUILDER

Matching

Match each term with the correct definition.

1. _____ vomitus
2. _____ difficulty swallowing
3. _____ excessive perspiration
4. _____ excessive fluid retention
5. _____ substances used by the body's cells
6. _____ food energy that comes from plants
7. _____ building blocks that make up protein
8. _____ lack of sufficient fluid in body tissues
9. _____ food energy that comes from animals
10. _____ breaking down of food into substances
11. _____ substances that regulate body processes
12. _____ fluid taken in and eliminated by the body
13. _____ diet made up of water and carbohydrates
14. _____ liquids and semisolid foods that are easy to digest
15. _____ diet prepared to address a specific health problem
16. _____ nutrient that can make new cells and rebuild tissues
17. _____ food that is blended until it is the consistency of pudding
18. _____ foods that are ground to the consistency of hamburger
19. _____ food, water, gastric contents enter the trachea and lungs
20. _____ type of diet made up of liquids thicker than water

a. amino acids
b. aspiration
c. carbohydrates
d. clear liquid diet
e. dehydration
f. diaphoresis
g. digestion
h. dysphagia
i. edema
j. emesis
k. fats
l. full liquid diet
m. intake & output
n. mechanical soft
o. nutrients
p. protein
q. pureed diet
r. soft diet
s. therapeutic diets
t. vitamins

CHAPTER REVIEW

Fill-in-the-Blank

Complete the following statements in the spaces provided.

1. The well-nourished person will have a well-developed _____ and body weight appropriate to _____.

2. Water is a(n) _____ nutrient.

3. A consistent carbohydrate diet may be ordered for a patient with _____.

4. Carbohydrates and fats are called _____ foods because the body uses them to produce heat and vitality.

© 2022 Cengage Learning. All Rights Reserved. May not be scanned, copied or duplicated, or posted to a publicly accessible website, in whole or in part.

5. Proteins are composed of _____ acids.

6. Select lean cuts of meat whenever possible to limit the amount of _____ fats in your diet.

7. Following surgery, a _____ diet is served.

8. The first postoperative intake usually permitted is _____ or sips of water.

9. The clear liquid diet does not irritate the bowel or encourage _____.

10. The daily intake of fluid (water) should be _____ glasses.

11. A patient with a fever should be given a(n) _____ diet.

12. The exchange lists are used in preparing a(n) _____ diet.

13. The exchange lists are based on standard _____ measurements.

14. If a patient is on I&O and you serve beverages, you must _____ _____

15. Before serving a tray, be sure to clear away anything that is _____ _____

16. When feeding the dependent patient, hold the spoon at a _____ to the patient's mouth.

17. Nutritional supplements are ordered by the physician and have _____.

18. A mechanically altered diet may be served to patients who have problems _____ or _____.

19. A pureed diet is commonly served to patients who have difficulty _____.

20. When a patient has an order for a calorie count, all food intake is accurately _____ at the end of each meal.

21. Patients with _____ have difficulty swallowing fluids and food and are at high risk of aspiration.

22. The speech-language pathologist may order addition of _____ to liquids for patients who have swallowing problems.

23. Sodium-restricted diets are some of the _____ diets for patients to follow.

True/False

Mark the following true or false by circling T or F.

1. T F Patients who are unable to swallow without aspiration require alternative nutrition.

2. T F Enteral feedings are introduced into smaller veins in the arm.

3. T F Gastrostomy feedings enter the stomach through a nasogastric tube.

4. T F Enteral feedings are usually controlled by an automatic device.

5. T F Oral hygiene may safely be omitted when patients receive enteral feedings because food does not enter the mouth.

6. T F Nausea or vomiting must be reported immediately to the nurse.

7. T F The head of the bed should be flat during feedings and remain in that position for half an hour after the feeding.

© 2022 Cengage Learning. All Rights Reserved. May not be scanned, copied or duplicated, or posted to a publicly accessible website, in whole or in part.

8. T   F   Patients must not be permitted to lie on enteral tubes.

9. T   F   Inform the nurse if tape is causing irritation.

10. T   F   Liquid nutritional supplements should be served at mealtime.

11. T   F   Completing a food intake or calorie count study requires a team effort.

12. T   F   Patients with dysphagia are at high risk of developing malnutrition and dehydration.

Short Answer

Complete the assessment in the space provided.

1. What are the names of three health care facility diets?

    a. _____

    b. _____

    c. _____

2. Why is an unhurried attitude important when feeding a patient?

    _____

3. What is meant by the order to "force fluids"?

    _____

4. Name two alternative methods of providing nutrients.

    a. _____

    b. _____

5. Three functions of nutrients are

    a. _____

    b. _____

    c. _____

6. The six basic nutrients are

    a. _____

    b. _____

    c. _____

    d. _____

    e. _____

    f. _____

7. Four examples of complete proteins are

    a. _____

    b. _____

    c. _____

    d. _____

© 2022 Cengage Learning. All Rights Reserved. May not be scanned, copied or duplicated, or posted to a publicly accessible website, in whole or in part.

8. Four examples of incomplete proteins are

   a. _____

   b. _____

   c. _____

   d. _____

9. Six minerals needed in any person's daily diet include the following:

   a. _____

   b. _____

   c. _____

   d. _____

   e. _____

   f. _____

10. Four functions of vitamins are to:

    a. _____

    b. _____

    c. _____

    d. _____

11. Six vitamins needed by the body are

    a. _____

    b. _____

    c. _____

    d. _____

    e. _____

    f. _____

12. Name the five "P" foods to be avoided in a low-sodium diet.

    a. _____

    b. _____

    c. _____

    d. _____

    e. _____

13. What are the amounts of average servings?

    a. Fruit _____

    b. Cooked fruit or vegetable _____

    c. Meat _____

    d. Pasta/bread _____

14. A person who is receiving a consistent carbohydrate diet receives about:

    a. _____% of the daily calories from fat.

    b _____% of the daily calories from protein.

    c. _____% of the daily calories from carbohydrate.

© 2022 Cengage Learning. All Rights Reserved. May not be scanned, copied or duplicated, or posted to a publicly accessible website, in whole or in part.

5. What is the purpose of serving nutritional supplements?

_____

_____

16. Explain the difference between supplements and nourishments.

_____

_____

_____

_____

17. Hot foods must be served at _____°F or above, and cold foods must be served at _____°F or below.

18. Explain why the food cart must be separated from the soiled linen hamper and housekeeping cart by at least one room's width in the hallways.

_____

_____

_____

_____

19. List three things you can do to maintain food temperature when the food cart arrives on the unit.

a. _____

b. _____

c. _____

20. Explain the difference between a PEG tube and a nasogastric tube, and state the purpose of each tube.

_____

_____

21. Intake and output records are kept for six special circumstances when specifically ordered, such as in patients who:

a. _____

b. _____

c. _____

d. _____

e. _____

f. _____

22. Output that must be recorded includes the following:

a. _____

b. _____

c. _____

d. _____

e. _____

f. _____

© 2022 Cengage Learning. All Rights Reserved. May not be scanned, copied or duplicated, or posted to a publicly accessible website, in whole or in part.

23. What does intake include?

   _____

24. What does output include?

   _____

25. In what unit of measurement are intake and output recorded?

   _____

CERTIFICATION REVIEW

Complete the following multiple-choice assessments.

1. Which food item is naturally high in oil?

   a. Fish

   b. Banana

   c. Avocado

   d. Pineapple

2. Which item will the nursing assistant remove from the tray of a patient prescribed a clear liquid diet?

   a. Tea

   b. Broth

   c. Ice cream

   d. Apple juice

3. Which food item is absent from an exchange list?

   a. Cake

   b. Steak

   c. Grapes

   d. Muffin

4. Which action will the nursing assistant take when providing a patient with a liquid nutritional supplement?

   a. Serve it with lunch.

   b. Provide it with dinner.

   c. Select one that is cold.

   d. Deliver it on the breakfast tray.

5. Which action will the nursing assistant take when adding thickener to a patient's beverage?

   a. Limit its use to cold beverages.

   b. Pour the thickener from the container.

   c. Mix the thickener for several minutes.

   d. Wait one minute after adding the thickener.

© 2022 Cengage Learning. All Rights Reserved. May not be scanned, copied or duplicated, or posted to a publicly accessible website, in whole or in part.

6. Which action will be taken when filling a patient's water pitcher?

    a. Place the scoop in the pitcher.

    b. Fill the pitcher to the rim with ice.

    c. Take the cover off of the pitcher in the patient's room.

    d. Ensure that the pitcher is labeled with the patient's name.

7. Which action will be taken to assist a patient who can self-feed a meal?

    a. Assist with oral hygiene.

    b. Place the tray on the patient's lap.

    c. Position the overbed table next to a wall.

    d. Pick up the tray when providing p.m. care.

8. In which way will the nursing assistant check the temperature of food?

    a. Blow on the food.

    b. Place a small amount on the wrist.

    c. Use an oral temperature measuring device.

    d. Provide the patient with a small bite and ask if it is the correct temperature.

9. Which action should be taken if a patient begins to cough while eating?

    a. Call for help.

    b. Move the tray.

    c. Observe the patient.

    d. Perform the Heimlich maneuver.

10. Which action should be taken if a patient receiving a tube feeding begins to cough?

    a. Turn patient on their side.

    b. Observe the patient.

    c. Lower the head of the bed.

    d. Perform the Heimlich maneuver.

CHAPTER APPLICATION

Matching

Identify each type of vitamin.

1. _____ vitamin A

2. _____ vitamin B complex

3. _____ vitamin C

4. _____ vitamin D

5. _____ vitamin E

6. _____ vitamin K

a. water-soluble

b. fat-soluble

© 2022 Cengage Learning. All Rights Reserved. May not be scanned, copied or duplicated, or posted to a publicly accessible website, in whole or in part.

Complete the Chart

Complete the chart in the spaces provided.

1. Write the names of the food groups at the top of the columns below. Write the names of each of the following foods in the column under the proper food group.

apples	bacon	beef	bread	butter	cereal
cheese	chicken	cottage cheese	fish	flour	honey
ice cream	liver	milk	olive oil	pasta	pears
peas	rice	spinach	yogurt		

Group 1	Group 2	Group 3	Group 4	Group 5	Group 6

Clinical Situations

Briefly describe how a nursing assistant should react to the following situations.

1. Your patient is on I&O and you picked up the lunch tray. _____

_____

2. You serve a tray to a blind person who is able to feed himself or herself. _____

_____

3. Your patient's chart includes an order to force fluids. _____

_____

4. The patient receiving an IV has 25 mL of fluid left in the bag. _____

_____

5. Your patient is on a strict kosher diet and the tray has a shrimp salad as an entrée.

_____

_____

© 2022 Cengage Learning. All Rights Reserved. May not be scanned, copied or duplicated, or posted to a publicly accessible website, in whole or in part.

Conversions

Convert the following values into milliliters. Show your work.

1. a. 2 (8 oz) cups of coffee _____ mL

   b. 1 (6 oz) bowl of soup _____ mL

   c. 3 (8 oz) glasses of water _____ mL

   d. 2 (4 oz) glasses of ice chips _____ mL

   e. 2 (4 oz) dishes of gelatin _____ mL

Complete the Form

1. Keep a diary of your food intake for 24 hours. Include everything you eat. Then determine if you have achieved an adequate intake of nutrients by answering the following questions.

Dietary Chart

Time	Food	Amount

Time	Food	Amount

Answer the following questions by entering Yes or No in the space provided.

_____ Did you include two or three servings from the meat group?

_____ Did you include six to eleven servings from the bread, cereal, rice, and pasta group?

_____ Did you include two or more glasses of milk or its equivalent in dairy products?

_____ Did you include at least one serving of a food high in vitamin C?

© 2022 Cengage Learning. All Rights Reserved. May not be scanned, copied or duplicated, or posted to a publicly accessible website, in whole or in part.

_____ Did you make sure there was some roughage in your diet?

_____ Did you include three to five servings of the vegetable group?

_____ Are there things in your diet that you think should be eliminated?

2. List four conditions in which dysphagia is commonly seen.

   a. _____

   b. _____

   c. _____

   d. _____

3. Complete an intake and output sheet that reflects the following information.
   The patient, John Rodriquez, is in Room 404B. During the day he felt fairly well. He drank about 50 mL of water after he brushed his teeth at 7:15 a.m. He also voided 550 mL of yellow urine. Breakfast arrived and he had a pot of tea (240 mL). Early morning nourishments arrived and he selected and consumed 120 mL of cranberry juice followed by 80 mL of water at lunch (11:15 a.m.) with 120 mL of orange sherbet for dessert. He voided again, 400 mL yellow urine, at 2:30 p.m. In the afternoon he had 240 mL of tea with a visitor. Dinner arrived and he had 180 mL of milk, 180 mL of soup, and 120 mL of gelatin. He asked for a urinal and voided 375 mL of urine. At 9:30 p.m. he tried to eat some gelatin, approximately 50 mL, and within minutes vomited 400 mL. He continued to feel nauseated and vomited 200 mL at 11:15 p.m., 150 mL at 12:00 a.m., and 80 mL at 2:30 a.m. At 5.30 a.m., 500 mL D/W was started IV. Mr. Rodriquez voided 300 mL at this time. The urine was pink-tinged.

WASHINGTON GENERAL HOSPITAL
FLUID INTAKE AND OUTPUT

Name _____   Room _____

Date	Time	Method of Adm.	Intake			Output		
			Solution	Amounts Rec'd	Time	Urine Amount	Others Kind	Others Amount
Total								

© 2022 Cengage Learning. All Rights Reserved. May not be scanned, copied or duplicated, or posted to a publicly accessible website, in whole or in part.

4. Identify each food group based on the MyPlate picture here.

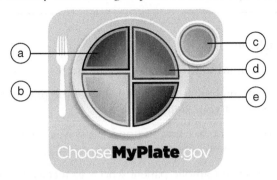

Balancing Calories

- Enjoy your food, but eat less.
- Avoid oversized portions.

Foods to Increase

- Make half your plate fruits and vegetables.
- Make at least half your grains whole grains.
- Switch to fat-free or low-fat (1%) milk.

Foods to Reduce

- Compare sodium in foods like, soup, bread, and frozen meals—and choose the foods with lower numbers
- Drink water instead of sugary drinks.

a. _____

b. _____

c. _____

d. _____

e. _____

RELATING TO THE NURSING PROCESS

Write the step of the nursing process that is related to each nursing assistant action.

Nursing Assistant Action	Nursing Process Step
1. The nursing assistant carefully checks the patient's identification band against the diet slip.	_____
2. The nursing assistant reports to the nurse that the patient ate only one-third of the soft diet ordered.	_____
3. The nursing assistant documents that the patient refused lunch because he felt nauseated.	_____
4. The nursing assistant carefully records the fluids taken by the patient who has an order for I&O.	_____
5. The nursing assistant checks with the team leader to be sure gelatin should be recorded as fluid intake.	_____
6. The nursing assistant makes a special note during report that their patient is on I&O.	_____

© 2022 Cengage Learning. All Rights Reserved. May not be scanned, copied or duplicated, or posted to a publicly accessible website, in whole or in part.

DEVELOPING GREATER INSIGHT

1. Make a statement to the class about the actions you would take if:

   a. Your patient is on I&O and you find a container of milk one-third full when you pick up trays.

   b. Your patient is on I&O and has perspired so much during the night that you had to change the pillowcase and bottom sheet. Describe what you will monitor for the rest of your shift.

2. Try to identify the feelings you might experience if you were an Orthodox Jew and pork roast was served to you.

3. Think through what action you might take while caring for a Roman Catholic patient who is to receive Communion at 8:00 a.m., when breakfast is served at 7:00 a.m.

4. Working in groups, plan how you would modify the regular diet for an 82-year-old, 110-pound woman who has trouble chewing because her dentures are loose.

5. Practice feeding and being fed. Wear a clothing protector. Discuss your feelings during the experience. Consider adding a blindfold to the person being fed. Describe your experience feeding a "blind" person. Describe how it felt to be unable to see what you were eating.

6. Sample each of your facility's diets (including pureed) and supplements.

© 2022 Cengage Learning. All Rights Reserved. May not be scanned, copied or duplicated, or posted to a publicly accessible website, in whole or in part.

Special Care Procedures

CHAPTER **27**

Warm and Cold Applications

OBJECTIVES

After completing this chapter, you will be able to:

27-1 Spell and define terms.

27-2 List the physical conditions requiring the use of heat and cold.

27-3 Name types of heat and cold applications.

27-4 Describe the effects of local cold applications.

27-5 Describe the effects of local heat applications.

27-6 List safety concerns related to application of heat and cold.

27-7 Demonstrate the following procedures:

- Procedure 75: Applying an Ice Bag or Gel Pack (Expand Your Skills)
- Procedure 76: Applying a Disposable Cold Pack (Expand Your Skills)
- Procedure 77: Giving a Sitz Bath (Expand Your Skills)

© 2022 Cengage Learning. All Rights Reserved. May not be scanned, copied or duplicated, or posted to a publicly accessible website, in whole or in part.

VOCABULARY BUILDER

Matching

Match each definition with the correct term.

1. _____ normal operating temperature that is in the deep structures of the center of the body
2. _____ blood vessels become smaller in diameter
3. _____ a type of bath that submerges the pelvic area
4. _____ a waterproof device filled with distilled water to warm or cool parts of the body
5. _____ lowering body temperature to 95°F or below
6. _____ excessive blood loss
7. _____ blood vessels become larger in diameter
8. _____ immersion of a body part in water that is approximately 105°F
9. _____ reusable waterproof container filled with ice; used for treatment on a single area of the body
10. _____ treatment using heat

a. aquathermia
b. core
c. diathermy
d. hemorrhage
e. hypothermia
f. ice bag
g. sitz
h. vasoconstrict
i. vasodilate
j. warm

CHAPTER REVIEW

Short Answer

Complete the following statements in the spaces provided.

1. Two types of hot and cold applications are _____ and _____.
2. Examples of hot applications are _____, _____, and _____.
3. Examples of cold applications are _____, _____, and _____.
4. An ice bag should be filled _____.
5. When filling an ice bag, pressing the hand against the flat surface expels the _____.
6. No application of heat or cold can be given without _____.
7. The Aquamatic K-Pad control unit should be filled with _____.
8. Apply the principles of _____ when applying heat and cold treatments.
9. Check the skin under a warm or cold application at least every _____ minutes.
10. Warm and cold applications should not be left in place for more than _____ minutes.
11. A thermal blanket used to reduce body temperature is known as a(n) _____.
12. Applications of cold to a sprained ankle can reduce _____ and numb the sensation of _____.
13. Warm applications cause blood vessels to _____.
14. Never set the whirlpool above _____°F without first checking with the nurse.
15. Heat should not be applied to the head because it can cause _____.

© 2022 Cengage Learning. All Rights Reserved. May not be scanned, copied or duplicated, or posted to a publicly accessible website, in whole or in part.

'6. If the patient might have appendicitis, _____ should not be applied to the abdomen.

17. Check all areas to which cold is applied for _____ and _____.

18. Before fastening the cap of an ice bag securely, expel all _____.

19. The metal cap of an ice bag should always be positioned _____ from the patient.

20. To activate a commercial cold pack, _____ or squeeze the pack.

21. Patients should never be allowed to _____ on an Aquamatic K-Pad.

22. The prescribed temperature for an arm or foot soak is about _____°F.

23. For accuracy, the temperature of all warm or cold treatments should be checked with a

_____.

24. Before applying a moist compress, always remove _____.

25 The Aquamatic K-Pad cord must be plugged into a(n) _____ for the unit to operate.

26. Always check a warm water bottle for _____ before applying.

27. A warm water bottle should always be _____ before application.

28. Aquamatic K-Pads are _____ used in a health care facility.

29. Four reasons for applying heat or cold are to:

a. _____

b. _____

c. _____

d. _____

30. List six conditions in which heat treatments should not be used.

a. _____

b. _____

c. _____

d. _____

e. _____

f. _____

31. List six conditions in which cold treatments should not be used.

a. _____

b. _____

c. _____

d. _____

e. _____

f. _____

32. List four complications of heat or cold therapy about which the nurse should be notified.

a. _____

b. _____

c. _____

d. _____

© 2022 Cengage Learning. All Rights Reserved. May not be scanned, copied or duplicated, or posted to a publicly accessible website, in whole or in part.

33. Two ways to apply dry cold are by:

    a. _____

    b. _____

34. Moist cold is applied through a wet compress.

35. List six complications of using the hypothermia blanket about which the nurse should be notified immediately.

    a. _____

    b. _____

    c. _____

    d. _____

    e. _____

    f. _____

36. List the information needed to document a warm or cold treatment.

    a. _____

    b. _____

    c. _____

    d. _____

    e. _____

CERTFICATION REVIEW

Complete the following multiple-choice assessments.

1. Which temperature for hot water should be the upper limit in a health care facility?

    a. 95°F

    b. 100°F

    c. 110°F

    d. 120°F

2. Which patient should receive extra care when applying heat or cold?

    a. 30-year-old female with an infiltrated IV

    b. 40-year-old male with a broken ankle

    c. 50-year-old female with muscle cramps

    d. 60-year-old male with peripheral vascular disease

3. Which item is used to induce hypothermia?

    a. Ice pack

    b. Ice bath

    c. Cold pack

    d. Thermal blanket

© 2022 Cengage Learning. All Rights Reserved. May not be scanned, copied or duplicated, or posted to a publicly accessible website, in whole or in part.

4. What should be done with a gel pack that is used for a patient who is to receive cold applications every 6 hours while awake?

   a. Drain in the sink.

   b. Throw in the trash.

   c. Empty in the toilet.

   d. Place in the freezer.

5. What should be done with the cover of a cold pack when it is removed from a patient?

   a. Throw in the trash.

   b. Flush down the toilet.

   c. Place in a laundry hamper.

   d. Place with biohazard waste.

6. Where will a patient receive a sitz bath?

   a. In bed

   b. In a chair

   c. On the toilet

   d. In the bathtub

7. What can occur if there is an air pocket inside of a K-Pad?

   a. Leaking

   b. Hot spot

   c. Cold spot

   d. Lower temperature

8. Where should the irrigation bag for a sitz bath be placed?

   a. On the floor

   b. On an IV pole

   c. Next to the patient

   d. On the back of the toilet

9. Which route should be used to measure the temperature of a patient who has hypothermia?

   a. Oral

   b. Rectal

   c. Axillary

   d. Tympanic

10. How often will the temperature be monitored for a patient who has an aquathermia blanket?

    a. Every 15 to 30 minutes

    b. Every hour

    c. Every 4 hours

    d. Once a shift

© 2022 Cengage Learning. All Rights Reserved. May not be scanned, copied or duplicated, or posted to a publicly accessible website, in whole or in part.

CHAPTER APPLICATION

Clinical Situations

Briefly describe how a nursing assistant should react to the following situations.

1. You found an ice bag without a cloth cover being used on a patient.

   _____

   _____

2. The patient receiving a cold treatment is shivering and complains of numbness in the part being treated.

   _____

   _____

RELATING TO THE NURSING PROCESS

Write the step of the nursing process that is related to each nursing assistant action.

Nursing Assistant Action	Nursing Process Step
1. The nursing assistant is instructed to apply an ice bag to the patient's arm. They is unsure of how long to leave it in place and asks the nurse.	_____
2. The nursing assistant covers the ice bag with a towel so that the bag is not directly against the patient's skin.	_____
3. The nursing assistant reports the patient's reaction to the placement of a warm water bag.	_____
4. The nursing assistant uses tape to secure the Aquamatic K-Pad in place over the patient's leg.	_____

DEVELOPING GREATER INSIGHT

1. Explain why air should be removed from an ice bag before application.
2. Describe the danger of not removing the patient's leg from the soaking basin before adding hot water to a foot soak.
3. Assist the nurse with application of a hypothermia blanket. Think of reasons this treatment might be administered.
4. Discuss with classmates the dangers of improperly applied treatments of heat and cold.

© 2022 Cengage Learning. All Rights Reserved. May not be scanned, copied or duplicated, or posted to a publicly accessible website, in whole or in part.

CHAPTER 28

Assisting with the Physical Examination

OBJECTIVES

After completing this chapter, you will be able to:

28-1 Spell and define terms.

28-2 Describe the responsibilities of the nursing assistant during the physical examination.

28-3 Name the various positions for physical examinations.

28-4 Drape the patient for the various positions.

28-5 Name the basic instruments necessary for physical examinations.

VOCABULARY BUILDER

Spelling

Each line has four different spellings of a word. Circle the correctly spelled word.

1. litotomy	lithotomy	lythotomy	lithotome
2. autoscope	otascop	otoscope	otascope
3. speculum	specalum	spiculum	specolom
4. opthalomoscope	ophthalmoscope	ophtalmoscope	ophtholmascope

© 2022 Cengage Learning. All Rights Reserved. May not be scanned, copied or duplicated, or posted to a publicly accessible website, in whole or in part.

Definitions

Define the following words.

1. dorsal recumbent _____

2. drape _____

3. flexed _____

4. ophthalmoscope _____

5. otoscope _____

6. speculum _____

CHAPTER REVIEW

Fill-in-the-Blank

Complete the following statements in the spaces provided.

1. When in the lithotomy position, the patient's knees are _____.

2. When in the dorsal recumbent position, the patient lies on his or her _____.

3. When in the knee–chest position, the patient should never be _____.

4. When in the prone position, the patient lies on his or her _____.

5. When in Sims' position, the patient lies on his or her _____ side.

6. The basic examination position is _____.

7. The position used for a pelvic examination is _____.

8. The position sometimes used for a rectal examination is the _____.

9. Patients are usually draped in cloth or paper _____.

10. However the draping is done, it is important that the patient _____ covered.

11. The most common position for head and neck examination is _____.

12. Name the positions pictured.

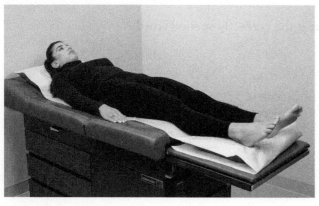

a. _____

© 2022 Cengage Learning. All Rights Reserved. May not be scanned, copied or duplicated, or posted to a publicly accessible website, in whole or in part.

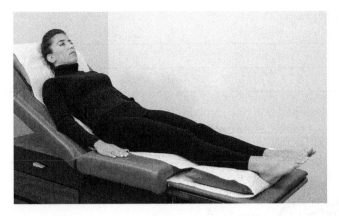

b. _____

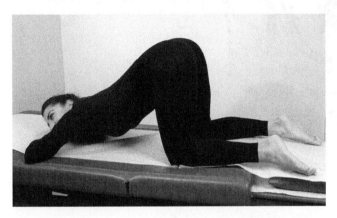

c. _____

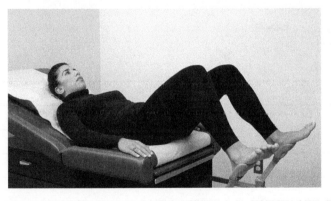

d. _____

Short Answer

Complete the assessment in the space provided.

1. Explain the role of the nursing assistant during a physical examination.

   _____

   _____

   _____

© 2022 Cengage Learning. All Rights Reserved. May not be scanned, copied or duplicated, or posted to a publicly accessible website, in whole or in part.

2. Explain how the physical examination helps the physician.

_____

_____

_____

3. Name the instruments and equipment in a physical examination and explain the use of each.

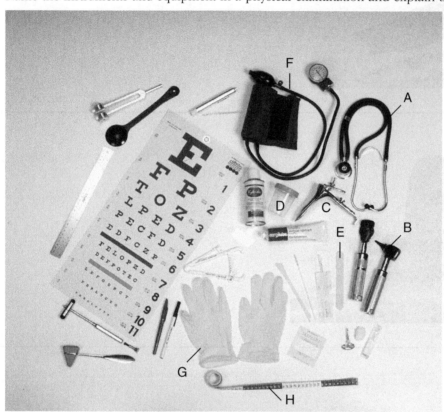

A. _____

B. _____

C. _____

D. _____

E. _____

F. _____

G. _____

H. _____

True/False

Mark the following true or false by circling T or F.

1 T F   A physical examination helps the physician establish a diagnosis.

2. T F   The nursing assistant examines the patient to make a nursing diagnosis.

3. T F   The nursing assistant should expose only the body part being examined.

© 2022 Cengage Learning. All Rights Reserved. May not be scanned, copied or duplicated, or posted to a publicly accessible website, in whole or in part.

4. T   F   The nursing assistant does not need to know how to operate the examination table because the physician will perform this task.

5. T   F   When in the horizontal recumbent position, the patient is placed on his or her abdomen.

6. T   F   The semi-Fowler's position is often used when the head and neck are to be examined.

7. T   F   Patients should void before a pelvic examination.

8. T   F   A Pap smear is usually taken with the patient in the semi-Fowler's position.

9. T   F   Provide privacy before the examination begins.

10. T   F   The nursing assistant should try to anticipate the examiner's needs.

CERTIFICATION REVIEW

Complete the following multiple-choice assessments.

1. What should be placed on the examination table?
    a. Blanket
    b. Disposable paper
    c. Medical record forms
    d. Equipment for the exam

2. In which way will a patient be helped to stay in a particular position for an extended period of time?
    a. Use pillows.
    b. Help the patient hold the position.
    c. Ask the examiner to help the patient.
    d. Ask another assistant to help the patient.

3. Which action should be taken when placing a patient into the dorsal recumbent position?
    a. Turn on the left side.
    b. Straighten the patient's legs.
    c. Loosen the gown at the neck.
    d. Place a pillow under the small of the patient's back.

4. Which action should be taken when placing a patient into the horizontal recumbent position?
    a. Flex the knees.
    b. Place feet flat on the table.
    c. Assist to lay on the right side.
    d. Place a pillow under the patient's head.

5. Which body position is used to assess hip extension?
    a. Sims'
    b. Prone
    c. Sitting
    d. Supine

© 2022 Cengage Learning. All Rights Reserved. May not be scanned, copied or duplicated, or posted to a publicly accessible website, in whole or in part.

6. Which body position is contraindicated for a patient with a respiratory condition?

  a. Sims'

  b. Supine

  c. Lithotomy

  d. Knee–chest

7. Which position increases circulation to the heart and brain?

  a. Prone

  b. Supine

  c. Knee–chest

  d. Trendelenburg

8. What action is taken when the Trendelenburg position is modified?

  a. Raise the head of the bed.

  b. Place the patient onto the left side.

  c. Turn the patient onto the right side.

  d. Elevate the legs higher than the heart.

9. Which position should not be assumed until the physician is in the room?

  a. Prone

  b. Supine

  c. Lithotomy

  d. Trendelenburg

10. Which position should be avoided for a patient with joint deformities?

  a. Sims'

  b. Prone

  c. Sitting

  d. Supine

CHAPTER APPLICATION

Clinical Situations

Briefly describe how a nursing assistant should react to the following situations.

1. The patient seems very nervous before a physical examination. _____

  _____

  _____

© 2022 Cengage Learning. All Rights Reserved. May not be scanned, copied or duplicated, or posted to a publicly accessible website, in whole or in part.

2. The physician wants to do a pelvic examination. _____

_____

_____

3. The nurse wants to examine the patient's throat and chest. _____

_____

_____

RELATING TO THE NURSING PROCESS

Write the step of the nursing process that is related to the nursing assistant action.

Nursing Assistant Action	Nursing Process Step
1. The nursing assistant helps the patient assume the dorsal lithotomy position for a pelvic examination.	_____
2. The nursing assistant records information as the health care provider carries out the examination.`	_____
3. The nursing assistant measures the patient's height and weight and passes instruments during the physical examination.	_____

DEVELOPING GREATER INSIGHT

1. Try positioning yourself in the knee–chest and lithotomy positions. Think carefully about how you feel. What might be done to increase your feelings of privacy and security?

2. Ask your instructor to let you try on a hospital or examination gown. Did you feel covered?

3. Examine the instruments used for the physical examination. Describe their purposes to your classmates.

© 2022 Cengage Learning. All Rights Reserved. May not be scanned, copied or duplicated, or posted to a publicly accessible website, in whole or in part.

The Surgical Patient

OBJECTIVES

After completing this chapter, you will be able to:

29-1 Spell and define terms.

29-2 Describe the concerns of patients who are about to have surgery.

29-3 List the various types of anesthesia.

29-4 Describe how to shave the area to be operated on.

29-5 Explain how to prepare the patient's unit for the patient's return from the operating room.

29-6 Explain how to give routine postoperative care when the patient returns to the room.

29-7 Describe the care and observations for surgical drains.

29-8 Assist the patient with deep breathing and coughing.

29-9 Apply elasticized stockings or bandages and pneumatic sleeves.

29-10 Demonstrate the following procedures:

- Procedure 78: Assisting the Patient to Deep Breathe and Cough (Expand Your Skills)
- Procedure 79: Applying Elasticized Stockings
- Procedure 80: Applying an Elastic Bandage (Expand Your Skills)
- Procedure 81: Assisting the Patient to Dangle (Expand Your Skills)

© 2022 Cengage Learning. All Rights Reserved. May not be scanned, copied or duplicated, or posted to a publicly accessible website, in whole or in part.

VOCABULARY BUILDER

Fill-in-the-Blank

Write each word being described.

1. artificial body part _____

2. walking _____

3. dizziness _____

4. hiccup _____

5. sitting with feet over bed edge _____

6. infection that develops in the hospital _____

7. collapse of lung tissue _____

8. removes hair _____

Matching

Match each term with the correct definition.

1. _____ opening into the body

2. _____ the period following surgery

3. _____ drawing foreign material into the lungs

4. _____ lack of adequate oxygen supply

5. _____ loss of feeling or sensation

6. _____ inflammation of veins that can cause blood clots

7. _____ dizziness

8. _____ moving blood clot

a. embolus

b. singultus

c. orifice

d. vertigo

e. thrombophlebitis

f. postoperative

g. hypoxia

h. aspiration

i. anesthesia

CHAPTER REVIEW

Short Answer

Complete the following statements in the spaces provided.

1. The three phases of care required by the surgical patient are

   a. _____

   b. _____

   c. _____

2. The purpose of anesthesia is _____.

© 2022 Cengage Learning. All Rights Reserved. May not be scanned, copied or duplicated, or posted to a publicly accessible website, in whole or in part.

3. When patients have general anesthesia, they are apt to _____ postoperatively.

4. With a local anesthetic, the patient may remain _____ during surgery.

5. When a spinal anesthetic is given, all sensations _____ the level of the injection are _____.

6. Intravenous anesthetics make the patient fall asleep _____.

7. Seven duties the nursing assistant may be assigned related to the preoperative patient are

   a. _____

   b. _____

   c. _____

   d. _____

   e. _____

   f. _____

   g. _____

8. Equipment left on the bedside table after the recovery bed is made includes the following:

   _____

9. When a patient vomits, their head should be _____ to prevent _____.

10. Spinal anesthesia is often given for abdominal surgery because it produces good

    _____

11. Patient questions should be referred to the _____.

12. The patient's position should be changed every _____ hours following surgery.

13. You should check the patient's _____ frequently as the patient dangles or ambulates for the first time.

14. Elasticized stockings or Ace bandages are applied postoperatively to help support the _____ of the legs.

15. Postoperative leg exercises should be performed _____ times every _____ hours.

In the spaces provided, complete the following statements regarding postoperative discomfort.

16. The patient complains of thirst. You should give special _____ care and check for signs of _____.

17. The patient has singultus. You should support the _____ area.

18. The patient complains of pain. You should report the _____, _____, and _____ of pain.

19. The patient's abdomen is distended. You should encourage increased _____ .

20. The patient has urinary retention. You should monitor _____ carefully.

21. The patient is hemorrhaging. You should keep the patient quiet and check

    _____

22. The patient may be going into shock. You suspect this because there is a fall in _____, the pulse is _____, the skin is _____, and the skin color is pale.

© 2022 Cengage Learning. All Rights Reserved. May not be scanned, copied or duplicated, or posted to a publicly accessible website, in whole or in part.

23. The patient is suffering from hypoxia. You should _____ to a sitting or _____ position and monitor oxygen if ordered.

24. The patient has suffered wound disruption. You should keep the patient _____ and _____ the incision area.

25. If a depilatory is used before surgery to remove hair, the nursing assistant should

_____.

26. If the skin area to which a depilatory has been applied becomes reddened, the nursing assistant should

_____.

27. Identify each of the following items.

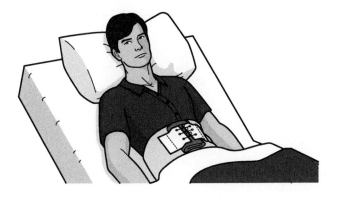

a. _____

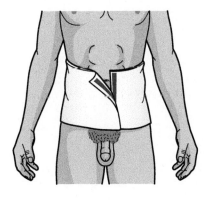

b. _____

© 2022 Cengage Learning. All Rights Reserved. May not be scanned, copied or duplicated, or posted to a publicly accessible website, in whole or in part.

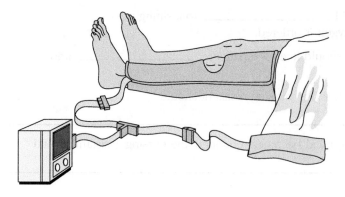

c. _____

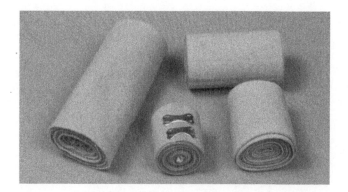

d. _____

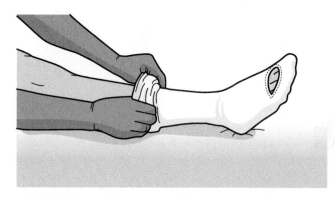

e. _____

© 2022 Cengage Learning. All Rights Reserved. May not be scanned, copied or duplicated, or posted to a publicly accessible website, in whole or in part.

28. State the name of each pulse.

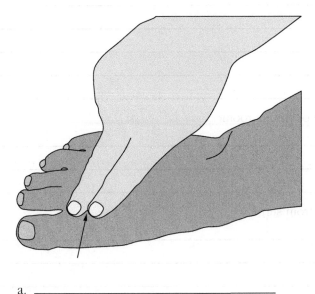

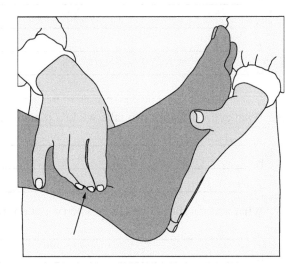

a. _____   b. _____

Short Answer

Answer the following questions.

1. What is needed for pain sensations to be realized?

    a. _____

    b. _____

    c. _____

2. What information is taught to a patient before surgery?

    a. _____

    b. _____

    c. _____

3. Why must nosocomial infections be prevented?

    a. _____

    b. _____

    c. _____

4. What actions should you take before the final preoperative medication is given?

    a. _____

    b. _____

    c. _____

    d. _____

    e. _____

    f. _____

    g. _____

© 2022 Cengage Learning. All Rights Reserved. May not be scanned, copied or duplicated, or posted to a publicly accessible website, in whole or in part.

5. What actions should you take after the medication is given?

   a. _____

   b. _____

   c. _____

   d. _____

   e. _____

6. What actions would you take while a patient is in the operating room?

   a. _____

   b. _____

   c. _____

7. What actions should be taken when a patient returns from surgery?

   a. _____

   b. _____

   c. _____

   d. _____

   e. _____

8. What special precautions should be taken when drainage tubes are in place?

   a. _____

   b. _____

   c. _____

   d. _____

   e. _____

   f. _____

   g. _____

   h. _____

9. Examine the following surgical checklist. List the items that are direct nursing assistant responsibilities.

   1. _____

   2. _____

   3. _____

   4. _____

   5. _____

   6. _____

   7. _____

   8. _____

   9. _____

© 2022 Cengage Learning. All Rights Reserved. May not be scanned, copied or duplicated, or posted to a publicly accessible website, in whole or in part.

1. Admission sheet

2. Surgical consent

3. Sterilization consent (if necessary)

4. Consultation sheet (if necessary)

5. History and physical

6. Lab reports (pregnancy tests also, if necessary)

7. Surgery prep done and charted, if required

8. Latest TPR and blood pressure charted

9. Preoperative medication given and charted (if required)

10. Wrist identification band on patient

11. Fingernail polish and makeup removed

12. Metallic objects removed (rings may be taped, if permitted)

13. Dentures removed

14. Other prostheses removed (such as artificial limb or eye)

15. Bath blanket and head cap in place

16. Bed in high position and side rails up after preop medication is given

17. Patient has voided

10. Define perioperative hypothermia and explain why it occurs. Describe what must happen before temperature stabilizes and approximately how long this takes. State the implications of this condition for nursing assistant care.

_____

_____

_____

_____

_____

_____

11. Describe how to determine which size of anti-embolism hosiery should be used for a patient and explain why having the correct size is important.

_____

_____

_____

_____

© 2022 Cengage Learning. All Rights Reserved. May not be scanned, copied or duplicated, or posted to a publicly accessible website, in whole or in part.

True/False

Mark the following true or false by circling T or F.

1. T   F   Vital signs should be taken every 2 hours during the immediate postoperative period.

2. T   F   Many facilities view pain as the fifth vital sign.

3. T   F   Bandages are used to cover a wound.

4. T   F   Dressings are wrapped around bandages to hold them in place.

5. T   F   Montgomery straps are long adhesive strips with ties to hold dressings in place.

6. T   F   Sequential compression therapy is used to prevent blood clots.

7. T   F   Check the brachial and femoral pulses before applying pneumatic hosiery.

8. T   F   Pneumatic hosiery may be applied over anti-embolism hose.

9. T   F   Pneumatic hosiery should be removed every 6 hours for 30 minutes.

10. T   F   Deep vein thrombosis and pulmonary embolus (blood clot in the lungs) are serious postoperative complications.

11. T   F   Binders may be used to hold dressings in place.

12. T   F   Caring for wound drains involves the use of sterile technique.

13. T   F   The skin surrounding a drain is usually very red.

CERTIFICATION REVIEW

Complete the following multiple-choice assessments.

1. Which body system should be monitored closely in a patient recovering from inhalation anesthesia?

    a. Respiratory

    b. Neurological

    c. Cardiovascular

    d. Musculoskeletal

2. Which action will be taken to support a patient psychologically before surgery?

    a. Focus on physical needs.

    b. Complete tasks in silence.

    c. Limit contact with the patient.

    d. Report signs of fear to the nurse.

3. Which action should be taken if a patient recovering from surgery is sleeping soundly?

    a. Lower the side rails.

    b. Enter the room quietly.

    c. Provide a fresh water pitcher.

    d. Limit checking on the patient.

© 2022 Cengage Learning. All Rights Reserved. May not be scanned, copied or duplicated, or posted to a publicly accessible website, in whole or in part.

Chapter 29 • The Surgical Patient

4. For which reason will a patient recovering from spinal anesthesia need to lie supine without a pillow for 8 to 12 hours?

    a. Enhance healing of the surgical site.

    b. Reduce the need for pain medication.

    c. Improve recovery from the anesthetic.

    d. Prevent the development of a headache.

5. Which action should be taken if a patient develops atelectasis as a postoperative complication?

    a. Turn every hour.

    b. Monitor pulse oximeter.

    c. Elevate the head of the bed.

    d. Check for abdominal distention.

6. Which action should be taken if a patient's surgical drain is leaking around the insertion site?

    a. Change the dressing.

    b. Disconnect the drain.

    c. Notify the nurse immediately.

    d. Place the drain higher that the surgical site.

7. Which item covers a wound?

    a. Binder

    b. Dressing

    c. Ace bandage

    d. Montgomery straps

8. For which patient will deep breathing and coughing be contraindicated after surgery?

    a. Patient who had appendix removed

    b. Patient recovering from spinal fusion surgery

    c. Patient who had a total hip replacement surgery

    d. Patient who had a stent placed in a coronary vessel

9. What has to occur before a patient recovering from surgery on the legs can perform leg exercises?

    a. Patient had a bowel movement.

    b. Physician has to write an order.

    c. Patient needs to be fully awake.

    d. Patient has to receive instructions.

10. What can be done to make applying anti-embolism stockings easier?

    a. Apply lotion to the legs.

    b. Wash the legs with soap and water.

    c. Have the patient dangle for 10 minutes.

    d. Lightly dust the legs with baby powder.

© 2022 Cengage Learning. All Rights Reserved. May not be scanned, copied or duplicated, or posted to a publicly accessible website, in whole or in part.

CHAPTER APPLICATION

Clinical Situations

Briefly describe how a nursing assistant should react to the following situations.

1. You are assigned to do a pubic prep, and your patient's pubic hair is very long.

   _____

   _____

2. You are assisting a patient with initial ambulation, and the patient faints.

   _____

   _____

3. You find that the anti-embolism stockings your patient is wearing are wrinkled and have slipped down their leg.

   _____

   _____

4. Your postoperative patient's blood pressure has dropped and their pulse is rapid and weak. Their skin is cold and moist. _____

   _____

5. Your postoperative patient is anxious, has a feeling of heaviness in their chest, and is cyanotic.

   _____

   _____

RELATING TO THE NURSING PROCESS

Write the step of the nursing process that is related to each nursing assistant action.

Nursing Assistant Action   **Nursing Process Step**

1. The nursing assistant listens to and reports to the nurse
   the patient's concerns about scheduled surgery.   _____

2. The nursing assistant helps the patient bathe or shower
   with surgical soap.   _____

3. The nursing assistant checks with the nurse to determine
   the specific area to be shaved for surgery.   _____

4. Following shaving, the nursing assistant removes unattached hairs
   by gently pressing the sticky side of surgical tape against them.   _____

5. The nursing assistant makes sure there are no wrinkles in
   elasticized stockings once they are applied.   _____

6. The nursing assistant finds that the patient's pulse rate has
   increased more than 10 bpm after initial standing. The nursing
   assistant returns the patient to bed and reports to the nurse.   _____

© 2022 Cengage Learning. All Rights Reserved. May not be scanned, copied or duplicated, or posted to a publicly accessible website, in whole or in part.

DEVELOPING GREATER INSIGHT

1. Discuss ways you can assist a patient to support himself or herself when they tries to cough and deep breathe following surgery.

2. Discuss ways you can contribute to the prevention of nosocomial infections.

3. With so many people having short-term surgery today, your contact with surgery patients may be limited. Think about ways you can make these contacts the most beneficial to the patient.

4. Optional: Your instructor will inform you if completing this figure is part of your assignment.

Surgical Prep Areas

Use colored pencil or crayon to shade in the surgical prep areas that are to be shaved before surgery.

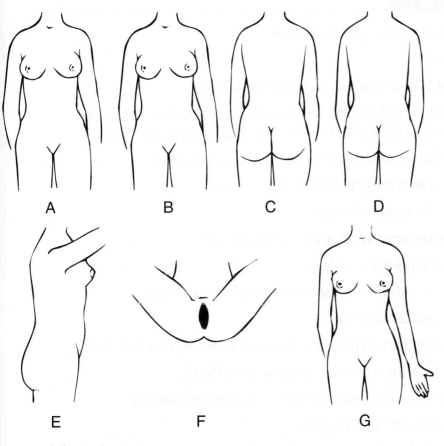

a. abdominal surgery

b. breast surgery—anterior

c. breast surgery—posterior

d. back surgery

e. kidney surgery

f. vaginal, rectal, and perineal surgery

g. left arm surgery

© 2022 Cengage Learning. All Rights Reserved. May not be scanned, copied or duplicated, or posted to a publicly accessible website, in whole or in part.

CHAPTER **30**

Caring for the Emotionally Stressed Patient

OBJECTIVES

After completing this chapter, you will be able to:

30-1 Spell and define terms.

30-2 Explain mental health and the process of adaptations.

30-3 Describe bipolar affective disorder, schizoaffective disorder, seasonal affective disorder, borderline personality disorder, and depression.

30-4 Give an overview of anorexia nervosa and bulimia nervosa.

30-5 Explain how physical and mental health are related.

30-6 Define and discuss substance abuse.

30-7 Describe the care of persons who are in withdrawal.

30-8 Identify common defense mechanisms.

30-9 Describe ways to help patients cope with stressful situations.

30-10 Define and discuss mental illness.

30-11 Describe the care of persons with adaptive and maladaptive behavior.

30-12 Describe methods of caring for the demanding patient.

30-13 List at least 10 guidelines for dealing with a violent individual.

30-14 Describe bullying behavior and triggers.

30-15 List steps to prevent being the target of a bully.

234

© 2022 Cengage Learning. All Rights Reserved. May not be scanned, copied or duplicated, or posted to a publicly accessible website, in whole or in part.

VOCABULARY BUILDER

Definitions

In the space provided, define each word.

1. adaptation
   _____

2. affective
   _____

3. agitation
   _____

4. alcoholism
   _____

5. anorexia
   _____

6. anxiety
   _____

7. bulimia
   _____

8. compulsion
   _____

9. coping
   _____

10. delusions
    _____

11. denial
    _____

12. depression
    _____

13. disorientation
    _____

14. DT
    _____

15. hypochondriasis
    _____

16. obsession
    _____

© 2022 Cengage Learning. All Rights Reserved. May not be scanned, copied or duplicated, or posted to a publicly accessible website, in whole or in part.

17. panic

_____

18. paranoia

_____

19. phobia

_____

20. projection

_____

21. repression

_____

22. SAD

_____

23. stressors

_____

24. suicide

_____

25. suppression

_____

CHAPTER REVIEW

Fill-in-the-Blank

Complete the following statements in the spaces provided.

1. Mental health means exhibiting behaviors that reflect a person's _____ to the multiple stresses of life.

2. A situation that makes a person anxious about their well-being is called a _____.

3. Poor mental health is demonstrated by _____.

4. Physical and mental health are _____.

5. A word used to mean handling stress is _____ with stress.

6. People use _____ mechanisms to protect their self-esteem.

7. Demanding patients are usually only expressing their own _____.

8. Some people turn to alcohol as a means of _____.

9. Alcohol _____ brain activity.

10. Alcohol is a drug that mixes _____ with other drugs.

11. Agitation is defined as inappropriate vocal or _____ activity due to causes other than confusion or need.

12. An extreme maladaptive response in which the person feels everyone is against him or her is called _____.

© 2022 Cengage Learning. All Rights Reserved. May not be scanned, copied or duplicated, or posted to a publicly accessible website, in whole or in part.

13. Patients often show their frustrations by being very _____.

14. A _____ is a purposeful, repetitive activity such as handwashing that is done many times each day and is beyond the person's control.

15. _____ is a condition in which the person has nightmares or flashbacks and may have trouble with normal emotional responses. It is common in survivors of major trauma.

16. A _____ is an unfounded, recurring fear that causes the person to feel panic.

True/False

Mark the following true or false by circling T or F.

1. T F   You can help patients cope with stress by being a good listener.
2. T F   You should try to make patients see situations from your point of view.
3. T F   It is all right to argue the point if you know the patient is wrong.
4. T F   Panic attacks are mental illnesses involving anxiety reactions in response to stress.
5. T F   Disorientation and depression may be associated with both physical and mental disorders.
6. T F   The most common functional disorder in the geriatric age group is depression.
7. T F   Some properly used drugs can cause a person to feel depressed.
8. T F   A proper approach to a depressed patient is to let him or her know how sorry you feel for him or her.
9. T F   A person who threatens suicide never attempts it.
10. T F   An elderly person who has just lost a spouse is at risk for suicide.
11. T F   A suicidal patient needs help in restoring their feelings of self-esteem.
12. T F   Agitation is a significant problem for the elderly, their families, and the nursing staff.
13. T F   A patient who is agitated has a prolonged attention span.
14. T F   One way to help a depressed patient is to reinforce their self-concept as a valued member of society.
15. T F   A disoriented person may show disorientation to time, person, or place.
16. T F   Labeling a behavior implies passing judgment.
17. T F   Speaking to others in the same way your supervisor speaks to you is a form of compensation.
18. T F   OCD is one form of anxiety disorder.
19. T F   PTSD most commonly occurs in children and young teens.
20. T F   Panic attacks seldom recur.
21. T F   A compulsion is a thought that makes no sense.
22. T F   Phobias may cause a person to panic.
23. T F   Snakes, spiders, and rats are common fears that may cause a person to feel panic.
24. T F   Affective disorders are seldom characterized by a disturbance in mood.
25. T F   Patients with bipolar disorder have mood swings ranging from elation to severe depression.
26. T F   Patients with schizoaffective disorder may have delusions and hallucinations.
27. T F   Patients with borderline personality disorder are often very manipulative.
28. T F   People with BPD are often indecisive and prefer that others take charge.

© 2022 Cengage Learning. All Rights Reserved. May not be scanned, copied or duplicated, or posted to a publicly accessible website, in whole or in part.

29. T F One positive aspect of BPD is that persons with this condition usually maintain stable, long-term relationships.

30. T F Females with eating disorders may stop having menstrual periods.

31. T F Males do not develop eating disorders.

32. T F Males with some mental health conditions lose interest in sex.

33. T F Substance abuse may cause impaired judgment and maladaptive behavior.

34. T F Culture affects a person's feelings about mental illness.

35. T F DTs usually occur when individuals withdraw from illegal drugs; they seldom occur as a result of use of substances such as alcohol, which can be legally purchased.

36. T F Suicide precautions are measures and practices a facility follows if a patient is at risk of harming himself or herself.

37. T F Suicide precautions are seldom necessary with persons who are mentally ill.

38. T F Signs and symptoms of delirium tremens include hallucinations and tremors.

Short Answer

Complete the assessment in the space provided.

1. Explain each of the following defense mechanisms.

   a. projection _____

   _____

   b. denial _____

   _____

   c. identification _____

   _____

   d. fantasy _____

   _____

   e. compensation _____

   _____

2. List four ways to deal successfully with a demanding patient.

   a. _____

   b. _____

   c. _____

   d. _____

3. List five ways a nursing assistant can assist an alcoholic patient.

   a. _____

   b. _____

   c. _____

   d. _____

   e. _____

© 2022 Cengage Learning. All Rights Reserved. May not be scanned, copied or duplicated, or posted to a publicly accessible website, in whole or in part.

CERTIFICATION REVIEW

Complete the following multiple-choice assessments.

1. Which is the most common anxiety disorder?

    a. Phobia

    b. Agitation

    c. Panic disorder

    d. Generalized anxiety

2. Which condition causes mood swings ranging from elation to severe depression?

    a. Schizoaffective disorder

    b. Bipolar affective disorder

    c. Seasonal affective disorder

    d. Borderline personality disorder

3. Which action should be taken to help a patient who is anxious?

    a. Confront the patient.

    b. Leave the patient alone.

    c. Avoid engaging in activities.

    d. Encourage to sit in a rocking chair.

4. Which is a characteristic of a patient with bulimia nervosa?

    a. Limits food intake

    b. Binge eats

    c. Views the body as fat

    d. Engages in excessive exercise

5. Which drug can cause alcohol poisoning if taken while drinking alcohol?

    a. Xanax

    b. Ritalin

    c. Salicylates

    d. Barbiturates

6. Which condition causes a patient to imagine or magnify a physical ailment?

    a. Paranoia

    b. Psychosis

    c. Depression

    d. Hypochondriasis

© 2022 Cengage Learning. All Rights Reserved. May not be scanned, copied or duplicated, or posted to a publicly accessible website, in whole or in part.

7. Which action enables a patient's disruptive behavior?

  a. Keep secrets about the patient.

  b. Report behavior issues to the nurse.

  c. Set limits on the patient's behavior.

  d. Refuse to give a patient money when requested.

8. Which action can be taken to prevent violence in the workplace?

  a. Disable door alarms.

  b. Prop security doors open.

  c. Walk with the head down.

  d. Avoid taking valuables to work.

9. Which action should be taken if a patient becomes violent?

  a. Place hands on the hips.

  b. Move toward the patient.

  c. Stare directly at the patient.

  d. Stand at a right angle to the patient.

10. Which situation can be a trigger for bullying?

  a. Receiving a promotion

  b. Calling people by name

  c. Showing respect for others

  d. Helping others when asked

CHAPTER APPLICATION

Clinical Situations

Briefly describe how a nursing assistant should react to the following situations.

1. Mrs. Sears has trouble sleeping, seems lethargic, and frequently dabs tears from her eyes.

  a. _____

  b. _____

  c. _____

2. Mr. Osborn is recovering from a head injury sustained in a fall down stairs. He insists that the patient in the next room is his daughter and tries to see her.

  a. _____

  b. _____

  c. _____

  d. _____

© 2022 Cengage Learning. All Rights Reserved. May not be scanned, copied or duplicated, or posted to a publicly accessible website, in whole or in part.

3. Mrs. Bell is pacing in the corridor. The nurse said in report that she may be experiencing delirium. She repeatedly asks the same question to the staff. She sometimes bites and spits at others. Explain the factors that contribute to her agitation.

a. _____

b. _____

c. _____

d. _____

e. _____

f. _____

RELATING TO THE NURSING PROCESS

Write the step of the nursing process that is related to each nursing assistant action.

Nursing Assistant Action

Nursing Process Step

1. The nursing assistant listens but does not argue, even though the patient's belief is clearly wrong.

   _____

2. The nursing assistant reports the patient's use of profanity without labeling his behavior.

   _____

3. The nurse observes the way the patient says words and the body language they uses at the time.

   _____

4. The nursing assistant reports to the nurse about ways they has found to help the patient deal with stress.

   _____

5. The nursing assistant acts in a positive way when a patient is depressed.

   _____

6. The nursing assistant reports that the patient is having crying spells.

   _____

7. The nursing assistant gives instructions slowly and clearly, in simple words, to a disoriented person.

   _____

© 2022 Cengage Learning. All Rights Reserved. May not be scanned, copied or duplicated, or posted to a publicly accessible website, in whole or in part.

DEVELOPING GREATER INSIGHT

1. Complete the chart to demonstrate your understanding of the concept of how people cope with stress. Discuss this with your classmates. Think carefully about your own coping mechanisms. Could you find more appropriate ways of dealing with stress?

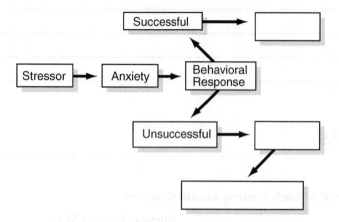

2. Look around your facility or clinical area. Try to identify anything that might be a safety hazard for a disoriented person.

3. Role-play with classmates the proper way to manage an agitated patient. Have one student act as the patient.

4. Think about your relationships with your teacher and classmates. Can you identify any situation in which you used one of the defense mechanisms described in this unit?

5. Discuss with the class ways you personally have found that help reduce stress.

© 2022 Cengage Learning. All Rights Reserved. May not be scanned, copied or duplicated, or posted to a publicly accessible website, in whole or in part.

Caring for the Bariatric Patient

OBJECTIVES

After completing this chapter, you will be able to:

31-1 Spell and define terms.

31-2 Define overweight, obesity, and morbid obesity, and explain how these conditions differ from each other.

31-3 Explain why weight affects life span (longevity) and health.

31-4 Define comorbidities and explain how they affect a person's health.

31-5 Briefly state how obesity affects the cardiovascular and respiratory systems.

31-6 Explain how stereotyping and discrimination affect persons with obesity.

31-7 List some team members and their responsibilities in the care of the bariatric patient.

31-8 Explain why environmental modifications are needed for bariatric patient care.

31-9 Describe observations to make and methods of meeting bariatric patients' ADL needs.

31-10 List precautions to take when moving and positioning bariatric patients.

31-11 List at least five complications of immobility in bariatric patients.

31-12 Describe nursing assistant responsibilities in the postoperative care of patients who have had bariatric surgery.

© 2022 Cengage Learning. All Rights Reserved. May not be scanned, copied or duplicated, or posted to a publicly accessible website, in whole or in part.

VOCABULARY BUILDER

Definitions

In the space provided, write a definition of each word.

1. advocate

2. bariatrics

3. BMI

4. comorbidities

5. (gastric) bypass

6. hyperventilation

7. IBW

8. (minimally) invasive (surgery)

9. morbid (obesity)

10. obesity

11. overweight

12. panniculus

13. reflux

© 2022 Cengage Learning. All Rights Reserved. May not be scanned, copied or duplicated, or posted to a publicly accessible website, in whole or in part.

14. stenosis

_____

15. stricture

_____

16. trapeze

_____

CHAPTER REVIEW

True/False

Mark the following true or false by circling T or F.

1. T F A person who is overweight has a BMI over 50.
2. T F Most obese people eat an enormous amount of food and lack willpower.
3. T F Obesity negatively affects every system of the body.
4. T F Obesity is commonly hereditary; environmental factors have no effect on weight.
5. T F Obesity is considered a chronic condition.
6. T F The BMI is diagnostic of an individual's health status.
7. T F Comorbidities are diseases and medical conditions that morbid obesity either causes or contributes to.
8. T F Persons with obesity are at increased risk for cancer.
9. T F Adipose tissue is poorly nourished and less resistant to injury than the tissues of a smaller person.
10. T F The weight of an obese person's chest makes breathing more difficult.
11. T F The bariatric nurse specialist writes the dietary plan of care and supervises the menu.
12. T F Because of the nutrient stores in the adipose tissue, the bariatric patient cannot develop malnutrition or dehydration.
13. T F Bariatric patients often sweat profusely.
14. T F Gore-Tex and nylon sheets have a slippery surface that reduces friction and shear and makes it easier to move the patient.
15. T F If the patient is too large for the regular scale, obtain a freight scale or laundry scale from the maintenance department.
16. T F The patient advocate's main responsibility is protecting the bariatric patient's dignity.
17. T F Do not ask a patient what works for their care, because it will appear that you do not know what you are doing.
18. T F A regular washcloth and towel may be very irritating to the skin of some bariatric patients.

© 2022 Cengage Learning. All Rights Reserved. May not be scanned, copied or duplicated, or posted to a publicly accessible website, in whole or in part.

19. T   F   Bariatric patients may need extra fluids to support their body's needs.

20. T   F   A condom catheter is commonly used for male bariatric patients because it is easier than inserting a regular catheter, stays in place well, and requires less frequent peri care.

21. T   F   Bariatric patients seldom develop pressure injuries because of the extra padding over bony prominences.

22. T   F   One staff person should never lift or move more than 55 pounds of body weight without extra help or a mechanical device.

23. T   F   Two or more nursing assistants are often needed to assist the bariatric patient with personal hygiene procedures.

24. T   F   Using the Trendelenburg position when moving the bariatric patient up in bed makes the job easier and reduces the risk of injury.

Short Answer

Complete the assessment in the space provided.

1. When a patient is positioned on their side, you should _____

    _____

2. Why does an obese patient walk with a wide-based gait? _____

    _____

3. The nurse may instruct you to apply an abdominal binder before moving a bariatric patient. Why is this done?

    _____

    _____

4. If a standing bariatric patient begins to fall to the floor, what is the most important action to take?

    _____

    _____

    _____

5. Identify the three most common complications of bariatric surgery.

    a. _____

    b. _____

    c. _____

6. What is the primary goal of the postoperative care given to a person who has had bariatric surgery?

    _____

    _____

    _____

© 2022 Cengage Learning. All Rights Reserved. May not be scanned, copied or duplicated, or posted to a publicly accessible website, in whole or in part.

7. Explain why a patient is permitted to have only very small amounts of food or fluid after bariatric surgery.

_____

_____

_____

8. List at least five potentially serious signs and symptoms of postoperative complications that should be reported to the nurse promptly.

a. _____

b. _____

c. _____

d. _____

e. _____

CERFITICATION REVIEW

Complete the following multiple-choice assessments.

1. Which BMI is considered normal weight?

   a. 16.5

   b. 22

   c. 28

   d. 34

2. What needs to be stabilized before bariatric surgery is done?

   a. Weight

   b. Appetite

   c. Leg strength

   d. Comorbidities

3. Which musculoskeletal problem is a comorbidity related to obesity?

   a. Fractures

   b. Scoliosis

   c. Achilles tendon rupture

   d. Carpal tunnel syndrome

4. Which therapy may be prescribed for a bariatric patient to improve the respiratory status?

   a. Chest physiotherapy

   b. Supplemental oxygen

   c. Nasotracheal suctioning

   d. Expectorant medications

© 2022 Cengage Learning. All Rights Reserved. May not be scanned, copied or duplicated, or posted to a publicly accessible website, in whole or in part.

5. What is an advantage of a bariatric bed?

   a. Has removable side rails

   b. Can be raised to waist level

   c. Can be used as a transport vehicle

   d. Prevents the development of pressure injuries

6. What can be done to facilitate providing a bariatric patient with personal care?

   a. Ask the patient to assist.

   b. Schedule routine showers.

   c. Use a binder to hold skin back.

   d. Cleanse the areas that can be accessed.

7. Which action absorbs moisture between skin folds?

   a. Apply lotion to the areas.

   b. Wash the skin with soap and hot water.

   c. Sprinkle the area with baby powder or corn starch.

   d. Place a piece of a flannel blanket between the folds.

8. Which action facilitates cleaning a bariatric patient after using the bathroom?

   a. Give the patient privacy.

   b. Sprinkle powder over the perineum.

   c. Use two people to cleanse the patient.

   d. Use alcohol pads to cleanse the areas.

9. Which action will the nursing assistant take before moving a bariatric patient?

   a. Review the care plan.

   b. Provide a complete bath.

   c. Collect linen to change the bed.

   d. Complete as much as possible with the patient in bed.

10. Which bariatric surgical procedure is most commonly performed?

    a. Gastric bypass

    b. Gastric banding

    c. Sleeve gastrectomy

    d. Partial gastrectomy

© 2022 Cengage Learning. All Rights Reserved. May not be scanned, copied or duplicated, or posted to a publicly accessible website, in whole or in part.

CHAPTER APPLICATION

Identification

1. Identify this item and describe why it is used.

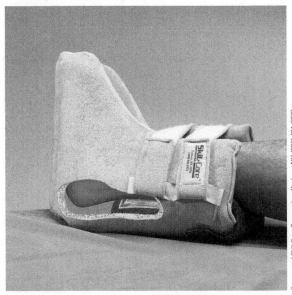

Courtesy of Skil-Care Corporation, Yonkers, NY: (800) 431-2972

2. Identify this item and describe when it should be used.

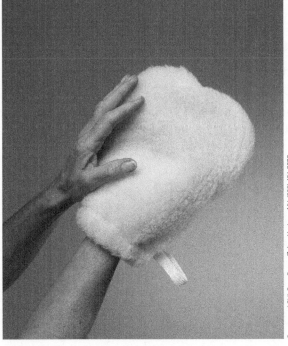

Courtesy of Skil-Care Corporation, Yonkers, NY: (800) 431-2972

© 2022 Cengage Learning. All Rights Reserved. May not be scanned, copied or duplicated, or posted to a publicly accessible website, in whole or in part.

RELATING TO THE NURSING PROCESS

Write the step of the nursing process that is related to each nursing assistant action.

Nursing Assistant Action   **Nursing Process Step**

1. The nursing assistant finds that the patient's blood pressure
   is 180/106, so they rechecks it. Finding the same value,
   they seeks out the nurse to report their findings.   _____

2. The nurse has given Mr. Mulvaney an insulin injection.
   They instructs the nursing assistant to monitor for
   signs of hypoglycemia, to recheck the blood sugar in
   2 hours, and to report the value.   _____

3. Mr. Romcevich's plan of care is not working and the
   patient is dissatisfied. The nurse asks the nursing
   assistant about care plan approaches that have been
   effective and which approaches have not worked.   _____

4. The nursing assistant notifies the nurse that Mr. Turpel,
   a recent bariatric surgery patient, is vomiting.   _____

5. The nursing assistant gets another assistant to help him or her
   perform peri care on Mrs. Evert.   _____

DEVELOPING GREATER INSIGHT

1. Think carefully about obese people you have known or seen in public. Identify problems and needs that nor-mal-sized individuals do not experience. List as many as you can and report them to the class.

2. Patients often view the day of their bariatric surgery as the first day of the rest of their lives. Why do you think this is?

3. Why should you avoid making unsolicited comments, such as "you don't look like you need this (weight loss) surgery" or "but you really do carry your weight well"? Think carefully about your answer and report your findings to the class. What can we learn from this?

© 2022 Cengage Learning. All Rights Reserved. May not be scanned, copied or duplicated, or posted to a publicly accessible website, in whole or in part.

CHAPTER **32**

Death and Dying

OBJECTIVES

After completing this chapter, you will be able to:

32-1 Spell and define terms.

32-2 Discuss the five stages of grief.

32-3 Describe differences in how people handle the process of death and dying.

32-4 Describe the spiritual preparations for death practiced by various religions.

32-5 State the purpose of the Patient Self-Determination Act.

32-6 Discuss Physician Orders for Life-Sustaining Treatment (POLST).

32-7 Describe the nursing assistant's responsibilities for providing supportive care.

32-8 Describe the hospice philosophy and method of care.

32-9 List the signs of approaching death.

32-10 Demonstrate the following procedure:

• Procedure 82: Giving Postmortem Care (Expand Your Skills)

© 2022 Cengage Learning. All Rights Reserved. May not be scanned, copied or duplicated, or posted to a publicly accessible website, in whole or in part.

VOCABULARY BUILDER

Spelling

Each line has four different spellings of a word. Circle the correctly spelled word.

1. critical	cretical	critecal	creticale
2. posmortum	postmartem	postmortem	postmortom
3. hopice	hopise	hospise	hospice
4. terminale	terminal	termanel	termanal
5. danial	deniel	denial	deniale
6. morabund	moribund	moreband	moribond
7. awtopsie	awtopsy	autopse	autopsy
8. bargaining	bargenan	bargainin	bergaining
9. rigor mortis	rigor mortus	rigger mortis	regor mortos

CHAPTER REVIEW

Fill-in-the-Blank

Complete the statements in the spaces provided.

1. When the patient's condition is critical, the _____ places the patient's name on the critical list.

2. Sacrament of the Sick is requested for the patient of the _____ faith.

3. Hospice care is based on the philosophy that death is a _____ process.

4. Hospice care is provided for people with a life expectancy of _____.

5. Hospice care is provided by _____ who work with the patient and the family.

6. As death approaches, body functions _____.

7. The last sense lost is the sense of _____.

8. As death approaches, the pulse becomes _____ and progressively _____.

9. The time of death is determined by the _____.

10. Under no circumstances should the _____ inform the family of the patient's death.

11. As a nursing assistant, you have a unique opportunity to be a source of _____ and _____ to the dying patient and the family.

12. During the dying period, you must provide the family and patient with _____.

13. The nursing assistant must realize that dying is a(n) _____ each person must make _____.

© 2022 Cengage Learning. All Rights Reserved. May not be scanned, copied or duplicated, or posted to a publicly accessible website, in whole or in part.

True/False

Mark the following true or false by circling T or F.

1. T   F   A patient goes through each stage of grieving in a sequential order.

2. T   F   Once they has moved on to another stage of the grieving process, the patient never returns to a former stage.

3. T   F   All patients go through each stage of grieving at the same rate.

4. T   F   The nursing assistant must have an understanding attitude during each stage of the grieving process.

5. T   F   The family members may go through the same five stages of the grieving process.

6. T   F   The nursing assistant should reflect the patient's statements during the stage of denial.

7. T   F   If the patient seems depressed, it is best to leave him or her alone to work it out himself or herself.

8. T   F   The patient in the stage of acceptance has no fear.

9. T   F   The stage of depression is often filled with expression of regrets.

10. T   F   The patient who has reached the stage of acceptance may try to assist those around him or her to deal with their death.

11. T   F   The Patient Self-Determination Act goes into effect as soon as a patient is admitted to a health care facility.

12. T   F   Supportive care for terminally ill patients does not include life-sustaining treatments.

13. T   F   The POLST document must be revised each time the patient's location changes.

14. T   F   The POLST document does not affect the advance directive.

Short Answer

Complete the assessment in the space provided.

1. List the five stages of grief as outlined by E. Kübler-Ross.

    a. _____

    b. _____

    c. _____

    d. _____

    e. _____

2. What are the goals of hospice programs?

    a. _____

    b. _____

    c. _____

3. As a member of the hospice team, how can you promote the hospice philosophy?

    a. _____

    b. _____

    c. _____

    d. _____

© 2022 Cengage Learning. All Rights Reserved. May not be scanned, copied or duplicated, or posted to a publicly accessible website, in whole or in part.

4. What are five moribund changes?

a. _____

b. _____

c. _____

d. _____

e. _____

5. What items would you expect to find in a morgue kit?

a. _____

b. _____

c. _____

d. _____

e. _____

6. What should you do before moving the body to the morgue, to prevent upsetting other patients?

_____

_____

7. Why is the use of standard precautions necessary when performing postmortem care?

_____

_____

CERTIFICATION REVIEW

Complete the following multiple-choice assessments.

1. Which action should be taken when a terminally ill patient expresses concerns about dying?

   a. Actively listen.

   b. Change the subject.

   c. Leave the patient alone.

   d. Tell the nurse about the conversation.

2. Which type of grief occurs before a person dies?

   a. Normal

   b. Accepted

   c. Anticipatory

   d. Complicated

3. Which behavior indicates that staff are aware of a patient dying?

   a. Exhibiting false cheerfulness

   b. Skipping doses of medications

   c. Spending more time with the patient

   d. Removing the water pitcher from the room

© 2022 Cengage Learning. All Rights Reserved. May not be scanned, copied or duplicated, or posted to a publicly accessible website, in whole or in part.

4. Which action should be taken if a resident asks about another that has died?

    a. Withhold information because it violates HIPAA.

    b. Suggest the resident not focus on the topic of death.

    c. Allow the resident to reminisce about the person who died.

    d. Remind the resident that the one who passed away was really sick.

5. Which type of care is typically absent when giving supportive care?

    a. Routine

    b. Comfort

    c. Standard

    d. Life-sustaining

6. Which action should be taken if a patient wants to change information on an advance directive?

    a. Report it to the nurse.

    b. Explain that the change would not prolong life.

    c. Explain that the advance directive cannot be changed.

    d. Ask the patient why they want to change the directive.

7. Which action should be taken if a family member wants to stay overnight with a dying patient?

    a. Offer a pillow and a blanket.

    b. Suggest they sit in the visitor's lounge.

    c. Remind the family of the visiting hours.

    d. Inform security that a family member won't leave.

8. In which way does hospice support the family of a dying patient?

    a. Provides care instead of the family

    b. Instructs the family on the dying process

    c. Provides care free of charge to the family

    d. Offers bereavement counseling after the death

9. Which action should be taken when providing care to a dying patient who is comatose?

    a. Provide care in silence.

    b. Encourage the patient to wake up.

    c. Move the patient as little as possible.

    d. Provide the same level of care as before.

10. Which action prevents staining of the face with blood after death?

    a. Position on the left side of the body.

    b. Position on the right side of the body.

    c. Place the patient flat without a pillow.

    d. Elevate the head of the bed 30 degrees in the semi-Fowler position.

© 2022 Cengage Learning. All Rights Reserved. May not be scanned, copied or duplicated, or posted to a publicly accessible website, in whole or in part.

CHAPTER APPLICATION

Clinical Situations

Briefly describe how a nursing assistant should react to the following situations.

1. Your terminal patient, who had been crying earlier, suddenly appears cheerful and talks about a trip he is planning for next year.

   _____

   _____

2. The patient expresses a desire to see their clergyperson.

   _____

3. The physician has pronounced the patient deceased, and you are to prepare the patient for the return of the family.

   a. _____

   b. _____

   c. _____

   d. _____

   e. _____

4. The patient has an order for supportive care only. What care does this include?

   a. _____

   b. _____

   c. _____

   d. _____

5. The patient has both a living will and a durable power of attorney. Write the name of the document that assigns responsibility for handling the patient's personal affairs and making health care decisions for the patient.

   _____

6. A patient has a no-code order. State how this order influences care if the patient experiences respiratory and cardiac arrest.

   _____

© 2022 Cengage Learning. All Rights Reserved. May not be scanned, copied or duplicated, or posted to a publicly accessible website, in whole or in part.

RELATING TO THE NURSING PROCESS

Write the step of the nursing process that is related to each nursing assistant action.

Nursing Assistant Action   **Nursing Process Step**

1. The nursing assistant promptly reports complaints of pain
   by the terminally ill patient to the nurse.   _____

2. During the postmortem period, the nursing assistant cares
   for the body with dignity.   _____

3. The nursing assistant checks the dying patient frequently.   _____

4. The nursing assistant offers quiet support to the family of
   the dying patient by listening.   _____

DEVELOPING GREATER INSIGHT

1. Share with classmates any special traditions or practices that your family carries out when someone dies.

2. Invite members of different faiths to share some of their experiences with dying people.

3. Invite a nursing assistant or nurse who works in a hospice organization to come and share some of his or her experiences with the class.

4. Think how you might feel if you were giving care to a patient who is terminally ill and has an order for supportive care only.

© 2022 Cengage Learning. All Rights Reserved. May not be scanned, copied or duplicated, or posted to a publicly accessible website, in whole or in part.

Other Health Care Settings

C H A P T E R **33**

Providing Care for Special Populations: Elderly, Chronically Ill, Alzheimer Disease, Intellectual Disabilities, and Developmental Disabilities

OBJECTIVES

After completing this chapter, you will be able to:

33-1 Spell and define terms.

33-2 Describe the services provided by the various types of long-term care facilities.

33-3 Discuss how culture change is transforming long-term care services.

33-4 Identify the expected changes of aging.

33-5 Identify residents who are at risk for malnutrition and dehydration.

33-6 List measures to promote sufficient intake.

© 2022 Cengage Learning. All Rights Reserved. May not be scanned, copied or duplicated, or posted to a publicly accessible website, in whole or in part.

33-7 Discuss how to meet the hygiene and grooming needs of long-term care residents.

33-8 Give an overview of at least eight diseases that cause dementia.

33-9 Briefly describe each of the three main stages of Alzheimer disease.

33-10 Explain how delirium differs from dementia.

33-11 List potential signs and symptoms of delirium to report.

33-12 Describe the nursing assistant's care for persons with cognitive impairment, disorientation, dementia, and wandering.

33-13 State the purpose of animal-assisted therapy, music therapy, reality orientation, reminiscing, and validation therapy.

33-14 List three criteria that must be present for a developmental disability diagnosis.

33-15 Define intellectual disability.

33-16 Discuss the care of persons with intellectual and other common developmental disabilities.

33-17 State the difference between a congenital developmental disability and an acquired developmental disability, and give examples of each.

33-18 Describe the nursing assistant's care and communication guidelines for persons with developmental disabilities.

VOCABULARY BUILDER

Definitions

Define the following words.

1. Medicaid _____

2. pigmentation _____

3. debilitating _____

4. assisted living _____

5. sundowning _____

6. reminiscing _____

7. diverticulitis_____

8. chronologic_____

9. dementia _____

10. long-term care _____

© 2022 Cengage Learning. All Rights Reserved. May not be scanned, copied or duplicated, or posted to a publicly accessible website, in whole or in part.

Matching

Match each term with the correct definition.

1. _____ excessive gas in stomach or intestines

2. _____ condition in which a person has 47 chromosomes

3. _____ weakening

4. _____ craving to eat nonfood items

5. _____ results from lack of oxygen during labor and delivery

6. _____ rate at which an illness occurs in a given population

7. _____ weakened places in intestinal wall

a. pica

b. cerebral palsy

c. morbidity

d. diverticula

e. debilitating

f. Down syndrome

g. flatulence

CHAPTER REVIEW

Matching

Match each problem with the system affected.

1. _____ blood vessels less elastic

2. _____ constipation

3. _____ incontinence

4. _____ less flexibility

5. _____ diminished hearing

6. _____ decreased primary taste sensation

7. _____ flatulence

8. _____ slower movements

9. _____ diminished depth perception

10. _____ loss of hair color

a. integumentary

b. nervous

c. musculoskeletal

d. urinary

e. digestive

f. cardiovascular

True/False

Determine which of the following are true statements about all elderly people.

1. T   F   They no longer contribute to society.

2. T   F   They have no interest in sex.

3. T   F   They are living in poverty.

4. T   F   They have sensory losses.

© 2022 Cengage Learning. All Rights Reserved. May not be scanned, copied or duplicated, or posted to a publicly accessible website, in whole or in part.

5. T   F   They are incompetent to make decisions.

6. T   F   They have short-term memory loss.

7. T   F   They undergo postural changes.

8. T   F   They are more prone to certain chronic conditions.

9. T   F   They have changed sleep patterns.

10. T   F   They are unable to learn.

11. T   F   They have the same rights as any citizen of the United States.

Fill-in-the-Blank

Complete the following statements in the spaces provided.

1. To be successful as a long-term care nursing assistant, you must have a sense of _____ and be able to _____ effectively.

2. Every resident must be treated with _____.

3. Most of the residents in long-term care are _____ and have _____ health problems.

4. The long-term care nursing assistant must be satisfied with _____ progress and _____ gains.

5. Each person moves from infancy to old age at a(n) _____ rate.

6. Some researchers believe that each person has an inborn biological _____.

7. Smell receptors and taste buds _____ with age.

8. Elderly people may not be _____ of their need for fluid.

9. Poor dental care and oral hygiene can result in loss of appetite and _____.

10. _____ maintains dignity by acknowledging memories and feelings.

11. Residents can and do develop _____, despite being served a balanced diet and having nutritional supplements available.

12. _____ is the most common type of dementia.

13. _____ is an acute state of confusion caused by reversible medical problems.

14. Another term for wandering away from the facility is _____.

15. Confused residents are very sensitive to the moods and _____ of staff members.

16. Seeing items associated with going outdoors may _____ wandering.

17. Persons with _____ repeat their actions or words.

18. Elderly people may develop an apathy about food that results in _____.

19. Lotions should be applied to _____ dry skin.

20. A _____ is the response of a person with dementia to overwhelming stimuli.

© 2022 Cengage Learning. All Rights Reserved. May not be scanned, copied or duplicated, or posted to a publicly accessible website, in whole or in part.

Short Answer

Complete the assessment in the space provided.

1. What are five changes frequently seen in the integumentary system of the elderly?

   a. _____

   b. _____

   c. _____

   d. _____

2. What are the four basic emotional needs of the elderly?

   a. _____

   b. _____

   c. _____

   d. _____

3. List the "fatal four" risks that are more common in people with developmental disabilities than in the general population.

   a. _____

   b. _____

   c. _____

   d. _____

4. Residents who are at greatest risk of malnutrition and unintentional weight loss are those who:

   a. _____

   b. _____

   c. _____

   d. _____

   e. _____

5. List five risks associated with pica.

   a. _____

   b. _____

   c. _____

   d. _____

   e. _____

6. What is meant by a "catastrophic reaction" relating to a person with dementia? _____

   _____

7. List five observations to make and report related to behavioral problems.

   a. _____

   b. _____

© 2022 Cengage Learning. All Rights Reserved. May not be scanned, copied or duplicated, or posted to a publicly accessible website, in whole or in part.

c. _____

d. _____

e. _____

8. List five triggers of wandering.

a. _____

b. _____

c. _____

d. _____

e. _____

True/False

Mark the following true or false by circling T or F.

1. T   F   Reminiscing is an inappropriate activity for elderly people.

2. T   F   Reminiscing helps people adapt to old age by allowing them to work through personal losses.

3. T   F   Reminiscing is a natural activity for people of all ages.

4. T   F   Reminiscing should be ignored because such remembrances have little relationship to today.

5. T   F   Clocks with large numbers should be placed around the facility.

6. T   F   Care for disoriented residents includes frequently asking residents to identify the date or the caregiver.

7. T   F   Treat adult residents as children when they act confused.

8. T   F   Call residents by cute or pet names so they will feel comfortable and at home.

9. T   F   Try to reason with a resident who is having a catastrophic reaction.

CERTIFICATION REVIEW

Complete the following multiple-choice assessments.

1. Skilled nursing care facilities:

    a. provide only assistance with activities of daily living.

    b. care only for acutely ill residents.

    c. provide care to residents with chronic conditions.

    d. employ only registered nurses.

2. Most residents in long-term care facilities:

    a. experience sundowning in the afternoon.

    b. have temporary acute conditions.

    c. require very little health care and supervision.

    d. have chronic, progressive conditions.

© 2022 Cengage Learning. All Rights Reserved. May not be scanned, copied or duplicated, or posted to a publicly accessible website, in whole or in part.

3. Which of the following applies to bathing the elderly?

   a. Full daily baths are essential.

   b. Bathing two to three times a week is fine.

   c. Frequent bathing is important.

   d. Use deodorants liberally.

4. Which of the following is true of nail care?

   a. Residents should never have dirty nails.

   b. Use a very stiff brush to clean nails.

   c. Clip fingernails at least once a week.

   d. Clean nails with a metal file.

5. A congenital condition:

   a. is acquired as a result of an accident.

   b. is present at the time of birth.

   c. develops between the ages of 8 and 22 years.

   d. results from lack of oxygen at birth.

6. Animal-assisted therapy has been shown to:

   a. relieve headaches.

   b. cause agitation.

   c. reduce the incidence of allergies.

   d. lower blood pressure.

7. Which is an advantage of using music as therapy?

   a. Improves mood

   b. Reduces stimulation

   c. Increases orientation

   d. Heightens emotional stress

8. At which time would a developmental disability be identified?

   a. Upon birth

   b. Before age 22

   c. When stressed

   d. Before middle-age

9. Which is a characteristic of a person with an intellectual disability?

   a. Complete inability to learn

   b. Commonly occurs with epilepsy

   c. Achieves economic independence

   d. Adapts socially to the environment

© 2022 Cengage Learning. All Rights Reserved. May not be scanned, copied or duplicated, or posted to a publicly accessible website, in whole or in part.

10. Which is a major characteristic of autism?

   a. More common in females

   b. Above average intelligence

   c. Difficulty with communication

   d. Caused by a missing chromosome

CHAPTER APPLICATION

Clinical Situations

Briefly describe how a nursing assistant should react to the following situations.

1. Mrs. Li, age 92, is withdrawn much of the time but occasionally complains and is hostile and demanding. Her family seldom visits, and her behavior is the same toward them.

   _____

   _____

   _____

   _____

2. Mrs. Preston reported drinking a lot of water, but the water carafe was still almost full.

   _____

   _____

   _____

   _____

3. Mrs. Gutierrez keeps trying to leave the facility and insists that she must hurry home to cook dinner for the children.

   _____

   _____

   _____

   _____

© 2022 Cengage Learning. All Rights Reserved. May not be scanned, copied or duplicated, or posted to a publicly accessible website, in whole or in part.

Hidden Picture

Identify the problems that require attention in the picture.

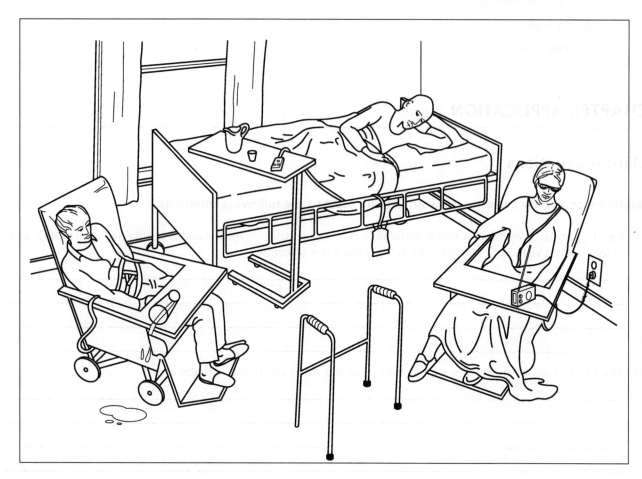

1. _____
2. _____
3. _____
4. _____
5. _____
6. _____
7. _____
8. _____

© 2022 Cengage Learning. All Rights Reserved. May not be scanned, copied or duplicated, or posted to a publicly accessible website, in whole or in part.

RELATING TO THE NURSING PROCESS

Write the step of the nursing process that is related to each nursing assistant action.

Nursing Assistant Action **Nursing Process Step**

1. The nursing assistant reassures the people in their care that they will not be abandoned. _____

2. The nursing assistant treats each resident with respect. _____

3. The nursing assistant reports that the resident has complained of feeling constipated. _____

4. The nursing assistant encourages the resident to feed himself or herself but is ready to assist if needed. _____

5. The nursing assistant encourages the resident to drink fluids frequently. _____

6. The nursing assistant patiently works with the intellectually disabled resident to meet their care plan goal. _____

7. The nursing assistant uses gestures to help communicate meaning when the resident has a hearing impairment. _____

DEVELOPING GREATER INSIGHT

1. Discuss with classmates the differences between reality orientation and validation therapy, including how each is appropriately used and the possible benefits to residents.

2. Explain ways to protect the resident who wanders.

© 2022 Cengage Learning. All Rights Reserved. May not be scanned, copied or duplicated, or posted to a publicly accessible website, in whole or in part.

CHAPTER **34**

The Organization of Home Care: Trends in Health Care

OBJECTIVES

After completing this chapter, you will be able to:

34-1 Spell and define terms.

34-2 Briefly outline the history of home care.

34-3 Describe the types of nursing services that are provided in the home.

34-4 Describe the benefits of working in home care.

34-5 List the qualifications for working as a nursing assistant in home care.

34-6 Identify members of the home health team.

34-7 State the purpose of the case manager.

34-8 State the purpose of the Outcome and Assessment Information Set (OASIS).

34-9 List guidelines for avoiding liability while working as a home health assistant.

34-10 Describe the types of information a home health assistant must be able to document.

34-11 Identify several time management techniques.

34-12 List ways in which the home health assistant can work successfully with client's families.

© 2022 Cengage Learning. All Rights Reserved. May not be scanned, copied or duplicated, or posted to a publicly accessible website, in whole or in part.

'OCABULARY BUILDER

Definitions

Write the definition for each of the following.

1. client care records _____

2. intermittent care _____

3. time/travel records _____

4. case manager _____

5. custodial _____

6. Outcome and Assessment Information Set (OASIS)_____

7. skilled home health nursing _____

CHAPTER REVIEW

Fill-in-the-Blank

¯omplete the following statements in the spaces provided by selecting the correct term from the list provided.

accuracy	assistance	calculations	complete
developed	home health care team	hospital	independence
insurance group	number	nurse	one
part-time	records	skilled nursing facility	taught

1. An advantage to working as a nursing assistant in the home is that there are opportunities for _____ employment.

2. In home care, there is the opportunity to give _____ care to _____ client at a time.

3. The home health care assistant has an opportunity to work with greater _____.

4. The care of the client is planned by the _____.

5. The services of the home nursing assistant may be implemented after a referral from a(n) _____.

6. It is important to keep accurate time and cost _____ of the care you give.

7. Most persons using home care have been discharged from a(n) _____ or _____ _____.

8. Clients may be in need of _____ with activities of daily living.

9. A nursing assistant may be assigned to care for a client for a(n) _____ of hours daily.

.0. The care plan is _____ with the client by the _____.

© 2022 Cengage Learning. All Rights Reserved. May not be scanned, copied or duplicated, or posted to a publicly accessible website, in whole or in part.

11. Liability can be avoided if the nursing assistant carries out actions as they was _____.

12. Keeping time/travel records requires _____ and _____.

Short Answer

Complete the assessment in the space provided.

1. Name three different types of home care providers.

   a. _____

   b. _____

   c. _____

2. List four advantages to working for a home health agency.

   a. _____

   b. _____

   c. _____

   d. _____

3. What are five time and cost values to record?

   a. _____

   b. _____

   c. _____

   d. _____

   e. _____

4. What are five ways to avoid liability when providing home care?

   a. _____

   b. _____

   c. _____

   d. _____

   e. _____

5. What are four types of activities that should be included in the client care record?

   a. _____

   b. _____

   c. _____

   d. _____

© 2022 Cengage Learning. All Rights Reserved. May not be scanned, copied or duplicated, or posted to a publicly accessible website, in whole or in part.

Matching

Match each activity or responsibility with the proper home health team member.

Activity/Responsibility   **Health Care Team**

1. _____ may or may not be supportive of client   a. client

2. _____ writes orders and acts as a consultant and guide   b. family

3. _____ provides direct client care   c. nursing assistant

4. _____ person in need of care   d. supervising nurse

5. _____ may act as alternate caregiver   e. physician

6. _____ provides for client's safety and comfort

7. _____ makes observations about care that was given

8. _____ teaches and supervises nursing assistants

9. _____ requires skilled services

10. _____ plans care

11. _____ may require assistance with ADLs

12. _____ completes periodic client assessments

13. _____ documents observations and care that was given

14. _____ may live in the client's home

CERTIFICATION REVIEW

Complete the following multiple-choice assessments.

1. Which factor increased the interest in home care?

   a. Lack of hospital beds

   b. Lower cost to provide care

   c. Increased number of musculoskeletal ailments

   d. Larger number of people with chronic illnesses

2. Which statement about skilled home health nursing care is incorrect?

   a. Recovery is desirable but not required.

   b. It is primarily for comfort and convenience.

   c. Instead of continued hospitalization, services are provided.

   d. Care is appropriate for the condition to reduce the risk of complications.

3. What is given that indicates a nursing assistant has permission to work in home health care?

   a. License

   b. Certificate

   c. Job description

   d. Procedure manual

© 2022 Cengage Learning. All Rights Reserved. May not be scanned, copied or duplicated, or posted to a publicly accessible website, in whole or in part.

4. What needs to be in place before a home health aid is assigned to provide care to a client in the home?

   a. Client is on Medicare.

   b. Client needs nursing care.

   c. Client has private insurance.

   d. Client needs 35 hours of care each week.

5. What is the first criteria to determine if a client is eligible for home care?

   a. Lives alone

   b. Needs teaching

   c. Homebound status

   d. Has a wound that needs care

6. Which health care professional coordinates the care of each home care client?

   a. Physician

   b. Charge nurse

   c. Social worker

   d. Case manager

7. Where is the Outcome and Assessment Information Set (OASIS) sent after it is completed?

   a. Physician

   b. Government

   c. Insurance provider

   d. Discharging hospital

8. At which time is the care plan for the client receiving home care reviewed?

   a. Weekly

   b. Once a month

   c. Every 62 days

   d. Every 3 months

9. Which action should be taken if a family member asks the nursing assistant to perform a task that is uncomfortable to complete?

   a. Contact the supervisor for direction.

   b. Complete the task after providing client care.

   c. Complete it with the family member's direction.

   d. Complete the task before completing client care.

10. Which action should be taken if a family member asks about the client's health problem?

   a. Answer the question.

   b. Refer the question to the case manager.

   c. Call the physician to have him or her answer the family's questions.

   d. Provide the family member with the medical record to read.

© 2022 Cengage Learning. All Rights Reserved. May not be scanned, copied or duplicated, or posted to a publicly accessible website, in whole or in part.

CHAPTER APPLICATION

Computations

Compute the time spent in each case. (Write the 24-hour time designation for each arrival and departure time in the space provided.)

Arrival Time	Departure Time	Time Spent
1. 8:15 a.m. _____	8:50 a.m. _____	_____
2. 10:05 a.m. _____	11:15 a.m. _____	_____
3. 11:20 a.m. _____	1:05 p.m. _____	_____
4. 2:10 p.m. _____	3:15 p.m. _____	_____
5. 3:45 p.m. _____	4:30 p.m. _____	_____

Clinical Situations

Briefly describe what the nursing assistant should do in the following home care settings.

1. Mary Johnson, who is 78 years of age, has diabetes mellitus. She requires a bed bath, change of linens, and a blood glucose level check. Your arrival time is 8:20 a.m. and you leave the client's home at 10:05. Your odometer read 42,738 miles when you left the agency and 42,743 miles when you arrived at the client's home. Compute the time spent with the client and the mileage from the agency to the client's home.

_____

_____

2. Mr. Alleandra is 58 and has a diagnosis of terminal cancer of the bone. Your assignment is to spend an entire evening shift with him. In addition to feeding the client and meeting his comfort needs, Mr. Alleandra is lonely and would like you to keep him company. He likes to play cards and dominoes and to watch TV. Describe your actions.

_____

_____

3. Mrs. Parks has congestive heart failure and tires so easily that she has difficulty carrying out her daily living activities. You are assigned to assist her for an entire shift. The family wants you to wash the floor and windows, vacuum, and do the laundry. These activities are not part of the nursing assistant's job description. Describe your actions.

_____

_____

© 2022 Cengage Learning. All Rights Reserved. May not be scanned, copied or duplicated, or posted to a publicly accessible website, in whole or in part.

RELATING TO THE NURSING PROCESS

Write the step of the nursing process that is related to each nursing assistant action.

Nursing Assistant Action	Nursing Process Step
1. The nursing assistant performs only skills they has been taught when providing home care.	_____
2. The nursing assistant and the supervisor discuss the exact care to be given to the homebound client.	_____
3. The nursing assistant keeps careful records of the length of time spent on specific activities when in the client's home.	_____

DEVELOPING GREATER INSIGHT

1. You are assigned to work the night shift in Mrs. Lawrence's home. The client sleeps most of the night but must be awakened to take her medication at 12 midnight and 4:00 a.m. Think about what activities you might engage in while the client sleeps.

2. Discuss with classmates the reasons why clients might prefer to have home care rather than remain in a long-term care facility.

3. Invite a nursing assistant who works in home care to share their experiences with you.

© 2022 Cengage Learning. All Rights Reserved. May not be scanned, copied or duplicated, or posted to a publicly accessible website, in whole or in part.

CHAPTER 35

The Nursing Assistant in Home Care

OBJECTIVES

After completing this chapter, you will be able to:

35-1 Spell and define terms.

35-2 Summarize the four levels of hospice care.

35-3 Define core values and explain why they are important.

35-4 Describe the characteristics that are especially important to the nursing assistant who provides home care.

35-5 List at least 10 methods of protecting your personal safety when working as a home care assistant in the community.

35-6 Describe the duties of the nursing assistant who works in the home setting.

35-7 Describe appropriate circumstances for assisting clients with medications and list the "Six Rights" of medication administration.

35-8 Describe the duties of the homemaker assistant.

35-9 Explain how to carry out home care activities needed to maintain a safe and clean environment.

VOCABULARY BUILDER

Definitions

Define the following terms.

1. core values _____

2. home health assistant _____

3. homemaker aide _____

4. homemaker assistant _____

5. respite care _____

© 2022 Cengage Learning. All Rights Reserved. May not be scanned, copied or duplicated, or posted to a publicly accessible website, in whole or in part.

CHAPTER REVIEW

Fill-in-the-Blank

Complete the following statements in the spaces provided.

1. The nursing assistant contributes to the planning step of the nursing process by actively participating in _____.

2. The client should, if able, make decisions about food _____.

3. The client's bathroom should be cleaned _____.

4. Before _____ the client's appliances, seek _____ from a family member.

5. Before storing clothes that have been laundered, check for needed _____.

6. Drip-dry fabrics should be washed _____ so they can be hung and folded.

7. The primary role of the home health assistant is to _____.

8. The major responsibility of the homemaker assistant is to provide _____.

9. In some cases, the nursing assistant who provides health care may be asked to carry out _____ chores.

10. Because home health assistants handle money, they must be _____ people.

11. The home health care assistant's activities are planned around the _____.

12. To save costs, _____ enema equipment may be substituted for disposable enema equipment.

13. Statements by the client that reflect neglect or abuse should be _____.

14. Chemicals such as household cleaning supplies and insecticides should be kept locked up when the client is _____.

15. Dust, dirty dishes, and improper care of foods contribute to the spread of _____.

Short Answer

Briefly answer the following questions in the spaces provided.

1. What are three areas to report that support the assessment process?
   a. _____
   b. _____
   c. _____

2. What are two ways to support the implementation portion of the nursing process?
   a. _____
   b. _____

3. What are two ways to promote the evaluation part of the nursing process?
   a. _____
   b. _____

© 2022 Cengage Learning. All Rights Reserved. May not be scanned, copied or duplicated, or posted to a publicly accessible website, in whole or in part.

4. What are three household duties the nursing assistant frequently performs?

 a. _____

 b. _____

 c. _____

5. What are three household cleaning duties not included in the nursing assistant's responsibilities?

 a. _____

 b. _____

 c. _____

6. What are four kinds of telephone numbers to be kept close to the phone during home care?

 a. _____

 b. _____

 c. _____

 d. _____

7. What action should the nursing assistant take when cleaning laundry soiled by blood?

 _____

8. What are 10 ways of maintaining your personal safety when working in home care?

 a. _____

 b. _____

 c. _____

 d. _____

 e. _____

 f. _____

 g. _____

 h. _____

 i. _____

 j. _____

True/False

Mark the following true or false by circling T or F.

1. T F Household duties may be part of the home nursing assistant's responsibilities.

2. T F Caring for food properly is part of your responsibility.

3. T F It is all right to leave dirty dishes in the sink after the client eats.

4. T F Cleaning the client's bathroom and kitchen are part of the nursing assistant's responsibilities.

5. T F Dirty dishes left to accumulate will contribute to infection.

6. T F Loose scatter rugs are safe to use in the home if the client knows where they are placed.

7. T F Electrical outlets that have multiple cords plugged in could cause fires.

8. T F Hospice is a philosophy of care that may be given in many locations.

9. T F Short-term respite care is available for persons receiving hospice services.

© 2022 Cengage Learning. All Rights Reserved. May not be scanned, copied or duplicated, or posted to a publicly accessible website, in whole or in part.

10. T F   The home care agency is responsible for assessing each client's core values.

11. T F   The home care nursing assistant is permitted to administer oral medications.

12. T F   Document the reason and response when the client takes a PRN (as needed) medication.

CERTIFICATION REVIEW

Complete the following multiple-choice assessments.

1. Which statement is correct about hospice care?

   a. It is a philosophy of care.

   b. It is provided to cure an illness.

   c. It is provided as an inpatient service only.

   d. It provides a limited amount of care.

2. Which information is least likely to be found in the folder of information left in the home of a patient receiving home care?

   a. Care notes

   b. Scope of services

   c. Advance directives

   d. HIPAA information

3. Which item can be used to cleanse dirty feet?

   a. Soap

   b. Baby oil

   c. Pumice stone

   d. Shaving cream

4. In which location should soiled dressing materials be discarded?

   a. Agency trash

   b. Outside trash

   c. Trash in the home

   d. Personal trash at home

5. For which reason would the nursing assistant decide to not enter a client's home?

   a. Client is bedbound.

   b. Client is home alone.

   c. Client is using oxygen.

   d. Client is holding a gun.

6. Which action should be taken if a client is having an argument with a family member?

   a. Leave the home.

   b. Take the side of the patient.

   c. Take the side of the family member.

   d. Perform care without giving an opinion.

© 2022 Cengage Learning. All Rights Reserved. May not be scanned, copied or duplicated, or posted to a publicly accessible website, in whole or in part.

7. Which item can be used to cleanse crusted areas around the eyes?

   a. Bar soap

   b. Alcohol pads

   c. Baby shampoo

   d. Waterless cleanser

8. In which way will a nursing assistant help a client at home take medications?

   a. Open the container.

   b. Give the client a dose.

   c. Instruct the client to take a dose.

   d. Read the label of the medication.

9. Which should be done if a client reports a medication "did not go down" when swallowing a dose?

   a. Give the client more water.

   b. Encourage the client to cough.

   c. Perform the Heimlich maneuver.

   d. Give the client a piece of a banana to eat.

10. Which item should be cleansed first when washing a client's dishes in the home?

    a. Dishes

    b. Glasses

    c. Silverware

    d. Pots and pans

CHAPTER APPLICATION

Clinical Situations

Briefly describe what the nursing assistant could do to address the following situations in the home setting.

1. The bed is not flexible and the client needs to be in a semi-Fowler's position.

   _____

2. The client has sprained an ankle and there is no ice bag to apply cold.

   _____

3. The client needs to remain in bed and likes to do puzzles to pass the time.

   _____

4. The client is very heavy and there is no trapeze to help with lifting and moving.

   _____

5. You must give a bed bath and there is no bath blanket.

   _____

6. The client must remain in bed, so all care must be given on a regular-height twin bed.

   _____

© 2022 Cengage Learning. All Rights Reserved. May not be scanned, copied or duplicated, or posted to a publicly accessible website, in whole or in part.

7. The client is a child who, though in traction, has many toys, crayons, and books scattered over the bed.

_____

8. You need a place to put soiled laundry as you give care.

_____

9. The client occasionally needs an enema, and disposable enema equipment is too expensive.

_____

10. The client has an upper respiratory infection, and you must safely dispose of soiled tissues.

_____

11. You are visiting Mrs. Morrison regularly as part of your assignment. This morning you notice a bruise on her arm, and she tells you that she and her daughter, who lives with her, quarreled last evening. What action should you take?

_____

_____

_____

12. Mary Schroeder is 91 years old and is very frail. She has been diagnosed with emphysema, CHF, and diabetes. She is being cared for by her sister, who is 93 years old. You are assigned to provide personal hygiene care three mornings each week. Ms. Schroeder is in a regular bed that is low to the floor and cannot have its position changed. The client is incontinent. You must adapt her low-income environment to provide proper care.

_____

_____

_____

RELATING TO THE NURSING PROCESS

Write the step of the nursing process that is related to each nursing assistant action.

Nursing Assistant Action   **Nursing Process Step**

1. The nursing assistant reports to their supervisor about improvement in the homebound client's appetite.   _____

2. The nursing assistant reports that the client receiving home care is now able to function independently.   _____

3. The nursing assistant informs the supervisor that stress between the client and their daughter about the client's planned activities is interfering with the client's recovery.   _____

DEVELOPING GREATER INSIGHT

1. Think back to a time when you were under extreme stress. Did you strike out physically or verbally and then were sorry afterward?

2. Make out a shopping list for meals for one day for two people who are on unrestricted diets but limited income. Look through newspapers for coupons and sales that could save money.

3. Look carefully around your own home and try to identify safety factors that could be changed if health care were needed.

© 2022 Cengage Learning. All Rights Reserved. May not be scanned, copied or duplicated, or posted to a publicly accessible website, in whole or in part.

CHAPTER 36

Subacute Care

OBJECTIVES

After completing this chapter, you will be able to:

36-1 Spell and define terms.

36-2 Describe the purpose of subacute care.

36-3 Explain the differences between acute care, subacute care, and long-term care.

36-4 Describe special procedures provided in the subacute care unit.

36-5 Describe the responsibilities of the nursing assistant when caring for patients using subacute care.

36-6 Define sterile technique and explain why it is used.

36-7 List the guidelines for sterile procedures.

36-8 Describe the purpose of a sterile field.

36-9 Demonstrate how to establish a sterile field.

36-10 Explain when to use sterile gloves.

36-11 Describe how to use sterile gloves without contamination.

36-12 Describe the care of surgical drains.

36-13 Describe continuous sutures, interrupted sutures, and staples.

36-14 Demonstrate the following procedures:

- Procedure 83: Applying and Removing Sterile Gloves
- Procedure 84: Applying a Dry Sterile Dressing (Expand Your Skills)

© 2022 Cengage Learning. All Rights Reserved. May not be scanned, copied or duplicated, or posted to a publicly accessible website, in whole or in part.

VOCABULARY BUILDER

Matching

Match each term with the correct definition.

1. _____ care and treatment of persons with cancer

2. _____ drugs given to relieve severe pain

3. _____ additional bag of fluid added to the main IV line

4. _____ subacute care

5. _____ sudden, frequent, involuntary muscle contractions that impair function

6. _____ mild, harmless electrical current that blocks the transmission of pain to the brain

a TENS

b. spasticity

c. narcotic analgesics

d. oncology

e. piggyback

f. transitional care

CHAPTER REVIEW

Fill-in-the-Blank

Complete the following statements in the spaces provided by selecting the proper terms from the list provided.

approaches	areas	consistency	emotional
goals	hyperalimentation	participate	peripheral
skilled nursing	transitional	three to four weeks	

1. Subacute care is sometimes referred to as _____ care.

2. Subacute care units are usually located in _____ facilities.

3. Most subacute care units provide specialized care in one or two primary _____ of practice.

4. Nursing assistants _____ in special inservice education to meet the needs of subacute care patients.

5. Nursing assistants work with other team members to provide for the _____ well-being of the patients.

6. To give proper care, the nursing assistant must know that _____ have been established.

7. The key to successful rehabilitation is _____.

8. IV therapy refers to fluids and medications given directly into a(n) _____ vein.

9. TPN is also called _____.

© 2022 Cengage Learning. All Rights Reserved. May not be scanned, copied or duplicated, or posted to a publicly accessible website, in whole or in part.

Short Answer

Complete the assessment in the space provided.

1. What is the purpose of subacute care?

   _____

   _____

2. Where do patients continue their care after discharge from a subacute care unit?

   a. _____

   b. _____

   c. _____

3. What are five expectations of a nursing assistant who works on a subacute care unit?

   a. _____

   b. _____

   c. _____

   d. _____

   e. _____

4. Name three types of patients who may require intensive rehabilitation.

   a. _____

   b. _____

   c. _____

5. What are two reasons IV therapy is administered via a central venous catheter?

   a. _____

   b. _____

6. What do the letters PICC stand for?

   _____

7. What are four actions the nursing assistant must not take when caring for a patient with an IV?

   a. _____

   b. _____

   c. _____

   d. _____

8. Explain why sterile technique must be used when caring for a wound drain and state whether standard precautions are or are not necessary.

   _____

   _____

9. What are four important observations to report about a patient who is receiving epidural catheter pain relief?

   a. _____

   b. _____

   c. _____

   d. _____

© 2022 Cengage Learning. All Rights Reserved. May not be scanned, copied or duplicated, or posted to a publicly accessible website, in whole or in part.

Fill-in-the-Blank

Complete the following related to care of the patient receiving an IV.

1. Know the _____ rate.

2. Notify the nurse if the drip chamber is _____.

3. Avoid twisting or pulling _____.

4. Make sure the patient does not _____ on the tubing.

5. Observe the needle insertion site for signs of _____.

6. Make sure all _____ in the tubing are secure.

7. Note signs of moisture that might indicate _____.

8. Report signs of _____, _____, or chest or back pain.

True/False

Mark the following true or false by circling T or F.

1. T F Some patients may feel very uncertain when in a subacute care unit.

2. T F Hyperalimentation allows the bowel to rest.

3. T F Inability to move the legs is normal immediately after a spinal medication pump is implanted.

4. T F Never allow the bag of IV fluid to be lower than the patient's arm.

5. T F The dosage for PCA is controlled by equipment that is preset by the nurse.

6. T F An epidural catheter is implanted under the skin near the elbow to administer a local anesthetic.

7. T F The T-tube will drain 300–500 mL of blood-tinged bile in the first 24 hours after surgery.

8. T F Tongue piercings are harmless fashion statements.

9. T F TENS is a nondrug method of pain relief.

10. T F Patients with implantable medication pumps must always be moved with a transfer belt.

11. T F Cancer may be treated with surgery, radiation, chemotherapy, or a combination of any of these.

CERTIFICATION REVIEW

Complete the following multiple-choice assessments.

1. What should the nursing assistant expect to be withheld from a patient receiving multi-sensory stimulation?

    a. Pain

    b. Smell

    c. Meals

    d. Touch

© 2022 Cengage Learning. All Rights Reserved. May not be scanned, copied or duplicated, or posted to a publicly accessible website, in whole or in part.

2. Which action should be taken if a blood pressure measurement is to be completed on a patient recovering from a bilateral mastectomy?

   a. Use the patient's thigh.

   b. Ask the nurse what to do.

   c. Use the patient's nondominant arm.

   d. Use the patient's dominant arm.

3. How much of a border is to be around a sterile field?

   a. One-half inch

   b. One inch

   c. Two inches

   d. Three inches

4. What should be done after a sterile field is established?

   a. Leave the room.

   b. Stand facing the field.

   c. Move to the side of the field.

   d. Place the field against a wall.

5. Which part of the first glove should be touched when applying a sterile glove?

   a. The cuff

   b. The palm

   c. The fingers

   d. The back of the glove

6. Into which body area is the tip of a central venous catheter placed?

   a. Right atrium

   b. Subclavian vein

   c. Inferior vena cava

   d. Internal jugular vein

7. Which item is used to prevent air from entering the circulation in a patient with a central venous catheter?

   a. Paper tape

   b. Safety pin

   c. Kelly clamp

   d. Rubber band

8. For which adverse effect should a patient receiving patient-controlled analgesia be assessed?

   a. Pain

   b. Cough

   c. Constipation

   d. Muscle cramps

© 2022 Cengage Learning. All Rights Reserved. May not be scanned, copied or duplicated, or posted to a publicly accessible website, in whole or in part.

9. Which finding would be expected after an epidural catheter is placed in a patient?

    a. Extreme thirst

    b. Increased urination

    c. Increased blood pressure

    d. Leg weakness for 24 hours

10. For which reason is a T-tube clamped before and after meals?

    a. Reduces pain

    b. Improves appetite

    c. Prevents infection

    d. Supports digestion

CHAPTER APPLICATION

Clinical Situations

Briefly describe how a nursing assistant should react to the following situation.

1. Mrs. Johns's wound appears red and swollen, and it has increased foul-smelling drainage.

   _____

   _____

RELATING TO THE NURSING PROCESS

Write the step of the nursing process that is related to each nursing assistant action.

Nursing Assistant Action	Nursing Process Step
1. The nursing assistant reports that their patient, who is receiving chemotherapy by IV, has a reddened area at the needle insertion site.	_____
2. The nursing assistant reports that the patient, who has an epidural catheter for pain relief, is complaining of numbness in their right leg.	_____
3. The nursing assistant carefully monitors the patient's vital signs following their return from surgery.	_____

DEVELOPING GREATER INSIGHT

1. Invite a nursing assistant who works in subacute care to discuss their experiences with you.

2. Visit a subacute care unit. If possible:

    a. Observe a working assistant.

    b. Identify the types of patients on the unit.

    Return to the classroom and discuss your experiences with your classmates and instructor.

© 2022 Cengage Learning. All Rights Reserved. May not be scanned, copied or duplicated, or posted to a publicly accessible website, in whole or in part.

Alternative, Complementary, and Integrative Approaches to Patient Care

OBJECTIVES

After completing this chapter, you will be able to:

37-1 Spell and define terms.

37-2 Define alternative medicine.

37-3 Differentiate alternative practices from complementary and integrative practices.

37-4 List five categories of alternative and complementary therapies.

37-5 Define holistic care.

37-6 List at least three ways in which the nursing assistant supports patients' spirituality.

VOCABULARY BUILDER

Matching

Match each term with the correct description.

1. _____ promotes proper nervous system function by using spinal adjustments

2. _____ uses tiny, thin needles inserted into the body to correct imbalances

3. _____ natural system of medicine that originated in India 2,000 years ago

4. _____ a method of rubbing on the body to stimulate circulation, promote relaxation, and enhance pain relief

a. qigong

b. hypnotherapy

c. visualization

d. Ayurveda

© 2022 Cengage Learning. All Rights Reserved. May not be scanned, copied or duplicated, or posted to a publicly accessible website, in whole or in part.

5. _____ creates a state of altered consciousness in which the mind is more open to suggestion

6. _____ involves exposing patients to special lights, in which ultraviolet rays are blocked

7. _____ retraining the mind to control physical problems and stress

8. _____ physical and mental activities to channel the body's energy

9. _____ stimulation of certain areas in hands and feet to treat illness and reduce stress

10. _____ using warm glass jars to create suction over various parts of the body

11. _____ burning herbal substances on or near the body

12. _____ using the imagination to create images

e. chiropractic

f. cupping

g. reflexology

h. light therapy

i. massage therapy

j. moxibustion

k. acupuncture

l. biofeedback

CHAPTER REVIEW

Fill-in-the-Blank

Complete the following statements in the spaces provided using the words below.

chelation	empowered	guided imagery
herbal therapy	holistic	mind
modalities	osteopathy	physician
privilege	supplements	yoga

1. Complementary and alternative therapies should be used only under _____ supervision.

2. A doctor of _____ combines manipulative therapy with traditional medical treatment.

3. _____ is an alternative practice that employs breath control, postures, and relaxation.

4. Caring for patients during very private moments is a(n) _____.

5. _____ uses medicines made from plants.

6. Practitioners of _____ believe that positive changes can be helped to occur by focusing on and visualizing these changes.

7. _____ are nutritional substances used to make up a deficiency.

8. Using CAM therapy may involve different types of treatments, or _____.

9. Practices that consider the whole person are _____.

10. _____ is an intravenous injection of amino acid to improve blood flow in the legs.

11. One principle of integrative health care is that each individual can be _____ to bring greater wellness and healing into their own life.

12. Practitioners of some CAM therapies believe that the _____ has a powerful effect on the body's healing process.

© 2022 Cengage Learning. All Rights Reserved. May not be scanned, copied or duplicated, or posted to a publicly accessible website, in whole or in part.

Short Answer

Complete the assessment in the space provided.

1. List five ways in which the nursing assistant can help support the patient's spirituality.

   a. _____

   b. _____

   c. _____

   d. _____

   e. _____

2. Explain why some individuals use CAM therapy.

   _____

   _____

   _____

3. List at least four risks associated with using herbs and nutritional supplements.

   a. _____

   b. _____

   c. _____

   d. _____

4. List the five complementary and alternative medicine categories and give a brief explanation of each.

   a. _____

   b. _____

   c. _____

   d. _____

   e. _____

5. Explain why nursing care is holistic.

   _____

   _____

   _____

True/False

Mark the following true or false by circling T or F.

1. T F When a CAM program is used, the patient is a passive participant.

2. T F Complementary therapies can be used to support and strengthen overall health.

3. T F All individuals using a CAM program will receive identical treatment.

4. T F Anthroposophically extended medicine (AEM) treats the whole person, not just the disease or symptoms.

5. T F Ayurveda uses essential oils to stimulate the patient's sense of smell.

© 2022 Cengage Learning. All Rights Reserved. May not be scanned, copied or duplicated, or posted to a publicly accessible website, in whole or in part.

6.   T   F   The hands do not touch the body directly during therapeutic touch.

7.   T   F   TCM restores the balance between the body and the elements of earth, fire, water, wood, and metal.

8.   T   F   Acupuncture is painful in certain areas of the body.

9.   T   F   Some vitamins and herbs can be toxic.

10.   T   F   Chiropractic adjustments and osteopathic manipulation are identical treatments.

11.   T   F   Dance therapy focuses on use of the senses and self-expression.

12.   T   F   Color therapy affects the mood and emotions.

13.   T   F   Moxibustion is one form of treatment used in TCM.

CERTIFICATION REVIEW

Complete the following multiple-choice assessments.

1. Which treatment regimen combines alternative practices with conventional health care?

   a. Aromatherapy

   b. Guided imagery

   c. Energy therapies

   d. Complementary medicine

2. Which therapy is an example of energy therapy?

   a. Reiki

   b. Ayurveda

   c. Meditation

   d. Chiropractic adjustments

3. Which therapy harmonizes the relationship of body, mind, and spirit?

   a. Art

   b. Chelation

   c. Chiropractic

   d. Anthroposophically extended medicine

4. According to Chinese medicine, what is the cause of pain and illness?

   a. Muscle tension

   b. Blocking of chi

   c. Misaligned vertebrae

   d. Nutritional deficiency

5. Which step is least likely to be completed when meditating?

   a. Merging

   b. Visualizing

   c. Preparation

   d. Concentration

© 2022 Cengage Learning. All Rights Reserved. May not be scanned, copied or duplicated, or posted to a publicly accessible website, in whole or in part.

6. Which additional approach is often used with meditation?

    a. Prayer

    b. Massage

    c. Homeopathy

    d. Light therapy

7. Which vitamin contributes to a loss of appetite?

    a. A

    b. B1

    c. B12

    d. C

8. Which food item is a source of vitamin A?

    a. Carrots

    b. Salmon

    c. Bananas

    d. Asparagus

9. Which alternative therapy approach believes that body ailments can be healed by manipulating the feet?

    a. Reflexology

    b. Acupuncture

    c. Moxibustion

    d. Therapeutic touch

10. In which way does chiropractic care differ from osteopathic care?

    a. Osteopathic care focuses on a higher power.

    b. Osteopathic care focuses on muscles and joints.

    c. Chiropractic care focuses on the body, mind, and spirit.

    d. Chiropractic care focuses on the balance on body energies.

CHAPTER APPLICATION

Matching

Match each characteristic with the correct type of therapy.

1. _____ stimulates sense and emotions

2. _____ uses an injection of an amino acid

3. _____ uses plants to treat pain and illness

4. _____ stimulates and improves circulation

a. chelation

b. color

c. electromagnetic

d. herbal

© 2022 Cengage Learning. All Rights Reserved. May not be scanned, copied or duplicated, or posted to a publicly accessible website, in whole or in part.

5. _____ analyzes the diet to maximize health   e. hypnotherapy

6. _____ used to treat mood and sleep disorders   f. light

7. _____ creates an altered state of consciousness   g. massage

8. _____ uses nonaerobic exercise and breath control   h. movement

9. _____ corrects imbalances in electrical and magnetic fields   i. nutrition

RELATING TO THE NURSING PROCESS

Write the step of the nursing process that is related to each nursing assistant action.

Nursing Assistant Action   **Nursing Process Step**

1. The nursing assistant checks the care plan to determine
   how to assist the patient with meditation.   _____

2. The nursing assistant informs the nurse that a patient who is
   using herbal therapy thinks they may be pregnant.   _____

3. The nursing assistant provides privacy when the patient is praying.   _____

4. The nursing assistant attends a care conference and describes
   how she calmed the patient when she found the patient crying
   in their room in the dark.   _____

5. The nursing assistant reports that the patient said the OMT
   and massage helped relieve their pain.   _____

6. The nursing assistant follows the care plan when the patient
   returns from their radiation treatment.   _____

7. The nursing assistant reports to the nurse that the patient
   vomited following their chemotherapy, so they did not
   take their herbs.   _____

DEVELOPING GREATER INSIGHT

1. Visit a health food store and get information on the use of herbal products and nutritional supplements.
   Report your findings to the class.

2. Ask a practitioner of a CAM therapy to speak to the class about the advantages and disadvantages of the
   treatment.

3. Discuss religion and spirituality with your classmates. How are they alike? How are they different?

© 2022 Cengage Learning. All Rights Reserved. May not be scanned, copied or duplicated, or posted to a publicly accessible website, in whole or in part.

Body Systems, Common Disorders, and Related Care Procedures

CHAPTER **38**

Integumentary System

OBJECTIVES

After completing this chapter, you will be able to:

38-1 Spell and define terms.

38-2 Review the function of the skin.

38-3 Describe some common skin lesions.

38-4 List three diagnostic tests associated with skin conditions.

38-5 Describe nursing assistant actions relating to care of patients with specific skin conditions.

38-6 Identify persons at risk for the formation of pressure injuries.

38-7 Describe measures to prevent pressure injuries.

38-8 Describe the stages of pressure injury formation and identify appropriate nursing assistant actions.

38-9 List nursing assistant actions in caring for patients with burns.

38-10 State how skin tears occur and describe prevention measures.

38-11 Describe the guidelines for caring for patients with negative pressure wound therapy.

38-12 Discuss precautions to use when assisting with a pulsatile lavage treatment.

38-13 Describe the importance of nutrition in healing wounds and burns.

38-14 List the guidelines for cleansing and observing a wound.

38-15 Demonstrate the following procedure:

- Procedure 85: Changing a Clean Dressing and Applying a Bandage (Expand Your Skills)

© 2022 Cengage Learning. All Rights Reserved. May not be scanned, copied or duplicated, or posted to a publicly accessible website, in whole or in part.

VOCABULARY BUILDER

Definitions

Define the following words.

1. cyanotic _____

2. crust _____

3. debride _____

4. obese _____

5. rubra _____

6. allergy _____

7. lesions _____

8. pallor _____

9. necrosis _____

Matching

Match each term with its definition.

1. _____ redness

2. _____ lukewarm

3. _____ having a bad smell

4. _____ outermost layer of the skin

5. _____ small knot-like protrusions

6. _____ injury from scraping the skin

7. _____ former term for pressure injury

8. _____ flat discolored spots like measles

9. _____ dead skin that is thick and leathery

10. _____ mass of blood confined to one area

11. _____ rubbing of the skin against a surface

12. _____ skin that is scraped or scratched away

13. _____ tissue that attaches the skin to the muscle

14. _____ injury caused by a blow causing a hemorrhage

15. _____ skin moves in one direction while underlying layers remain fixed

a. abrasion

b. contusion

c. decubitus

d. epidermis

e. eschar

f. excoriation

g. friction

h. hematoma

i. macule

j. malodorous

k. nodule

l. rubra

m. shearing

n. subcutaneous

o. tepid

© 2022 Cengage Learning. All Rights Reserved. May not be scanned, copied or duplicated, or posted to a publicly accessible website, in whole or in part.

CHAPTER REVIEW

Fill-in-the-Blank

Complete the following statements in the spaces provided.

1. Another name for allergic reactions is _____ reactions.

2. The most severe allergic reaction is called _____ shock.

3. _____ is a flexible connective tissue found in many areas of the body, such as the joints between bones, the rib cage, the ear, and the nose.

4. Patients with skin lesions must be handled _____ without _____ the skin.

5. Pressure injuries are more easily _____ than _____.

6. Pressure injuries are common in obese patients under the _____, in the abdominal folds, and between the folds of the _____.

7. Reddening of skin that does not fade in 30 minutes is a sign of the _____ stage of tissue breakdown.

8. If the epidermis is broken, it should be kept _____.

9. Indication of infection in a pressure injury might include _____ and a foul _____.

10. Early necrosis over a pressure point may be indicated by _____ discoloration.

11. In stage 2 breakdown, it is imperative that the _____ be relieved, or more serious damage will occur.

12. Patients who have pressure injuries are always at high risk of developing _____.

13. _____ is a purple or maroon area of intact skin or a blood blister caused by damage to underlying soft tissue from pressure or shear.

14. Crusts should not be removed from skin lesions without _____.

15. Shearing occurs when skin moves in one direction while structures underneath _____.

16. Patients with stage 4 pressure injuries experience _____ and _____ and are at great risk for infection.

17. In a technique called _____, pillows or props are used to relieve pressure on specific areas of the body.

18. _____ the heels from the surface of the bed to relieve pressure.

19. Patients with _____ fractures are at high risk of developing heel ulcers.

20. In a dark-skinned person, a stage 1 pressure injury will appear _____ or _____ in color.

21. _____ are injuries that result from scraping the skin.

22. _____ are mechanical injuries (usually caused by a blow) resulting in hemorrhage beneath the unbroken skin.

23. A bruise is also called a(n) _____.

24. A(n) _____ is a localized mass of blood that is confined to one area.

25. _____ are accidental breaks in the skin.

© 2022 Cengage Learning. All Rights Reserved. May not be scanned, copied or duplicated, or posted to a publicly accessible website, in whole or in part.

26. Dark purple bruises on the forearms and back of hands that commonly occur in elderly individuals are called _____.

27. A(n) _____ is an injury that separates the epidermis from underlying structures as a result of friction or shearing and is common in aging skin.

28. An unstageable ulcer is covered with _____ or _____.

29. A loud whistling sound from the NPWT system indicates a(n) _____.

30. Small, knot-like protrusions on the skin surface are called _____.

Short Answer

Complete the assessment in the space provided.

1. What clinical problem might you suspect because of these changes in skin?

    a. hot, dry, flushed _____

    b. darkish blue, cyanotic _____

    c. very dry _____

2. How could you best document the following skin lesions?

    a. flat discolored, as in measles _____

    b. skin appears scratched or scraped away _____

    c. raised spot filled with serous fluid _____

    d. areas of dried body secretions _____

3. List four types of patients who are at high risk for skin breakdown.

    a. _____

    b. _____

    c. _____

    d. _____

4. What are 12 ways to avoid the development of pressure ulcers?

    a. _____

    b. _____

    c. _____

    d. _____

    e. _____

    f. _____

    g. _____

    h. _____

    i. _____

    j. _____

    k. _____

    l. _____

© 2022 Cengage Learning. All Rights Reserved. May not be scanned, copied or duplicated, or posted to a publicly accessible website, in whole or in part.

5. What are the four goals of burn treatment?

    a. _____

    b. _____

    c. _____

    d. _____

6. What special care will the nursing assistant emphasize when assisting in the care of a burn patient?

    a. _____

    b. _____

    c. _____

    d. _____

    e. _____

    f. _____

7. List four actions that the nursing assistant should take when caring for a patient with a negative pressure wound therapy system.

    a. _____

    b. _____

    c. _____

    d. _____

8. Why is it important to prevent skin tears?

    a. _____

    b. _____

    c. _____

9. Mr. French is in fair physical condition. He is rather lethargic and is ambulatory with assistance. He has limited movement of his left arm and leg, is continent, and eats poorly. He has an open lesion over his left hip. What is his risk of pressure injury development?

    _____

    _____

CERTIFICATION REVIEW

Complete the following multiple-choice assessments.

1. Which body area should be avoided when applying lotion to the skin of an older client?

    a. Arms

    b. Back

    c. Lower legs

    d. Between the toes

© 2022 Cengage Learning. All Rights Reserved. May not be scanned, copied or duplicated, or posted to a publicly accessible website, in whole or in part.

2. Which type of skin condition can develop in a client with an HIV infection?

   a. Wheals

   b. Vesicles

   c. Excoriations

   d. Kaposi's sarcoma

3. Which treatment may be prescribed to treat a skin condition?

   a. Alcohol rubs

   b. Steroid cream

   c. Soap and water

   d. Colloidal oatmeal

4. Which condition increases the risk of developing a pressure injury?

   a. Stroke

   b. Diabetes

   c. Pneumonia

   d. Osteoarthritis

5. Which action should be taken if a client has a reddened area on the skin?

   a. Massage the area.

   b. Remove the pressure.

   c. Apply a cool compress.

   d. Apply lotion to the area.

6. Which is a characteristic of a stage 3 pressure injury?

   a. Red skin area

   b. Presence of a crater

   c. Obvious bone present

   d. Development of a blister

7. What should be done if eschar is covering a wound?

   a. Remove the eschar.

   b. Apply a sterile dressing.

   c. Keep the wound open to air.

   d. Cleanse the wound with soap and water.

8. What action will increase circulation to body tissues?

   a. Bathe every day.

   b. Provide a backrub.

   c. Encourage ambulation.

   d. Elevate the head of the bed.

© 2022 Cengage Learning. All Rights Reserved. May not be scanned, copied or duplicated, or posted to a publicly accessible website, in whole or in part.

9. What should be done when caring for a patient on a floatation mattress?

   a. Turn the client every two hours.

   b. Pin the blanket to the bed frame.

   c. Avoid tucking sheets around the mattress.

   d. Move the mattress when changing the linens.

10. What is an advantage of using a hydrocolloid dressing for a wound?

   a. Is ideal for skin tears

   b. Needs to be changed daily

   c. Must be covered to be effective

   d. Provides a moist environment for wound healing

CHAPTER APPLICATION

Identification

Name the areas indicated by writing their proper names in the spaces provided.

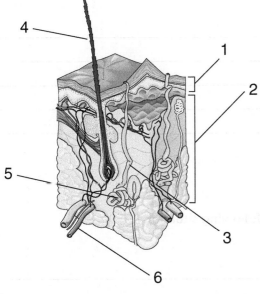

1. _____

2. _____

3. _____

4. _____

5. _____

6. _____

© 2022 Cengage Learning. All Rights Reserved. May not be scanned, copied or duplicated, or posted to a publicly accessible website, in whole or in part.

7. Complete the turning wheel to demonstrate your understanding of the principle of relieving pressure.

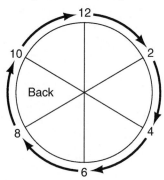

8. List the areas most subject to breakdown when the patient is in the position shown.

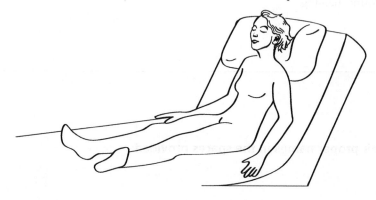

a. _____

b. _____

c. _____

d. _____

e. _____

Clinical Situations

Briefly describe how a nursing assistant should react to the following situations.

1. You burned your finger.

_____

_____

_____

2. You are assigned to give a bed bath and find that the patient has skin lesions.

_____

_____

_____

© 2022 Cengage Learning. All Rights Reserved. May not be scanned, copied or duplicated, or posted to a publicly accessible website, in whole or in part.

RELATING TO THE NURSING PROCESS

Write the step of the nursing process that is related to each nursing assistant action.

Nursing Assistant Action	**Nursing Process Step**
1. The nursing assistant charts the presence of excoriation on the patient's buttocks.	_____
2. The nursing assistant turns the patient who is in a low-air-loss bed every 90 minutes, following the nurse's orders.	_____
3. The nursing assistant reports seeing a pustule on the patient's thigh.	_____
4. The nursing assistant makes sure the dependent patient's position is changed at least every two hours.	_____
5. The nursing assistant uses a turning sheet to move dependent patients in bed.	_____
6. The nursing assistant reports an area of irritation around the entrance of the nasogastric tube into the patient's nose.	_____

DEVELOPING GREATER INSIGHT

1. What do the following patients have in common: a patient with a nasogastric tube, a patient with an indwelling catheter, and a patient who is able to move independently?

2. Discuss with classmates reasons why changes in the aging integumentary system make the elderly more prone to develop pressure ulcers.

© 2022 Cengage Learning. All Rights Reserved. May not be scanned, copied or duplicated, or posted to a publicly accessible website, in whole or in part.

Respiratory System

OBJECTIVES

After completing this chapter, you will be able to:

39-1 Spell and define terms.

39-2 Review the location of the respiratory organs.

39-3 Explain the function of the respiratory organs.

39-4 Describe some common diseases of the respiratory system.

39-5 List five diagnostic tests used to identify respiratory conditions.

39-6 Describe nursing assistant actions related to the care of patients with respiratory conditions.

39-7 Identify patients who are at high risk of poor oxygenation.

39-8 Describe the care of patients with a tracheostomy, a laryngectomy, or chest tubes.

39-9 List five safety measures for the use of oxygen therapy.

39-10 Describe the care of patients who have an endotracheal tube and are mechanically ventilated.

39-11 State the purpose of the oral airway and nasal airway.

39-12 Discuss the care of patients who have airways in place.

39-13 Discuss the use of the incentive spirometer.

39-14 Discuss the use of the nebulizer.

39-15 Explain (or discuss) the use of BiPAP and CPAP masks.

39-16 Demonstrate the following procedure:

  • Procedure 86: Collecting a Sputum Specimen (Expand Your Skills)

© 2022 Cengage Learning. All Rights Reserved. May not be scanned, copied or duplicated, or posted to a publicly accessible website, in whole or in part.

VOCABULARY BUILDER

Matching

Match each term with the correct definition.

1. _____ voice box
2. _____ gas needed for life
3. _____ difficulty breathing
4. _____ bring up material from lungs
5. _____ serious inflammation of the lungs
6. _____ inspiration followed by exhalation
7. _____ joins upper respiratory tract to lungs
8. _____ areas of the lungs where oxygen exchange occurs
9. _____ condition caused by narrowing and clogging of the bronchi

a. dyspnea
b. expectorate
c. ventilation
d. trachea
e. pneumonia
f. alveoli
g. asthma
h. oxygen
i. larynx

Definitions

Define the following terms and abbreviations.

1. biopsy

_____

2. sputum

_____

3. URI

_____

4. COPD

_____

5. cannula

_____

6. stoma

_____

© 2022 Cengage Learning. All Rights Reserved. May not be scanned, copied or duplicated, or posted to a publicly accessible website, in whole or in part.

CHAPTER REVIEW

Fill-in-the-Blank

Complete the following statements in the spaces provided.

1. The patient experiencing an asthmatic attack has dyspnea and wheezing because there is increased _____ production, spasm of the _____ tree, and swelling of the _____ lining the respiratory tract.

2. The person with bronchitis has _____ cough.

3. Common allergens include pollen, medications, dust, _____, and _____.

4. Symptoms of a URI include runny nose, watery eyes, and _____.

5. The tiny air sacs forming the lungs are called _____.

6. In emphysema, the alveoli lose some of their _____.

7. Changes in emphysema allow _____ to become trapped in the lungs.

8. A patient with emphysema has the most difficulty in the _____ phase of respiration.

9. It is important for the nursing assistant to know and read the _____ rate of oxygen for each patient.

10. _____ is a condition in which there is insufficient oxygen in the blood.

11. During oxygen administration, the area around the mask should be periodically _____ and _____.

12. The external opening of the tracheostomy is the _____.

13. If a patient has had a(n) _____, the larynx has been removed.

14. Avoid getting _____, _____, _____, or _____ near or in the stoma.

15. _____ are used after chest surgery to drain bloody fluid from the chest.

16. Being unable to _____ is very frightening.

Short Answer

Complete the assessment in the space provided.

1. What four practices should be taught to all patients with upper respiratory infections?

   a. _____

   b. _____

   c. _____

   d. _____

2. What are four observations regarding patients with respiratory disease that must be reported?

   a. _____

   b. _____

   c. _____

   d. _____

© 2022 Cengage Learning. All Rights Reserved. May not be scanned, copied or duplicated, or posted to a publicly accessible website, in whole or in part.

3. What are 10 important points about the care of patients with COPD?

    a. _____

    b. _____

    c. _____

    d. _____

    e. _____

    f. _____

    g. _____

    h. _____

    i. _____

    j. _____

4. What four precautions must be taken when a patient receives oxygen from a tank?

    a. _____

    b. _____

    c. _____

    d. _____

5. List five conditions that increase a patient's risk of hypoxemia.

    a. _____

    b. _____

    c. _____

    d. _____

    e. _____

6. List eight observations of a patient with chest tubes that require immediate nursing notification.

    a. _____

    b. _____

    c. _____

    d. _____

    e. _____

    f. _____

    g. _____

    h. _____

7. Give three characteristics of the orthopneic position.

    a. _____

    b. _____

    c. _____

8. What kind of breathing exercises might be ordered for a patient with COPD?

    _____

© 2022 Cengage Learning. All Rights Reserved. May not be scanned, copied or duplicated, or posted to a publicly accessible website, in whole or in part.

9. What is a technique used to loosen mucus and clear the air passageways?

_____

10. List four safety precautions specific to the use of liquid oxygen.

a. _____

b. _____

c. _____

d. _____

CERTIFICATION REVIEW

Complete the following multiple-choice assessments.

1. What must be done before checking a patient's capillary refill?

   a. Check the Kardex.

   b. Remove nail polish.

   c. Read the medical record.

   d. Lower the head of the bed.

2. Which symptom would be reported to the nurse for a patient with an upper respiratory infection?

   a. Dyspnea

   b. Sleepiness

   c. Runny nose

   d. Watery eyes

3. Which action can help prevent a patient with a weakened respiratory system from contracting an infection?

   a. Encourage bedrest.

   b. Use a plastic pillow cover.

   c. Limit exposure to other people.

   d. Reduce the amount of oral fluids.

4. Which action helps a patient with chronic obstructive pulmonary disease conserve energy?

   a. Pace activities.

   b. Assist with ambulation every hour.

   c. Encourage to perform pursed-lip breathing.

   d. Remind to raise arms over the head several times a day.

5. What should be done if a patient with a tracheostomy begins to cough sputum through the stoma tube?

   a. Elevate the head of the bed.

   b. Notify the nurse immediately.

   c. Turn the patient onto the right side.

   d. Cleanse the stoma with a disposable tissue.

© 2022 Cengage Learning. All Rights Reserved. May not be scanned, copied or duplicated, or posted to a publicly accessible website, in whole or in part.

6. Why is it important to limit dust from entering the stoma of a patient with a tracheostomy?

    a. Reduces the need for rest

    b. Limits the need for extra water

    c. Prevents pathogens from entering the lungs

    d. Eliminates the need to measure pulse oximetry

7. Which item needs to be at the bedside of a patient with chest tubes?

    a. Suction

    b. Tissues

    c. Emesis basin

    d. Water pitcher

8. Which fluid is used to refill a reusable humidifier?

    a. Tap water

    b. Sterile water

    c. Intravenous fluid

    d. Sterile normal saline

9. Which is the most common delivery system used to provide oxygen to a patient?

    a. Face mask

    b. Nasal cannula

    c. Endotracheal tube

    d. Tracheostomy tube

10. Which action needs to be corrected for a patient with an oxygen concentrator in the room?

    a. Alarm set

    b. Unit against a wall

    c. No smoking signs posted

    d. Unit plugged into the wall outlet

CHAPTER APPLICATION

Identification

Using a colored pencil or crayon, fill in the areas on the following figure through which oxygen must flow from the outside to the exchange area. Then name the parts in their proper order.

© 2022 Cengage Learning. All Rights Reserved. May not be scanned, copied or duplicated, or posted to a publicly accessible website, in whole or in part.

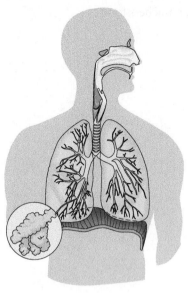

1. _____
2. _____
3. _____
4. _____
5. _____
6. _____

Hidden Picture

Carefully study the following picture and identify 7 rules of oxygen safety that have been violated. Write them in the spaces provided. (There are 11.)

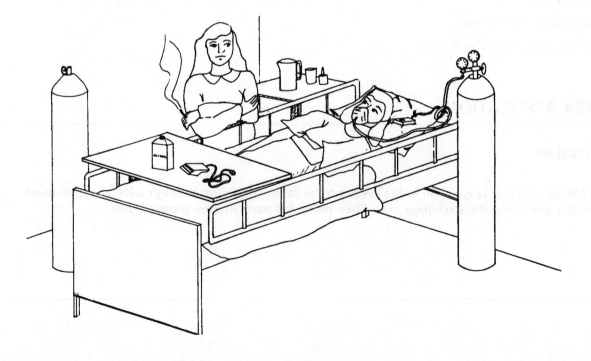

© 2022 Cengage Learning. All Rights Reserved. May not be scanned, copied or duplicated, or posted to a publicly accessible website, in whole or in part.

1. _____

2. _____

3. _____

4. _____

5. _____

6. _____

7. _____

Clinical Situations

Briefly describe how a nursing assistant should react to the following situations.

1. You enter a patient's room and find the patient receiving a higher level of oxygen than is ordered.

   _____

   _____

2. Your patient complains of mouth dryness while receiving oxygen therapy.

   _____

   _____

3. Your patient who is receiving oxygen therapy wants to shave with an electric razor.

   _____

   _____

4. You are assigned to collect a sputum specimen for culture and sensitivity. Before collecting a specimen, the patient should _____

   _____

5. Complete the following label, which is attached to a specimen container, using the following information: Mr. James Brown is a patient in Room 604. His medical record number is 689473. Dr. Smith has written an order to obtain a sputum specimen for culture and sensitivity testing today.

   Name _____   Room _____

   Date _____   Hospital Number _____

   Doctor _____   Examination _____

   Specimen _____

Matching

Match each term to the correct explanation.

1. _____ source of water to moisten oxygen

2. _____ extends from the nostril to the posterior pharynx

3. _____ tube that provides complete control over the airway

4. _____ should not be used for liter flows over 5

a. bag-valve-mask (BVM)

b. continuous positive airway pressure (CPAP)

c. endotracheal tube (ET tube)

d. humidifier

© 2022 Cengage Learning. All Rights Reserved. May not be scanned, copied or duplicated, or posted to a publicly accessible website, in whole or in part.

5. _____ rigid plastic suction device   e. incentive spirometer

6. _____ device used to manually ventilate a patient   f. liquid oxygen

7. _____ used only for unconscious patients   g. nasal cannula

8. _____ device used to mechanically ventilate a patient   h. nasopharyngeal airway

9. _____ delivers oxygen through the nose   i. nebulizer

10. _____ opening into the body   j. oropharyngeal airway

11. _____ treatment for sleep apnea   k. oxygen concentrator

12. _____ made by cooling oxygen gas   l. stoma

13. _____ delivers moisture or medication deep into the lungs   m. ventilator

14. _____ prevents atelectasis and pneumonia   n. Yankauer catheter

RELATING TO THE NURSING PROCESS

Write the step of the nursing process that is related to each nursing assistant action.

Nursing Assistant Action	Nursing Process Step
1. The nursing assistant makes sure the strap holding a mask delivering oxygen is not too tight.	_____
2. The nursing assistant periodically removes an oxygen delivery mask and carefully washes and dries the skin underneath it.	_____
3. The nursing assistant reports that the patient's respirations have become labored.	_____
4. The nursing assistant keeps the patient's face free of any nasal discharge when a nasal airway is in use.	_____
5. The nursing assistant positions pillows behind the patient's back to assist their breathing.	_____
6. The nursing assistant helps position the patient so the respiratory therapist can give a treatment.	_____
7. The nursing assistant informs the nurse that the oxygen flow meter is set lower than the level noted on the care plan.	_____

DEVELOPING GREATER INSIGHT

1. Try wearing an oxygen mask on your face for 20 minutes. Be sure the tubing is open so you have a continuous source of air. Describe your feelings when you remove the mask.

2. In the clinical area, practice identifying the number of liters on a flow meter, under supervision.

© 2022 Cengage Learning. All Rights Reserved. May not be scanned, copied or duplicated, or posted to a publicly accessible website, in whole or in part.

CHAPTER **40**

Circulatory (Cardiovascular) System

OBJECTIVES

After completing this chapter, you will be able to:

40-1 Spell and define terms.

40-2 Review the location of the organs of the circulatory system.

40-3 Describe the functions of the organs of the circulatory system.

40-4 Describe some common disorders of the circulatory system.

40-5 Describe nursing assistant actions related to care of patients with disorders of the circulatory system.

40-6 List five specific diagnostic tests for disorders of the circulatory system.

40-7 State the purpose of the pacemaker and implantable cardioverter defibrillator.

VOCABULARY BUILDER

Definitions

Define the following terms.

1. anemia _____

_____

2. embolus _____

_____

3. ischemia _____

_____

© 2022 Cengage Learning. All Rights Reserved. May not be scanned, copied or duplicated, or posted to a publicly accessible website, in whole or in part.

4. thrombus _____

_____

5. hypertrophy _____

_____

6. angina _____

_____

7. diuresis _____

_____

8. atheroma _____

_____

9. dyscrasias _____

_____

CHAPTER REVIEW

Fill-in-the-Blank

Complete the following statements in the spaces provided.

1. Patients who have long-standing cardiac disease often develop diseases of the _____ system.

2. Blood vessels that serve the outer parts of the body are called _____ blood vessels.

3. Blood abnormalities are referred to as blood _____.

4. Following prescribed exercises carefully can help promote _____ flow and _____ return.

5. The diet of the person who is hypertensive usually limits the amount of _____ intake.

6. Angioplasty is a surgical procedure to _____ blood vessels.

7. Coronary bypass is a surgical procedure that _____ blocked arteries.

8. When the coronary muscles are blocked, the heart tissue becomes _____.

Short Answer

Complete the assessment in the space provided.

1. List 10 nursing assistant responsibilities in caring for the feet of patients with peripheral vascular disease.

    a. _____

    b. _____

    c. _____

    d. _____

© 2022 Cengage Learning. All Rights Reserved. May not be scanned, copied or duplicated, or posted to a publicly accessible website, in whole or in part.

e. _____

f. _____

g. _____

h. _____

i. _____

j. _____

2. Which observations would be reported about patients with circulatory disorders?

a. _____

b. _____

c. _____

d. _____

e. _____

3. What six signs and symptoms indicate decreased circulation to an area?

a. _____

b. _____

c. _____

d. _____

e. _____

f. _____

4. To what part of the body do the vessels lead that are most commonly affected by atherosclerosis and the formation of atheromas?

a. _____

b. _____

c. _____

5. What seven conditions predispose a person to the development of atherosclerosis?

a. _____

b. _____

c. _____

d. _____

e. _____

f. _____

g. _____

6. What four factors are stressed in the treatment of a patient with atherosclerosis?

a. _____

b. _____

c. _____

d. _____

© 2022 Cengage Learning. All Rights Reserved. May not be scanned, copied or duplicated, or posted to a publicly accessible website, in whole or in part.

7. What four diagnostic medical terms are used to indicate a coronary heart attack?

a. _____

b. _____

c. _____

d. _____

8. What three special observations must the nursing assistant note when caring for a patient who is recovering from an MI?

a. _____

b. _____

c. _____

9. What four signs or symptoms might be noted and reported in a patient with CHF?

a. _____

b. _____

c. _____

d. _____

10. What seven nursing care procedures would the nursing assistant carry out for a patient with CHF?

a. _____

b. _____

c. _____

d. _____

e. _____

f. _____

g. _____

True/False

Mark the following true or false by circling T or F.

1. T F A rocking bed is used to lull the patient into relaxation.

2. T F A patient with peripheral vascular disease should avoid sitting with the legs crossed.

3. T F The safest way to supply warmth to a patient with peripheral vascular disease is to apply a heating pad.

4. T F People with poor peripheral circulation should avoid smoking.

5. T F In atherosclerosis, blood vessels become widely dilated.

6. T F Severe, crushing chest pain may be a symptom of an MI.

7. T F Heart failure is also known as PVD.

8. T F An anemic patient may require special mouth care.

9. T F An anemic person is pale and may experience exhaustion and dyspnea.

10. T F Sickle cell anemia is due to an inability to absorb vitamin B12.

11. T F The nursing care of a person with leukemia is similar to that given to a person with anemia.

© 2022 Cengage Learning. All Rights Reserved. May not be scanned, copied or duplicated, or posted to a publicly accessible website, in whole or in part.

12. T   F   A patient with a pacemaker must hold a cell phone or cordless phone on the opposite side of the body from the pacemaker.

13. T   F   Persons with pacemakers should not be in the same room with a microwave oven.

14. T   F   A pacemaker must be replaced every four years.

15. T   F   The nursing assistant will be shocked if they is touching a patient when an ICD delivers a shock.

16. T   F   Ventricular dysrhythmias occur in the lower chambers of the heart.

17. T   F   A stent keeps the arteries open.

18. T   F   Sickle cell anemia is seen most often in persons of Mediterranean descent.

CERTIFICATION REVIEW

Complete the following multiple-choice assessments.

1. Which blood component is a watery solution?

    a. Plasma

    b. Thrombocytes

    c. Red blood cells

    d. White blood cells

2. Which is an age-related change to the cardiovascular system?

    a. Heart rate slows.

    b. Blood pressure decreases.

    c. Blood vessels more elastic.

    d. Heart muscle becomes thinner.

3. What causes a person with heart disease to have a fever?

    a. Dehydration

    b. Undiagnosed infection

    c. Inflammatory response

    d. New onset of renal failure

4. Which part of the heart is affected when edema occurs?

    a. Aorta

    b. Valves

    c. Left heart

    d. Right heart

5. What causes varicose veins to develop?

    a. Weak leg veins

    b. Poor muscle tone

    c. Stiffening of the veins

    d. Buildup of fat in the veins

© 2022 Cengage Learning. All Rights Reserved. May not be scanned, copied or duplicated, or posted to a publicly accessible website, in whole or in part.

6. In which position should the legs of a patient with peripheral vascular disease be placed when sitting in a chair?

   a. Elevate the feet.

   b. Stretch the legs forward.

   c. Cross the legs at the knees.

   d. Cross the legs at the ankles.

7. A transient ischemic attack is a warning sign of which condition?

   a. Stroke

   b. Heart failure

   c. Diverticulitis

   d. Osteoarthritis

8. What should be done when checking the skin color of a patient with a heart condition?

   a. Turn on a light.

   b. Position in a chair.

   c. Offer to drink water first.

   d. Ask to empty the bladder.

9. What should be done first if a patient's implantable cardioverter defibrillator discharges while giving care?

   a. Call for help.

   b. Listen to heart rate.

   c. Measure blood pressure.

   d. Have the patient stop all activity.

10. What occurs when a patient is taking a drug to remove excess fluid from the body?

    a. Diuresis

    b. Elevated heart rate

    c. Irregular heart rhythm

    d. Increased blood pressure

CHAPTER APPLICATION

Identification

Name the valves located between:

1. The right atrium and the right ventricle _____

2. The left atrium and the left ventricle _____

3. The right ventricle and the pulmonary artery

4. The left ventricle and the aorta _____

5. Using colored pencils or crayons, color the venous blood blue and the arterial blood red in the following figure.

© 2022 Cengage Learning. All Rights Reserved. May not be scanned, copied or duplicated, or posted to a publicly accessible website, in whole or in part.

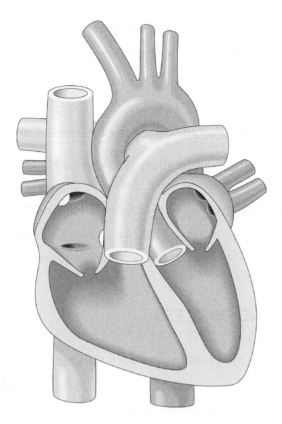

Explain the action that occurs at the four numbered areas on the diagram below.

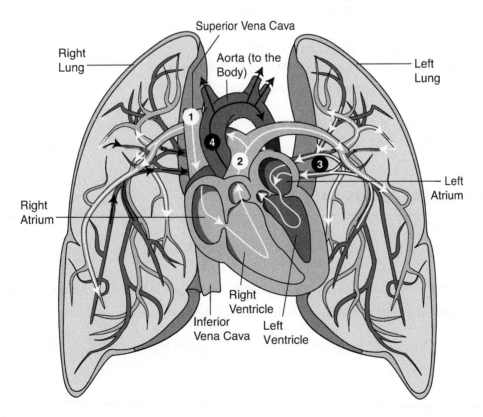

1. _____

2. _____

© 2022 Cengage Learning. All Rights Reserved. May not be scanned, copied or duplicated, or posted to a publicly accessible website, in whole or in part.

3. _____

4. _____

Clinical Situations

Briefly describe how a nursing assistant should react to the following situations.

1. Your patient, who has angina pectoris, is having an argument with a visitor.

2. You are passing out meal trays and find a salt packet on the tray of a patient who has congestive heart failure.

3. A patient with congestive heart failure has an erratic radial pulse rate of 72 beats per minute.

4. A patient with congestive heart failure has a fluid intake far in excess of output.

5. Your patient who has hypertension suddenly complains of blurred vision and their speech is slurred.

RELATING TO THE NURSING PROCESS

Write the step of the nursing process that is related to each nursing assistant action.

Nursing Assistant Action	Nursing Process Step
1. The nursing assistant reports that the resident's legs are pale and cool to the touch.	_____
2. The nursing assistant weighs the patient who has congestive heart failure daily.	_____
3. The nursing assistant completes the bath for the patient who has congestive heart failure, to lessen fatigue.	_____
4. The nursing assistant provides special mouth care for the patient with anemia.	_____
5. The nursing assistant reports that the patient who is anemic tires very easily.	_____

DEVELOPING GREATER INSIGHT

1. Think through reasons why a patient with peripheral vascular disease should wear properly fitting shoes when out of bed.

2. Discuss with classmates the kinds of concerns you might have if you were dependent on a pacemaker.

3. Practice finding and measuring the pulse in each of the following vessels:

   a. temporal

   b. carotid

   c. popliteal

   d. dorsalis pedis

4. Think through why people who cross their legs, sit long hours at work, or have the heavy weight of pregnancy in the abdomen tend to develop varicose veins.

© 2022 Cengage Learning. All Rights Reserved. May not be scanned, copied or duplicated, or posted to a publicly accessible website, in whole or in part.

CHAPTER 41

Musculoskeletal System

OBJECTIVES

After completing this chapter, you will be able to:

41-1 Spell and define terms.

41-2 Describe the location of the musculoskeletal system.

41-3 Explain the functions of the musculoskeletal system.

41-4 Describe some common conditions of the musculoskeletal system.

41-5 Describe nursing assistant actions related to the care of patients with conditions and diseases of the musculoskeletal system.

41-6 List at least seven specific diagnostic tests for musculoskeletal conditions.

41-7 Demonstrate the following procedure:

- Procedure 87: Performing Range-of-Motion Exercises (Passive)

VOCABULARY BUILDER

Spelling

Each line has four different spellings of a word. Circle the correctly spelled word.

1. barsitis	bursitis	bursites	buresitis
2. cartilage	cartalage	cartilege	catelage
3. comminnuted	cominuted	comminooted	comminuted
4. suppinachon	suppination	supination	suppinasion
5. virtebrae	vertabrae	vertebrae	vertobrae
6. extension	extinsion	extenchon	extention
7. aduction	adducsion	adduchon	adduction
8. dorsiflexion	dorseflexion	dorsiflextion	dorsifection

© 2022 Cengage Learning. All Rights Reserved. May not be scanned, copied or duplicated, or posted to a publicly accessible website, in whole or in part.

Matching

Match each term on the right with the correct description. Answers may be used more than once.

1. _____ collapses bone inward; seen only in the vertebrae of the spine

2. _____ involves only part of the cross-section of bone

3. _____ breaks completely across the bone

4. _____ occurs when the fragment from one bone is wedged into another bone

5. _____ shattering and splintering of the bone into more than three fragments

6. _____ seen only in fractures of the skull and face; collapses bone fragments inward

7. _____ runs at an angle across the bone

8. _____ twists around the bone

9. _____ fracture in a diseased bone

10. _____ occurs when a bone fragment is pulled off at the point of ligament or tendon attachment

11. _____ occurs when only one side of the bone is broken and the other side is bent; common in children

12. _____ break across the entire cross-section of the bone

13. _____ improperly aligned

14. _____ occurs when the skin is intact and not broken

15. _____ occurs when the skin over the fracture is broken

16. _____ an area containing many blood vessels that bleeds readily when a bone is fractured

a. spiral fracture

b. pathologic fracture

c. depressed fracture

d. avulsion fracture

e. complete fracture

f. oblique fracture

g. greenstick fracture

h. comminuted fracture

i. incomplete fracture

j. displaced

k. transverse fracture

l. closed fracture

m. compound fracture

n. impacted fracture

o. compression fracture

p. vascular

CHAPTER REVIEW

Fill-in-the-Blank

Complete the statements in the spaces provided.

1. To remain healthy, the musculoskeletal system must be _____ .

2. Abnormal shortening of muscles is called _____ .

3. Moving each toe away from the second toe is called _____ .

4. Moving each finger toward the middle finger is called _____ .

5. Touching the thumb to the little finger of the same hand is called _____ .

6. Rolling the hip in a circular motion toward the midline is called _____ .

7. Small fluid-filled sacs found around joints are called _____ .

8. Inflammation of a joint is called _____ .

9. Any break in the continuity of a bone is a _____ .

10. If a broken bone protrudes through the skin, it is called a(n) _____ fracture.

11. Traction that uses several weights and lines is called _____ traction.

© 2022 Cengage Learning. All Rights Reserved. May not be scanned, copied or duplicated, or posted to a publicly accessible website, in whole or in part.

Short Answer

Complete the assessment in the space provided.

1. What are four dangers of insufficient exercise?

   a. _____

   b. _____

   c. _____

   d. _____

2. What five special techniques should you use when carrying out ROM exercises?

   a. _____

   b. _____

   c. _____

   d. _____

   e. _____

3. What five techniques are used to treat chronic arthritis?

   a. _____

   b. _____

   c. _____

   d. _____

   e. _____

4. What are five ways to immobilize a fracture?

   a. _____

   b. _____

   c. _____

   d. _____

   e. _____

5. What two special beds are sometimes used when patients have multiple fractures?

   a. _____

   b. _____

6. What eight special nursing care procedures must be given to a patient who is in a fresh plaster leg cast?

   a. _____

   b. _____

   c. _____

   d. _____

   e. _____

   f. _____

   g. _____

   h. _____

© 2022 Cengage Learning. All Rights Reserved. May not be scanned, copied or duplicated, or posted to a publicly accessible website, in whole or in part.

7. What are four general factors to keep in mind as care is given to a patient who is in traction?

   a. _____

   b. _____

   c. _____

   d. _____

8. Define the following range-of-motion terms.

   a. extension

   _____

   b. abduction

   _____

   c. rotation: lateral

   _____

   d. eversion

   _____

   e. inversion

   _____

   f. pronation

   _____

   g. radial deviation

   _____

   h. ulnar deviation

   _____

   i. plantar flexion

   _____

   j. dorsiflexion

   _____

9. List two changes that may occur after a cast dries that suggest infection or ulceration under the cast.

   a. _____

   b. _____

10. List six general orders following hip surgery.

   a. _____

   b. _____

   c. _____

   d. _____

   e. _____

   f. _____

© 2022 Cengage Learning. All Rights Reserved. May not be scanned, copied or duplicated, or posted to a publicly accessible website, in whole or in part.

1. List four general orders following joint replacement surgery.

    a. _____

    b. _____

    c. _____

    d. _____

12. List six benefits of continuous passive motion therapy.

    a. _____

    b. _____

    c. _____

    d. _____

    e. _____

    f. _____

13. List four contraindications to CPM therapy.

    a. _____

    b. _____

    c. _____

    d. _____

14. List four observations that would cause you to stop a CPM device and promptly report to the nurse.

    a. _____

    b. _____

    c. _____

    d. _____

15. List 10 signs or symptoms of compartment syndrome.

    a. _____

    b. _____

    c. _____

    d. _____

    e. _____

    f. _____

    g. _____

    h. _____

    i. _____

    j. _____

© 2022 Cengage Learning. All Rights Reserved. May not be scanned, copied or duplicated, or posted to a publicly accessible website, in whole or in part.

CERTIFICATION REVIEW

Complete the following multiple-choice assessments.

1. Which type of muscle attaches to bones?

    a. Cardiac

    b. Visceral

    c. Voluntary

    d. Involuntary

2. Which is an age-related change to the musculoskeletal system?

    a. Height increases by two inches

    b. Spine becomes more flexible

    c. Lean muscle mass increases

    d. Posture becomes hunched over

3. What is the most common symptom of osteoarthritis?

    a. Fever

    b. Joint pain

    c. Deformities

    d. Swollen great toe

4. Which symptom is least likely to occur in a patient with fibromyalgia?

    a. Pain that affects the head

    b. Pain on both sides of the body

    c. Pain above and below the waist

    d. Pain affecting 11 of 18 body sites

5. What is another name for a body cast?

    a. Spica

    b. Plaster

    c. Fiberglass

    d. Removable

6. What is the difference between skin and skeletal traction?

    a. Skin traction can be removed for bathing.

    b. Skin traction requires a surgical procedure.

    c. Skeletal traction needs pins through the bone.

    d. Skeletal traction can be removed to make the bed.

© 2022 Cengage Learning. All Rights Reserved. May not be scanned, copied or duplicated, or posted to a publicly accessible website, in whole or in part.

7. What should be done when making the bed of a patient in traction?

    a. Roll the patient to each side.

    b. Assist the patient out of bed.

    c. Change the bottom sheet weekly.

    d. Change the bottom linen from top to bottom.

8. What device should be used when an ambulatory patient recovering from hip replacement surgery needs to void?

    a. Commode chair

    b. Fracture bedpan

    c. Bedside commode

    d. Elevated commode seat

9. In which location is compartment syndrome most likely to occur in an adult?

    a. Hip

    b. Tibia

    c. Radius

    d. Humerus

10. Which action will be taken when caring for a patient recovering from a lower extremity amputation?

    a. Flex the hip on the affected leg.

    b. Keep the head of the bed elevated.

    c. Assist to a prone position twice a day.

    d. Place a pillow under the amputated extremity.

© 2022 Cengage Learning. All Rights Reserved. May not be scanned, copied or duplicated, or posted to a publicly accessible website, in whole or in part.

CHAPTER APPLICATION

Identification

Using colored pencils or crayons, color in the following bones as indicated.

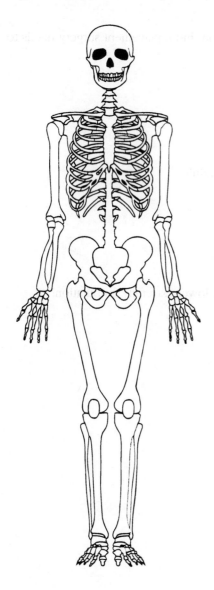

1. femur—red

2. humerus—blue

3. ribs—brown

4. ulna—green

5. radius—red

6. sternum—brown

7. pelvis—blue

8. cranium—green

9. tibia—yellow

© 2022 Cengage Learning. All Rights Reserved. May not be scanned, copied or duplicated, or posted to a publicly accessible website, in whole or in part.

Identification

1. Identify the fractures by writing the proper names in the spaces provided.

a. _____

c. _____

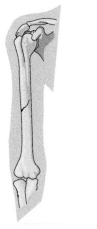

A

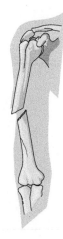

C

b. _____

d. _____

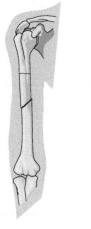

B

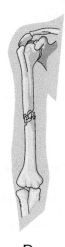

D

Differentiation

Contrast two forms of chronic arthritis.

Form	Tissue Affected	Possible Cause	Age Affected
Rheumatoid arthritis	_____ _____	_____ _____	_____ _____
Osteoarthritis	_____ _____	_____ _____	_____ _____

© 2022 Cengage Learning. All Rights Reserved. May not be scanned, copied or duplicated, or posted to a publicly accessible website, in whole or in part.

Identification

Figures A and B represent two patients who each have a new right hip prosthesis. Identify the incorrect behavior being demonstrated.

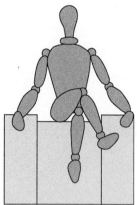

A. _____

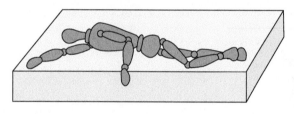

B. _____

Clinical Situations

Briefly describe how a nursing assistant should react to the following situations.

1. The toes of your patient in a leg cast felt cold and looked bluish. _____
   _____
   _____

2. Your patient has fibromyalgia. Despite receiving pain medication an hour ago, they is crying and says they has severe pain.
   _____
   _____
   _____

3. You find Mr. Lossero, an 82-year-old confused patient, on the floor. His right leg is shortened and externally rotated.
   _____
   _____
   _____

© 2022 Cengage Learning. All Rights Reserved. May not be scanned, copied or duplicated, or posted to a publicly accessible website, in whole or in part.

4. Mrs. Huynh has a short leg cast, which is dry. She has an order to take a shower.

_____

_____

_____

5. Your patient has an order for CPM therapy. You take their vital signs and discover that they has a fever and pulse of 104.

_____

_____

_____

6. Your patient has a fractured tibia and fractured radius. Both extremities are casted in plaster casts. You enter the room and the patient tells you that the pain in their tibia is agonizing—even worse than it was when she fell and broke it.

_____

_____

_____

7. Your patient complained of discomfort during range-of-motion exercises.

_____

_____

8. The patient has had a lower leg amputated below the knee. You must position the extremity.

_____

_____

RELATING TO THE NURSING PROCESS

Write the step of the nursing process that is related to each nursing assistant action.

Nursing Assistant Action	Nursing Process Step
1. The nursing assistant handles the wet cast with open palms.	_____
2. The nursing assistant supports each joint above and below while exercising that joint.	_____
3. The nursing assistant stops carrying out range of motion and reports to the nurse when the patient complains of pain.	_____
4. The nursing assistant carries out each ROM exercise five times.	_____
5. The nursing assistant reports the patient's feelings of numbness in the toes of the newly casted leg.	_____
6. The nursing assistant helps support the patient in a spica cast while another assistant changes the linen.	_____
7. The nursing assistant is very careful not to disturb the weights while caring for the patient with skeletal traction.	_____
8. The nursing assistant asks the nursing supervisor to review the traction lines on the skeletal traction before they begins to give care.	_____

© 2022 Cengage Learning. All Rights Reserved. May not be scanned, copied or duplicated, or posted to a publicly accessible website, in whole or in part.

DEVELOPING GREATER INSIGHT

1. Stand in front of a full-length mirror. Be sure you have something to hang onto for support. Raise one leg, bending it at the knee, and pretend that you have had an amputation. How do you feel about your body image now?

2. Wrap one leg in an Ace bandage so you will keep your knee straight, simulating a cast. Try to ambulate safely using crutches. Identify difficulties that a patient in a similar situation might have.

3. Put your dominant arm in a sling and try to carry out your activities of daily living. Did you feel frustrated by the experience?

4. Working in pairs, take turns being patient and nursing assistant, and practice passive ROM exercises.

© 2022 Cengage Learning. All Rights Reserved. May not be scanned, copied or duplicated, or posted to a publicly accessible website, in whole or in part.

CHAPTER 42

Endocrine System

OBJECTIVES

After completing this chapter, you will be able to:

42-1 Spell and define terms.

42-2 Review the location of the endocrine system.

42-3 Explain (or Describe) the functions of the endocrine system.

42-4 List five specific diagnostic tests associated with conditions of the endocrine system.

42-5 Describe some common diseases of the endocrine system.

42-6 Recognize the signs and symptoms of hypoglycemia and hyperglycemia.

42-7 Describe nursing assistant actions related to the care of patients with disorders of the endocrine system.

42-8 Perform blood tests for glucose levels if facility policy permits.

42-9 Perform the following procedure:

- Procedure 88: Obtaining a Fingerstick Blood Sugar (Expand Your Skills)

VOCABULARY BUILDER

Matching

Match each definition with the correct term.

1. _____ blood sugar
2. _____ sugar in the urine
3. _____ endocrine secretion
4. _____ male reproductive cell
5. _____ produced by the thyroid gland
6. _____ organs that secrete body fluids
7. _____ needed for production of thyroxine
8. _____ glands located on top of the kidneys

a. sperm
b. glands
c. iodine
d. glucose
e. adrenals
f. hormone
g. thyroxine
h. glycosuria

© 2022 Cengage Learning. All Rights Reserved. May not be scanned, copied or duplicated, or posted to a publicly accessible website, in whole or in part.

Definitions

Define the following terms or abbreviations in the spaces provided.

1. hypersecretion

_____

2. hypertrophy

_____

3. polydipsia

_____

4. tetany

_____

CHAPTER REVIEW

Fill-in-the-Blank

Complete the following statements in the spaces provided.

1. The role of glands in the body is to secrete _____.

2. The chemicals secreted by glands _____ body activities and growth.

3. A major contribution the nursing assistant can make to the care of a patient with hyperthyroidism is to keep the room _____ and be patient and calm.

4. The treatment for hyperthyroidism is to _____ the level of thyroxine production.

5. Hypothyroidism can occur even when the thyroid gland _____.

6. The role of parathormone is to regulate the electrolyte levels of _____ and
_____.

7. One of the severe effects of inadequate levels of parathormone is acute muscle spasm called
_____.

8. Hypersecretion of adrenal cortical hormones causes a disease syndrome called
_____

9. A patient with Addison's disease becomes dehydrated and has a low tolerance to
_____.

10. In addition to diet and insulin, an important part of diabetic therapy is _____.

11. Two medications given for diabetes mellitus are insulin and _____ drugs.

12. A patient with diabetes has a sweet, fruity odor to the breath, so you might suspect
_____

13. A patient with diabetes is feeling excited, nervous, and hungry, so you might suspect

© 2022 Cengage Learning. All Rights Reserved. May not be scanned, copied or duplicated, or posted to a publicly accessible website, in whole or in part.

4. Daily foot care for the diabetic patient includes washing, drying, and _____ the feet.

15. Toenails of the diabetic patient should be cut only by a _____.

16. Diabetic patients should never be permitted to go _____.

17. The radioactive iodine uptake test is performed to check _____.

18. Special care must be taken of the _____ of the patient with diabetes.

Short Answer

Briefly answer the following questions.

1. How might the person with hyperthyroidism look and behave?

   _____

   _____

2. Your patient has just returned from surgery following a partial thyroidectomy. What six things should you check for and report?

   a. _____

   b. _____

   c. _____

   d. _____

   e. _____

   f. _____

3. What five factors seem to play a role in the incidence of diabetes mellitus?

   a. _____

   b. _____

   c. _____

   d. _____

   e. _____

4. What seven complications are common to patients who suffer from uncontrolled diabetes mellitus for many years?

   a. _____

   b. _____

   c. _____

   d. _____

   e. _____

   f. _____

   g. _____

© 2022 Cengage Learning. All Rights Reserved. May not be scanned, copied or duplicated, or posted to a publicly accessible website, in whole or in part.

5. What role does diet play in care of the diabetic patient?

_____

6. What six factors can contribute to a hyperglycemic state?

    a. _____

    b. _____

    c. _____

    d. _____

    e. _____

    f. _____

7. What six factors can contribute to a hypoglycemic state?

    a. _____

    b. _____

    c. _____

    d. _____

    e. _____

    f. _____

8. What are the nine nursing assistant responsibilities in caring for a patient with insulin-dependent diabetes mellitus?

    a. _____

    b. _____

    c. _____

    d. _____

    e. _____

    f. _____

    g. _____

    h _____

    i. _____

9. What are four typical signs and symptoms associated with IDDM?

    a. _____

    b. _____

    c. _____

    d. _____

10. What does each abbreviation stand for?

    a. IDDM _____

    b. NIDDM _____

© 2022 Cengage Learning. All Rights Reserved. May not be scanned, copied or duplicated, or posted to a publicly accessible website, in whole or in part.

1. What daily care should be given to the feet of a patient with diabetes?

    a. _____

    b. _____

    c. _____

    d. _____

    e. _____

    f. _____

CERTIFICATION REVIEW

Complete the following multiple-choice assessments.

1. Which gland is considered the master gland?

    a. Pituitary

    b. Thyroid

    c. Pancreas

    d. Hypothalamus

2. Which gland is located on the top of the kidneys?

    a. Thyroid

    b. Adrenal

    c. Pituitary

    d. Pancreas

3. Which finding is associated with hyperthyroidism?

    a. Anxiety

    b. Sleepiness

    c. Slow heart rate

    d. Low blood pressure

4. Which gland regulates the amount of calcium in the blood?

    a. Adrenal

    b. Pancreas

    c. Parathyroid

    d. Hypothalamus

5. Which finding is associated with Cushing syndrome?

    a. Dehydration

    b. Low blood sugar

    c. High blood pressure

    d. Too much potassium

© 2022 Cengage Learning. All Rights Reserved. May not be scanned, copied or duplicated, or posted to a publicly accessible website, in whole or in part.

6. Which type of diet should a patient with diabetes follow?

   a. Keto

   b. Vegetarian

   c. No particular type

   d. Carbohydrate exchange

7. Which route is used to administer medication to a patient with type 1 diabetes?

   a. Oral

   b. Topical

   c. Injection

   d. Inhalation

8. In a patient with diabetes, what is a strong predictor of death from heart and kidney disease?

   a. Body weight

   b. Activity level

   c. Blood sugar level

   d. Periodontal disease

9. Which laboratory test is used to determine a patient's blood glucose level over a prolonged period of time?

   a. Hemoglobin A1c

   b. Fasting blood glucose

   c. Capillary blood glucose

   d. Two-hour post prandial glucose

10. What does an elevated urine ketone level indicate?

    a. Presence of infection

    b. Fat being burned for energy

    c. Insufficient glucose in the blood

    d. Patient receiving too much insulin

© 2022 Cengage Learning. All Rights Reserved. May not be scanned, copied or duplicated, or posted to a publicly accessible website, in whole or in part.

CHAPTER APPLICATION

Identification
Using colored pencils, color the glands as indicated.

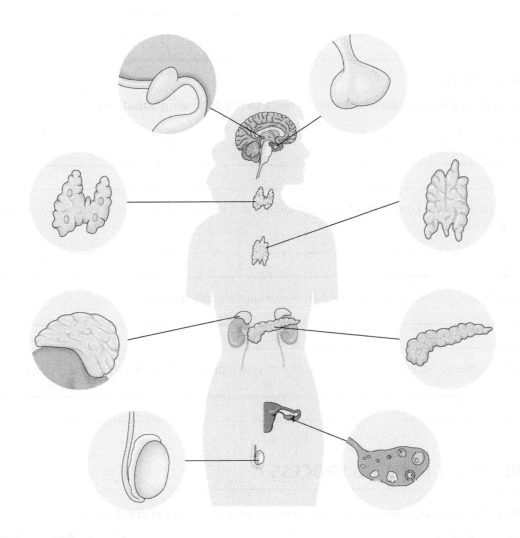

1. ovaries—red

2. thyroid—green

3. pituitary—blue

4. parathyroids—black

5. adrenals—brown

6. pancreas—red

7. pineal body—green

8. testes—yellow

© 2022 Cengage Learning. All Rights Reserved. May not be scanned, copied or duplicated, or posted to a publicly accessible website, in whole or in part.

Differentiation

Compare the signs and symptoms of diabetic coma and insulin shock.

	Diabetic Coma	**Insulin Shock**
Respirations	_____	_____
Pulse	_____	_____
Skin	_____	_____

Clinical Situations

Briefly describe how a nursing assistant should react to the following situations.

1. Your patient is to have a BMR at 8:00 a.m.

   _____

   _____

2. Your older obese patient complains of constant fatigue and burning on urination. They has a bruise on their leg that is healing poorly.

   _____

   _____

3. Your postoperative thyroidectomy patient has increasing difficulty speaking.

   _____

   _____

4. Your postoperative thyroidectomy patient has moved down in the bed so that their neck is hyperextended.

   _____

   _____

RELATING TO THE NURSING PROCESS

Write the step of the nursing process that is related to each nursing assistant action.

Nursing Assistant Action	**Nursing Process Step**
1. The nursing assistant reports that their patient, who has diabetes, has diarrhea.	_____
2. The nursing assistant makes sure the room of the patient with hyperthyroidism is kept cool and quiet.	_____
3. The nursing assistant documents the amount of fluid that the patient with diabetes is consuming.	_____
4. The nursing assistant reports that the patient with diabetes has pale, moist skin and seems nervous.	_____
5. The nursing assistant tests the patient's urine for acetone using the Ketostix strip test.	_____
6. The nursing assistant carefully washes and inspects the feet of the patient with diabetes daily.	_____

© 2022 Cengage Learning. All Rights Reserved. May not be scanned, copied or duplicated, or posted to a publicly accessible website, in whole or in part.

DEVELOPING GREATER INSIGHT

1. Make a list of ways your life would change if you were diagnosed with diabetes mellitus type 2. Share your list with the class.

2. Test your own urine for acetone using a Ketostix strip tape.

© 2022 Cengage Learning. All Rights Reserved. May not be scanned, copied or duplicated, or posted to a publicly accessible website, in whole or in part.

Nervous System

OBJECTIVES

After completing this chapter, you will be able to:

43-1 Spell and define terms.

43-2 State the location of the organs of the nervous system.

43-3 Describe the functions of the organs of the nervous system.

43-4 List five diagnostic tests used to determine conditions of the nervous system.

43-5 Describe 15 common conditions of the nervous system.

43-6 Describe nursing assistant actions related to the care of patients with conditions of the nervous system.

43-7 Explain the proper care and handling when caring for an artificial eye and mucous membranes in the eye socket.

43-8 Explain the proper care, handling, and insertion of a hearing aid.

VOCABULARY BUILDING

Matching

Match each term with the correct definition.

1. _____ within the skull
2. _____ paralysis affecting one limb only
3. _____ organ of hearing in the inner ear
4. _____ paralysis on one side of the body
5. _____ part of the eye in front of the lens
6. _____ abnormal, involuntary jerking movements
7. _____ portion of the neuron that carries the impulse of the cell
8. _____ paralysis affecting the same region on both sides of the body
9. _____ paralysis of the trunk (usually below the waist) and both legs

a. cochlea

b. chorea

c. nerve

d. neurotransmitter

e. hemiplegia

f. hemiparesis

g. diplegia

h. cornea

i. tremors

© 2022 Cengage Learning. All Rights Reserved. May not be scanned, copied or duplicated, or posted to a publicly accessible website, in whole or in part.

0. _____ weakness on one side of the body, usually caused by a stroke

11. _____ paralysis of the trunk (usually below the neck), both arms, and both legs

12. _____ specialized chemical messenger that sends a message from one nerve cell to another; the chemical needed for nerve transmission

13. _____ involuntary and rhythmic shaking movements in the muscles of parts of the body, usually the hands, feet, jaw, tongue, and head

14. _____ an enclosed, cable-like bundle of nerve fibers (axons and dendrites); part of the peripheral nervous system responsible for sending and receiving messages

j. intracranial

k. axon

l. monoplegia

m. tetraplegia

n. paraplegia

Definitions

Define the following terms or abbreviations in the spaces provided.

1. akinesia

_____

2. ossicles

_____

3. aphasia

_____

4. meninges

_____

5. tremors

_____

6. paralysis

_____

7. Lhermitte's sign

_____

8. tetraplegia

_____

9. nystagmus

_____

10. convulsion

_____

© 2022 Cengage Learning. All Rights Reserved. May not be scanned, copied or duplicated, or posted to a publicly accessible website, in whole or in part.

CHAPTER REVIEW

Fill-in-the-Blank

Complete the following statements in the spaces provided.

1. The pressure of tissue and fluid within the skull is called _____ pressure.
2. Other names for stroke are _____ or cerebrovascular accident.
3. The symptoms of a stroke depend on the area of _____ that is affected.
4. Left-brain damage often results in loss of _____.
5. Poststroke patients have a high level of _____.
6. TIAs are sometimes called _____.
7. The incidence of macular degeneration increases with _____.
8. Following cataract surgery, the patient should avoid _____.
9. Following cataract surgery, it is especially important to report _____ in the operative eye.
10. Otitis media is an infection of the _____ and may result in _____ of the ossicles, leading to deafness.
11. It is important not to let a hearing aid get _____.
12. Patients with post-polio syndrome are very sensitive to _____, particularly in the feet and legs.
13. Patients with post-polio syndrome need close _____ after surgery because they commonly experience complications.
14. Amyotrophic lateral sclerosis is a progressive neuromuscular disease that causes muscle weakness and _____.
15. _____ acuity is intact in patients with amyotrophic lateral sclerosis.
16. The most common cause of autonomic dysreflexia is _____.
17. Glaucoma is a condition in which the pressure is _____ within the eye.

Short Answer

Complete the assessment in the space provided.

1. What are six signs that the intracranial pressure is rising in a patient with a head injury?

   a. _____

   b. _____

   c. _____

   d. _____

   e. _____

   f. _____

© 2022 Cengage Learning. All Rights Reserved. May not be scanned, copied or duplicated, or posted to a publicly accessible website, in whole or in part.

2. In what four ways can the nursing assistant help an aphasic patient communicate?

   a. _____

   b. _____

   c. _____

   d. _____

3. What eight measures are carried out when caring for a patient in the acute phase of a cerebrovascular accident?

   a. _____

   b. _____

   c. _____

   d. _____

   e. _____

   f. _____

   g. _____

   h. _____

4. List eight signs and symptoms of post-polio syndrome.

   a. _____

   b. _____

   c. _____

   d. _____

   e. _____

   f. _____

   g. _____

   h. _____

5. List 10 things the nursing assistant must do in caring for a patient with ALS.

   a. _____

   b. _____

   c. _____

   d. _____

   e. _____

   f. _____

   g. _____

   h. _____

   i. _____

   j. _____

© 2022 Cengage Learning. All Rights Reserved. May not be scanned, copied or duplicated, or posted to a publicly accessible website, in whole or in part.

6. List six observations that should be reported to the nurse when a patient has had a seizure.

   a. _____

   b. _____

   c. _____

   d. _____

   e. _____

   f. _____

7. List at least 10 conditions that cause autonomic dysreflexia.

   a. _____

   b. _____

   c. _____

   d. _____

   e. _____

   f. _____

   g. _____

   h. _____

   i. _____

   j. _____

8. List 10 signs and symptoms of autonomic dysreflexia.

   a. _____

   b. _____

   c. _____

   d. _____

   e. _____

   f. _____

   g. _____

   h. _____

   i. _____

   j. _____

9. What are two important goals of nursing care for a patient during a seizure?

   a. _____

   b. _____

10. What are three ways to prevent contractures in a patient who has a spinal cord injury?

   a. _____

   b. _____

   c. _____

11. What two techniques can be learned to help communicate with someone who is deaf?

   a. _____

   b. _____

© 2022 Cengage Learning. All Rights Reserved. May not be scanned, copied or duplicated, or posted to a publicly accessible website, in whole or in part.

omplete the Chart

Type of Seizure	Description
1. absence	_____
2. generalized tonic-clonic	_____
3. status epilepticus	_____

True/False

Mark the following true or false by circling T or F.

1. T F Patients who are paralyzed are prone to pressure ulcers.

2. T F During a seizure, an airway is best maintained by keeping the head straight.

3. T F Parkinson disease is characterized by muscular rigidity and akinesia.

4. T F Intention tremors become worse as the individual tries to touch or pick up an object.

5. T F Multiple sclerosis is a progressive disease associated with inadequate levels of neurotransmitters in the cerebellum and brainstem.

6. T F Seizure syndrome is sometimes known as epilepsy.

7. T F Patients with spinal cord injuries need long-term nursing care.

8. T F Meningitis is an inflammation of the inner ear that may result in deafness.

CERTIFICATION REVIEW

Complete the following multiple-choice assessments.

1. What is an age-related change to the nervous system?

    a. Increased sensitivity to pressure

    b. Improved blood flow to the brain

    c. Changes in balance and coordination

    d. Reduced length of time for fine motor activities

2. Which part of the body has no blood supply?

    a. Skin

    b. Bones

    c. Lungs

    d. Cornea

3. What is an age-related change to the sensory organs?

    a. Improved hearing acuity

    b. Increased tear production

    c. Gradual decline in visual acuity

    d. Reduced risk of impacted ear wax

© 2022 Cengage Learning. All Rights Reserved. May not be scanned, copied or duplicated, or posted to a publicly accessible website, in whole or in part.

4. What is used to monitor neurologic problems after a stroke, illness, or injury?

    a. Heart rate

    b. Blood pressure

    c. Pulse oximeter

    d. Glasgow Coma Scale

5. Which finding is caused by a loss of autonomic nervous control in the patient with Parkinson disease?

    a. Tremors

    b. Drooling

    c. Muscle rigidity

    d. Shuffling when walking

6. Which information is true about Huntington disease?

    a. It has one cure.

    b. It causes one-sided paralysis.

    c. It is characterized by muscle tremors.

    d. It causes pain and pressure in the eyes.

7. Which is a finding associated with multiple sclerosis?

    a. Dyspnea

    b. Nystagmus

    c. Debilitating fatigue

    d. Joint and muscle pain

8. Which action should be taken when assisting a patient with amyotrophic lateral sclerosis with meals?

    a. Provide liquids with meals.

    b. Provide mouth care before meals.

    c. Explain where the food is on the tray.

    d. Check the mouth for pocketing of food.

9. Which action should be taken when caring for a patient who is taking phenytoin?

    a. Meticulous mouth care

    b. Range-of-motion exercises

    c. Careful assessment of the skin

    d. Strict measurement of intake and output

10. Which term may be used interchangeably with *quadriplegia*?

    a. Diplegia

    b. Flaccidity

    c. Tetraplegia

    d. Monoplegia

© 2022 Cengage Learning. All Rights Reserved. May not be scanned, copied or duplicated, or posted to a publicly accessible website, in whole or in part.

CHAPTER APPLICATION

Matching

Match each term to the correct description.

1. _____ 3 percent of strokes; blood fills the space surrounding the brain rather than inside of it.

2. _____ usually in the basal ganglia and thalamus; common in persons with diabetes and/or hypertension.

3. _____ clot forms in the brain; usually in a cerebral artery.

4. _____ sudden rupture of an artery; blood spills out, compressing brain structures.

5. _____ temporary period of diminished blood flow to the brain; precedes 15 percent of all strokes.

6. _____ most common type of stroke; about 87 percent of all strokes.

7. _____ clot develops elsewhere in the body, then travels to brain and lodges in small artery.

a. cerebral hemorrhage

b. embolic stroke

c. ischemic stroke

d. lacunar infarct

e. subarachnoid hemorrhage

f. thrombotic stroke

g. transient ischemic attack

Identification

Using colored pencils, markers, or crayons, color the functional areas of the brain as indicated.

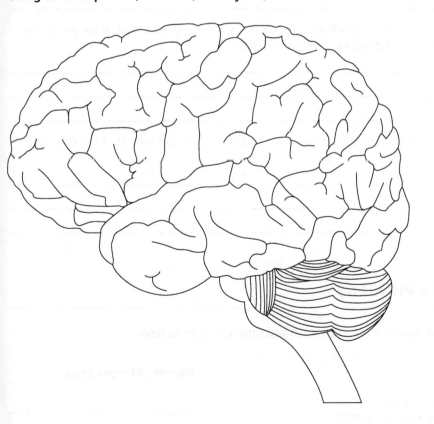

© 2022 Cengage Learning. All Rights Reserved. May not be scanned, copied or duplicated, or posted to a publicly accessible website, in whole or in part.

1. movement—red

2. hearing—yellow

3. pain and other sensations—green

4. seeing—brown

5. speech and language—blue

6. spinal cord—black

Clinical Situations

Briefly describe how a nursing assistant should react to the following situations.

1. The patient is on the floor convulsing.

   _____

   _____

   _____

2. You notice a change in the level of consciousness of your patient with a head injury.

   _____

   _____

   _____

3. Your patient in the private room has post-polio syndrome. The bed is on the opposite wall of the room from their bed at home. They is having trouble getting into and out of bed.

   _____

   _____

   _____

4. Mr. Herrera, an ALS patient, had difficulty swallowing his regular diet when you fed him. He kept coughing and choking.

   _____

   _____

   _____

RELATING TO THE NURSING PROCESS

Write the step of the nursing process that is related to each nursing assistant action.

Nursing Assistant Action   **Nursing Process Step**

1. The nursing assistant notes uncontrolled body
   movements in the patient with a head injury and
   calls this to the nurse's attention.   _____

© 2022 Cengage Learning. All Rights Reserved. May not be scanned, copied or duplicated, or posted to a publicly accessible website, in whole or in part.

2. The nursing assistant helps the nurse turn and
   position the patient who has had a stroke.   _____

3. The nursing assistant carries out ROM exercises for
   the patient who is paralyzed.   _____

4. The nursing assistant finds a patient who is convulsing.
   They calls for help but does not leave the patient alone.   _____

5. The nursing assistant uses a picture board to
   assist in communication with a patient who has aphasia.   _____

6. The nursing assistant pays particular attention when
   the patient with Parkinson disease ambulates,
   knowing that he is more apt to fall.   _____

7. The nursing assistant and all staff members try to
   maintain a calm environment for the patients
   with Parkinson disease.   _____

DEVELOPING GREATER INSIGHT

1. Put cotton balls in your ears and try to communicate with your classmates. Discuss your feelings and
   frustrations.

2. Try communicating your feelings and needs to a classmate without words and without the use of one hand
   and arm. Describe your feelings.

© 2022 Cengage Learning. All Rights Reserved. May not be scanned, copied or duplicated, or posted to a publicly accessible website, in whole or in part.

Gastrointestinal System

OBJECTIVES

After completing this chapter, you will be able to:

44-1 Spell and define terms.

44-2 Review the location of the organs of the gastrointestinal system.

44-3 Explain the functions of the organs of the gastrointestinal system.

44-4 List specific diagnostic tests associated with disorders of the gastrointestinal system.

44-5 Describe some common disorders of the gastrointestinal system.

44-6 Describe nursing assistant actions related to the care of patients with disorders of the gastrointestinal system.

44-7 Explain the purpose of the different types of enemas.

44-8 List the guidelines for caring for an ostomy.

44-9 Demonstrate the following procedures:

- Procedure 89: Collecting a Stool Specimen (Expand Your Skills)
- Procedure 90: Testing for Occult Blood Using Hemoccult and Developer (Expand Your Skills)
- Procedure 91: Inserting a Rectal Suppository (Expand Your Skills)
- Procedure 92: Giving a Soap-Solution Enema (Expand Your Skills)
- Procedure 93: Giving a Commercially Prepared Enema (Expand Your Skills)
- Procedure 94: Giving Routine Stoma Care (Colostomy) (Expand Your Skills)
- Procedure 95: Giving Routine Care of an Ileostomy (with Patient in Bed) (Expand Your Skills)

© 2022 Cengage Learning. All Rights Reserved. May not be scanned, copied or duplicated, or posted to a publicly accessible website, in whole or in part.

VOCABULARY BUILDER

Matching

Match each term with the correct definition.

1. _____ intestinal gas

2. _____ pertaining to the stomach

3. _____ removal of the stomach

4. _____ removal of the gall bladder

5. _____ another name for the large bowel

6. _____ eliminating feces through the anus

7. _____ a strong feeling of the need to eliminate

8. _____ collection of hardened feces in the rectum

9. _____ artificial opening made in the large bowel for fecal elimination

10. _____ protrusion of the intestines through a weakened area in the abdominal wall

a. cholecystectomy

b. gastrectomy

c. colostomy

d. defecation

e. colon

f. hernia

g. impaction

h. flatus

i. urgency

j. gastric

Definitions

Define the following terms or abbreviations.

1. HCl

2. cholelithiasis

3. peristalsis

4. herniorrhaphy

5. impaction

6. bolus

7. umami

8. inguinal

9. papillae

10. TWE

© 2022 Cengage Learning. All Rights Reserved. May not be scanned, copied or duplicated, or posted to a publicly accessible website, in whole or in part.

CHAPTER REVIEW

Fill-in-the-Blank

Complete the following statements in the spaces provided.

1. A(n) _____ of the gastrointestinal tract is often the first major sign of a tumor.

2. If a patient has a nasogastric tube in place, to prevent _____, you must be careful when moving the patient.

3. Following a bowel resection, it may be necessary to create an artificial opening called a(n) _____.

4. A patient with ulcerative colitis becomes dehydrated because of frequent _____.

5. A patient with ulcerative colitis should be eating a high-protein, high-calorie, _____ diet.

6. A patient with a duodenal ulcer is given medication to neutralize the _____ of the stomach, which causes additional trauma to the _____ area.

7. If a patient has an NPO order, special _____ should be given.

8. A patient with cholecystitis or cholelithiasis is usually placed on a low-_____ diet.

9. Following a cholecystectomy, _____ are often placed in the operative area.

10. In addition to routine postoperative care, a cholecystectomy patient should be placed in the _____ position.

11. Your patient is scheduled for a GB series, so you should check for orders regarding _____ or a special _____.

12. The solution used for a soap-solution enema is _____.

13. The best patient position for administration of an enema is the _____.

14. When possible, an enema should be given _____ giving the bath.

15. A _____ is required before giving an enema.

16. An oil-retention enema is retained and followed with a _____ enema.

17. The lubricated enema tube should be inserted _____ into the anus.

18. The enema solution container should be raised _____ above the level of the _____ while allowing the fluid to flow into the patient.

19. The rectal tube is used to relieve abdominal _____.

20. Commercially prepared chemical enema solutions drain fluid from the body to stimulate _____.

21. The chemical enema solution should be retained as _____.

22. Rectal tubes should be used no more than _____ in 24 hours.

23. Standard precautions require the use of _____ to protect the _____ from contamination during procedures involving the anus or rectum.

24. Antibiotics are given to control _____ that is involved in the development of gastric ulcers.

© 2022 Cengage Learning. All Rights Reserved. May not be scanned, copied or duplicated, or posted to a publicly accessible website, in whole or in part.

Short Answer

Complete the assessment in the space provided.

1. What are three important observations regarding your patient who has had a cholecystectomy that should immediately be reported to the nurse?

    a. _____

    b. _____

    c. _____

2. List 10 factors that affect bowel function and increase the risk of constipation.

    a. _____

    b. _____

    c. _____

    d. _____

    e. _____

    f. _____

    g. _____

    h. _____

    i. _____

    j. _____

3. List at least 10 signs and symptoms of fecal impaction.

    a. _____

    b. _____

    c. _____

    d. _____

    e. _____

    f. _____

    g. _____

    h. _____

    i. _____

    j. _____

4. What are five reasons that enemas are commonly given?

    a. _____

    b. _____

    c. _____

    d. _____

    c. _____

© 2022 Cengage Learning. All Rights Reserved. May not be scanned, copied or duplicated, or posted to a publicly accessible website, in whole or in part.

5. What information should be included when documenting an enema?

a. _____

b. _____

c. _____

d. _____

CERTIFICATION REVIEW

Complete the following multiple-choice assessments.

1. Which part of the mouth contains an enzyme that initiates carbohydrate digestion?

   a. Teeth

   b. Tongue

   c. Pharynx

   d. Salivary glands

2. What should be done if a patient with a nasogastric tube begins to vomit?

   a. Notify the nurse.

   b. Provide an emesis basin.

   c. Remove the nasogastric tube.

   d. Advance the nasogastric tube.

3. What is an age-related change to the gastrointestinal system?

   a. Food moves more quickly.

   b. The gag reflex is less effective.

   c. Taste buds are more sensitive.

   d. Saliva production increases.

4. Which symptom indicates a patient is severely impacted?

   a. Excessive flatus

   b. Loud bowel sounds

   c. Report of heartburn

   d. Vomiting fecal material

5. Which contributes to the development of constipation?

   a. Activity

   b. Narcotics

   c. Fluid intake

   d. High-fiber diet

© 2022 Cengage Learning. All Rights Reserved. May not be scanned, copied or duplicated, or posted to a publicly accessible website, in whole or in part.

6. When testing a stool specimen, which color indicates there is blood in the stool?

    a. Red

    b. Blue

    c. Green

    d. Yellow

7. Which position should be used to give an enema if the left Sims' position cannot be used?

    a. Prone

    b. Seated

    c. Supine

    d. Knee–chest

8. What should be done if a patient complains of cramping while receiving an enema?

    a. Stop the enema.

    b. Coach the patient to take deep breaths.

    c. Increase the flow of the solution.

    d. Raise the level of the solution bag.

9. Which type of colostomy will have solid formed feces in the appliance container?

    a. Sigmoid

    b. Ascending

    c. Transverse

    d. Descending

10. What should be done if a patient's abdominal stoma for an ostomy appears blue-red in color?

    a. Remove the appliance.

    b. Report the finding to the nurse.

    c. Cleanse the stoma with warm water.

    d. Cleanse the skin around the appliance.

© 2022 Cengage Learning. All Rights Reserved. May not be scanned, copied or duplicated, or posted to a publicly accessible website, in whole or in part.

CHAPTER APPLICATION

Identification

Using colored pencils or crayons, color the organs of the digestive system as indicated.

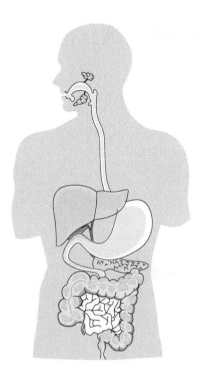

1. esophagus—blue
2. stomach—yellow
3. small intestine—green
4. liver—red
5. gallbladder—black
6. colon—blue
7. appendix—brown
8. pancreas—blue

Clinical Situations

Briefly describe how a nursing assistant should react to the following situations.

1. You have an order to give a soap-solution enema and the patient has just finished breakfast.

_____

_____

© 2022 Cengage Learning. All Rights Reserved. May not be scanned, copied or duplicated, or posted to a publicly accessible website, in whole or in part.

2. The patient complains of cramping while you are giving an enema.

_____

_____

3. Your patient has returned from surgery following a cholecystectomy. Drains are in place.

_____

_____

4. Your patient expresses concern about retaining a rectal suppository.

_____

_____

RELATING TO THE NURSING PROCESS

Write the step of the nursing process that is related to each nursing assistant action.

Nursing Assistant Action	Nursing Process Step
1. The nursing assistant carefully explains the procedure before administering an enema to the patient.	_____
2. The nursing assistant inserts a lubricating suppository beyond the rectal sphincter.	_____
3. The nursing assistant instructs the patient that an oil-retention enema must be retained for at least 20 minutes after introduction.	_____
4. The nursing assistant lubricates the tip of the enema tube well before insertion.	_____
5. The nursing assistant reports and records the results of the soap-solution enema.	_____

DEVELOPING GREATER INSIGHT

1. Tumors of the colon can often grow large before being detected. Give some reasons why you think this might be.

2. Discuss reasons enemas are given before a meal rather than after.

© 2022 Cengage Learning. All Rights Reserved. May not be scanned, copied or duplicated, or posted to a publicly accessible website, in whole or in part.

CHAPTER **45**

Urinary System

OBJECTIVES

After completing this chapter, you will be able to:

45-1 Spell and define terms.

45-2 Review the location of the urinary system.

45-3 Review the function of the urinary system.

45-4 List five diagnostic tests associated with conditions of the urinary system.

45-5 Describe some common diseases of the urinary system.

45-6 Describe nursing assistant actions related to the care of patients with urinary system diseases and conditions.

45-7 State the purpose of the renal dialysis.

45-8 Give an overview of the two types of dialysis.

45-9 Describe the care of a person with an indwelling catheter.

45-10 State the reasons for removing an indwelling catheter as soon as possible.

45-11 Demonstrate the following procedures:

- Procedure 96: Collecting a Routine Urine Specimen (Expand Your Skills)
- Procedure 97: Collecting a Clean-Catch Urine Specimen (Expand Your Skills)
- Procedure 98: Collecting a 24-Hour Urine Specimen (Expand Your Skills)
- Procedure 99: Collecting a Urine Specimen Through a Drainage Port (Expand Your Skills)
- Procedure 100: Routine Drainage Check (Expand Your Skills)
- Procedure 101: Giving Indwelling Catheter Care
- Procedure 102: Emptying a Urinary Drainage Unit
- Procedure 103: Disconnecting the Catheter
- Procedure 104: Connecting a Catheter to a Leg Bag
- Procedure 105: Emptying a Leg Bag
- Procedure 106: Removing an Indwelling Catheter
- Procedure 107: Ultrasound Bladder Scan

© 2022 Cengage Learning. All Rights Reserved. May not be scanned, copied or duplicated, or posted to a publicly accessible website, in whole or in part.

VOCABULARY BUILDER

Definitions

Define the following terms.

1. dysuria _____

2. hematuria _____

3. hydronephrosis _____

4. kidneys _____

5. retention _____

6. ureter _____

7. nephritis _____

8. cystitis _____

9. glomerulus _____

10. oliguria _____

11. renal calculi _____

12. IVP _____

13. suppression _____

14. catheter _____

Matching

Match each term with the correct definition.

1. _____ condition resulting from too much fluid on the kidney

2. _____ severe renal pain

3. _____ attaching a vein to an artery in the arm or leg

4. _____ kidney stones

5. _____ pain or burning on urination

6. _____ process of cleaning blood and removing accumulated wastes

7. _____ decreased urine production

8. _____ kidneys function at less than 10 percent of normal

9. _____ inability of kidneys to maintain fluid balance, excrete waste, and regulate essential body functions

10. _____ loss of control over urination

11. _____ inflammation of the urinary bladder

12. _____ synthetic material is used to connect artery and vein

13. _____ liquid substance used to clean blood

14. _____ inflammation of the kidney

a. CAPD

b. cystitis

c. dialysate

d. dialysis

e. dysuria

f. end-stage renal disease

g. fistula

h. graft

i. hematuria

j. hemodialysis

k. hydronephrosis

l. lithotripsy

m. nephritis

n. oliguria

© 2022 Cengage Learning. All Rights Reserved. May not be scanned, copied or duplicated, or posted to a publicly accessible website, in whole or in part.

15. _____ using sound waves to crush kidney stones

16. _____ uses artificial kidney machine

17. _____ administers dialysis through the abdominal cavity

18. _____ portable type of dialysis used at the bedside, long-term care facility, or the client's home

19. _____ blood in the urine

o. peritoneal dialysis

p. renal calculi

q. renal colic

r. renal failure

s. urinary incontinence

Fill-in-the-Blank

Complete the following statements in the spaces provided.

1. Cystitis is a fairly common problem in _____ because of the shortness of the urethra.

2. Patients with cystitis may find relief from a bladder spasm using a _____ bath.

3. Fluid intake should be _____ in cystitis patients.

4. You might expect the blood pressure of a patient with long-standing renal disease to be _____.

5. Edema is common in patients who have nephritis because of diminished ability of the kidneys to _____.

6. Renal calculi can cause _____ to the normal flow of urine.

7. The sudden intense pain associated with renal calculi is known as renal _____.

8. Because of the damage done by renal calculi, blood in the urine is common. This is known as _____.

9. All the urine of a patient with renal calculi should be _____.

10. A patient with renal calculi should have fluids _____.

11. Lithotripsy is a technique used to _____ renal calculi.

12. Destructive accumulation of fluid in the kidneys is called _____.

13. A Foley catheter has a _____ surrounding the neck so it can be retained in the bladder.

14. The insertion of a catheter is a _____ procedure and should be performed by the _____ or _____.

15. Urinary condoms can be used on _____ patients needing long-term drainage.

16. Avoid disconnecting the catheter from the _____s because doing so increases the risk of the patient developing a urinary infection.

17. Special care is needed when there are urinary conditions, because the urinary tract is a(n) _____ area.

18. Properties of a fresh urine specimen begin to change after _____ minutes.

19. If a sample of urine cannot be delivered to the laboratory immediately, it should be _____.

© 2022 Cengage Learning. All Rights Reserved. May not be scanned, copied or duplicated, or posted to a publicly accessible website, in whole or in part.

0. Approximately _____ of urine are sent to the laboratory as a routine specimen.

21. Before collecting a midstream urine specimen, always clean the area around the _____ and then allow some urine to be expelled.

22. The procedure for collection of a 24-hour urine specimen requires that the patient start the 24-hour interval with the bladder _____.

23. The last urine voided is _____ in the 24-hour specimen.

Short Answer

Complete the assessment in the space provided.

1. List four signs and symptoms of cystitis.

    a. _____

    b. _____

    c. _____

    d. _____

2. What four orders might be written for the patient who has severe nephritis?

    a. _____

    b. _____

    c. _____

    d. _____

3. What important nursing procedures must the nursing assistant carry out following removal of renal calculi? _____

4. Besides carefully reporting I&O, what are six other signs and symptoms that should be reported immediately in a patient following a nephrectomy?

    a. _____

    b. _____

    c. _____

    d. _____

    e. _____

    f. _____

5. What are the two types of catheters commonly used to drain the urinary bladder?

    a. _____

    b. _____

© 2022 Cengage Learning. All Rights Reserved. May not be scanned, copied or duplicated, or posted to a publicly accessible website, in whole or in part.

6. What are seven responsibilities the nursing assistant has when caring for a patient with urinary drainage?

   a. _____

   b. _____

   c. _____

   d. _____

   e. _____

   f. _____

   g. _____

7. If a urinary drainage system must be disconnected, what two parts must be protected against contamination?

   a. _____

   b. _____

CERTIFICATION REVIEW

Complete the following multiple-choice assessments.

1. What is an age-related change to the urinary system?

   a. Weaker bladder muscles

   b. Increased bladder capacity

   c. Reduced kidney function at rest

   d. Reduced size of the prostate gland

2. What should be reported to the nurse about a patient receiving peritoneal dialysis?

   a. Weight loss

   b. Request to have a snack

   c. Bloody dialysate solution

   d. Blood pressure 120/80 mm Hg

3. Which is a symptom of nephritis?

   a. Thirst

   b. Pyuria

   c. Cough

   d. Hunger

4. Which diagnostic test looks at the internal structures of the bladder?

   a. CT scan

   b. Ultrasound

   c. Cystoscopy

   d. Intravenous pyelogram

© 2022 Cengage Learning. All Rights Reserved. May not be scanned, copied or duplicated, or posted to a publicly accessible website, in whole or in part.

5. Where should the container for a 24-hour urine be stored?

    a. Refrigerator

    b. On ice in the bathroom

    c. Under the patient's bed

    d. In the dirty utility room

6. Which type of catheter is inserted surgically through the abdominal wall directly into the bladder?

    a. Foley

    b. Condom

    c. Suprapubic

    d. Intermittent

7. What does sediment in a catheter indicate?

    a. Diabetes

    b. Infection

    c. Dehydration

    d. Fluid overload

8. What is used to perform catheter care?

    a. Alcohol pads

    b. Soap and water

    c. Betadine solution

    d. Sterile normal saline

9. Where should the urinary collection bag be placed when the patient is in a wheelchair?

    a. On the patient's lap

    b. Under the wheelchair

    c. At the back of the seat

    d. Attached to the arm rest

10. At which time should a patient's condom catheter be changed?

    a. Every shift

    b. Once a week

    c. Every 24 hours

    d. When it becomes loose

© 2022 Cengage Learning. All Rights Reserved. May not be scanned, copied or duplicated, or posted to a publicly accessible website, in whole or in part.

CHAPTER APPLICATION

Identification
Using colored pencils, markers, or crayons, color the organs of the urinary system as indicated.

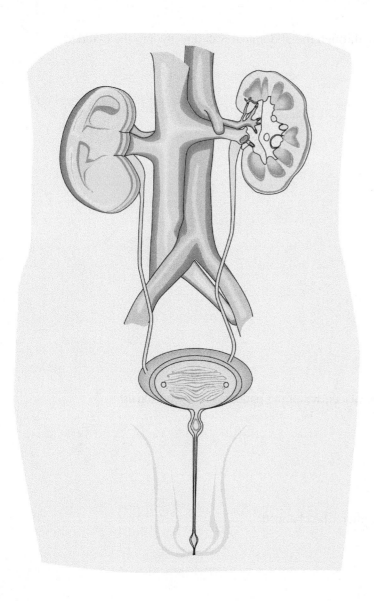

1. right kidney—red

2. ureters—blue

3. bladder—green

4. urethra—yellow

5. adrenal glands—brown

6. left kidney cortex—red

7. left kidney medulla—blue

8. left kidney pelvis—yellow

© 2022 Cengage Learning. All Rights Reserved. May not be scanned, copied or duplicated, or posted to a publicly accessible website, in whole or in part.

Clinical Situations

Briefly describe how a nursing assistant should react to the following situations.

1. Your patient has an indwelling catheter. Explain the daily care you will provide.

_____

_____

_____

2. Your patient uses condom drainage. List three responsibilities of the nursing assistant.

_____

_____

_____

3. Your patient is on I&O. Explain how to measure the drainage when the patient has an indwelling catheter.

_____

_____

_____

4. Your patient has urinary drainage into a leg bag. List four points to keep in mind while providing care.

a. _____

b. _____

c. _____

d. _____

RELATING TO THE NURSING PROCESS

Write the step of the nursing process that is related to each nursing assistant action.

Nursing Assistant Action	Nursing Process Step
1. The nursing assistant promptly reports that the patient is experiencing chills.	_____
2. The nursing assistant checks the drainage tubing to be sure it is fastened properly and is not obstructed.	_____
3. The nursing assistant is careful not to let the tip of the urine drainage tube touch the side of the graduate when the bag is emptied.	_____
4. The nursing assistant wears gloves when handling the patient's urinary drainage equipment.	_____
5. The nursing assistant strains all urine as ordered when the patient has renal calculi.	_____
6. If the patient is not circumcised, the nursing assistant makes sure to reposition the foreskin after giving indwelling catheter care.	_____
7. The nursing assistant maintains a positive attitude when changing the soiled linens of a patient who is incontinent.	_____

© 2022 Cengage Learning. All Rights Reserved. May not be scanned, copied or duplicated, or posted to a publicly accessible website, in whole or in part.

8. The nursing assistant uses standard precautions to collect and measure a urine specimen.   _____

9. All the nursing assistants add urine to a 24-hour collection from a single patient, even though the patient is the primary responsibility of one nursing assistant.   _____

DEVELOPING GREATER INSIGHT

1. Discuss with classmates why continence is so important to self-esteem.

2. Discuss with classmates why gloves are to be worn when handling bedpans or urine samples.

© 2022 Cengage Learning. All Rights Reserved. May not be scanned, copied or duplicated, or posted to a publicly accessible website, in whole or in part.

CHAPTER 46

Reproductive System

OBJECTIVES

After completing this chapter, you will be able to:

46-1 Spell and define terms.

46-2 Review the location of the organs of the female reproductive system.

46-3 Review the location of the organs of the male reproductive system.

46-4 Explain the functions of the organs of the female reproductive system.

46-5 Explain the functions of the organs of the male reproductive system.

46-6 Describe some common disorders and conditions of the male reproductive system.

46-7 Describe some common disorders and conditions of the female reproductive system.

46-8 List six diagnostic tests associated with conditions of the male and female reproductive systems.

46-9 Describe nursing assistant actions related to the care of patients with conditions and diseases of the reproductive system.

46-10 State the nursing precautions required for patients who have sexually transmitted infections.

VOCABULARY BUILDER

Matching

Match each term with the correct definition.

1. _____ womb

2. _____ infertility

3. _____ male sex glands

4. _____ lining of the uterus

a. endometrium

b. rectocele

c. genitalia

d. mastectomy

© 2022 Cengage Learning. All Rights Reserved. May not be scanned, copied or duplicated, or posted to a publicly accessible website, in whole or in part.

5. _____ excision of a breast   e. testes

6. _____ term for fallopian tube   f. uterus

7. _____ female organ of copulation   g. oviduct

8. _____ pouch that covers the testes   h. vagina

9. _____ inflammation of the vagina   i. scrotum

10. _____ external reproductive organs   j. sterility

11. _____ a sexually transmitted disease   k. gonorrhea

12. _____ protrusion of rectum into vagina   l. vaginitis

CHAPTER REVIEW

Fill-in-the-Blank

Complete the statements in the spaces provided.

1. A common enlargement of the prostate gland is called benign _____.

2. The tube-like organ passing through the center of the prostate gland is the _____.

3. A major problem for men suffering from the condition named in question 1 is urinary _____.

4. The prostate surgery during which an incision is made above the pubic bone is called a _____ prostatectomy.

5. A patient who is returning from prostate surgery will have a _____ in place.

6. Testicular self-examination should be performed at least once each _____.

7. The best time to perform testicular self-examination is during a _____.

8. A colporrhaphy is performed to tighten the _____ walls.

9. An uncomfortable and distressing problem associated with a cystocele is urinary _____.

10. Vulvovaginitis that is often caused by *Candida albicans* is a(n) _____ infection.

11. A simple test used to detect possible cancer of the cervix is the _____.

12. A _____ is a surgical procedure employed to help diagnose conditions of the uterus.

13. Removal of the fallopian tubes is known as a bilateral _____.

14. Following a mastectomy, bed linens should be checked, because blood may drain to the _____ of the dressing.

15. Vaginitis caused by *Trichomonas vaginalis* is associated with a foul-smelling discharge called _____.

16. In early stages, females infected with *Neisseria gonorrhea* are frequently _____ that they have been infected.

17. Chlamydia infections can cause serious _____.

18. Cancer of the testes may require removal by a surgical procedure called a(n) _____.

© 2022 Cengage Learning. All Rights Reserved. May not be scanned, copied or duplicated, or posted to a publicly accessible website, in whole or in part.

9. Prostate cancer may be treated with _____, a procedure in which radioactive pellets are implanted.

20. Although viruses cannot be eliminated, medications are available to stop the _____ of the virus in patients with herpes.

21. HIV disease destroys the _____.

22. There is no _____ for HIV/AIDS, but drugs can slow the damage to the body.

23. A _____ occurs when the uterus slips downward into the vaginal canal.

24. A 2007 study found that _____, a little-known and difficult-to-detect STD, was more prevalent than gonorrhea in U.S. adolescents.

Short Answer

Complete the assessment in the space provided.

1. What three functions do the male and female reproductive tracts have in common?

    a. _____

    b. _____

    c. _____

2. What special care should you give postoperatively when caring for the patient who has had a prostatectomy?

    a. _____

    b. _____

    c. _____

    d. _____

    e. _____

    f. _____

    g. _____

    h. _____

    i. _____

    j. _____

3. Why is an attempt made to leave at least part of an ovary when a hysterectomy is needed in a younger woman? _____

4. When and how should a woman check her breasts?

    a. _____

    b. _____

5. How often should the procedure for testicular self-examination be performed?

    _____

6. What are two problems associated with rectoceles?

    a. _____

    b. _____

© 2022 Cengage Learning. All Rights Reserved. May not be scanned, copied or duplicated, or posted to a publicly accessible website, in whole or in part.

7. Why is it important to maintain good circulation in the patient who has just experienced a panhysterectomy?

_____

8. What are six signs or symptoms of a breast tumor?

a. _____

b. _____

c. _____

d. _____

e. _____

f. _____

CERTIFICATION REVIEW

Complete the following multiple-choice assessments.

1. Which male reproductive organ produces sperm?

   a. Testes

   b. Epididymis

   c. Vas deferens

   d. Seminal vesicles

2. Which female reproductive organ produces estrogen?

   a. Ovary

   b. Uterus

   c. Vagina

   d. Fallopian tube

3. Which is an age-related change to the male reproductive system?

   a. Increased size of the testes

   b. Decreased risk of prostate cancer

   c. Enlargement of the prostate gland

   d. Rapid development of an erection

4. Which is an age-related change to the female reproductive system?

   a. Lengthening of vagina

   b. Cessation of menstrual periods

   c. Increased amount of vaginal secretions

   d. Increased hormones produced

© 2022 Cengage Learning. All Rights Reserved. May not be scanned, copied or duplicated, or posted to a publicly accessible website, in whole or in part.

5. For which reason will a patient recovering from prostate surgery have a three-way indwelling catheter?

    a. Drain urine.

    b. Drain blood.

    c. Irrigate the bladder.

    d. Remove excess tissue.

6. Which term describes difficulty or painful menstrual flow?

    a. Amenorrhea

    b. Menorrhagia

    c. Metrorrhagia

    d. Dysmenorrhea

7. Which action will be taken when caring for a patient recovering from a mastectomy?

    a. Position the patient on the operative side.

    b. Encourage independence with ambulation.

    c. Place the drain above the level of the incision.

    d. Measure blood pressure using the nonoperative side.

8. What is the most common cause for a prolapsed uterus?.

    a. Sexual activity

    b. Cervical cancer

    c. Vaginal infection

    d. Loss of muscle tone

9. What is the most common symptom of the third stage of syphilis?

    a. Rash

    b. Sore throat

    c. Chancre sore

    d. Cognitive impairment

10. What is the most common sexually transmitted infection (STI)?

    a. Gonorrhea

    b. Chlamydia

    c. Herpes simplex

    d. Venereal warts

© 2022 Cengage Learning. All Rights Reserved. May not be scanned, copied or duplicated, or posted to a publicly accessible website, in whole or in part.

CHAPTER APPLICATION

Identification

Male Tract. **Using colored pencils or crayons, color the organs of the male reproductive tract as indicated. In red, trace the pathway of sperm; move from the origin to leaving the body.**

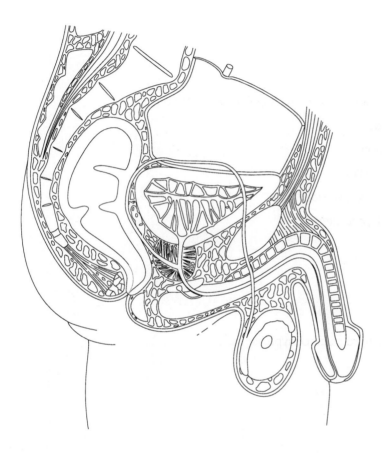

1. urinary bladder—yellow

2. penis—blue

3. testis—brown

4. prostate gland—green

© 2022 Cengage Learning. All Rights Reserved. May not be scanned, copied or duplicated, or posted to a publicly accessible website, in whole or in part.

Female Tract. **Using colored pencils or crayons, color the organs of the female tract as indicated. In red, trace the pathway of an egg from the point of origin to the uterus.**

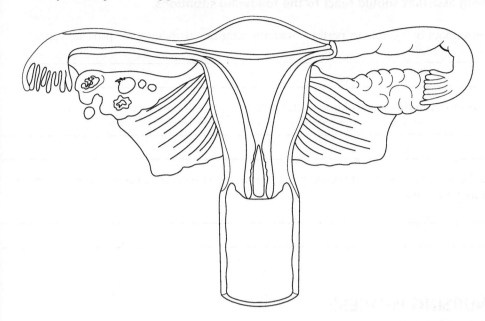

1. uterine walls—yellow

2. right ovary—blue

3. right oviduct—green

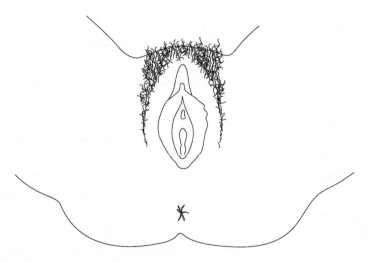

4. labia majora—red

5. clitoris—yellow

6. urinary meatus—green

7. labia minora—blue

© 2022 Cengage Learning. All Rights Reserved. May not be scanned, copied or duplicated, or posted to a publicly accessible website, in whole or in part.

Clinical Situations

Briefly describe how a nursing assistant should react to the following situations.

1. A patient expresses concern about being able to perform sexually after brachytherapy for prostate cancer.

   _____

   _____

2. A patient is to have a lumpectomy and wants to know if the entire breast will be removed.

   _____

   _____

3. Your patient is scheduled for a suprapubic prostatectomy. He expresses to you his concerns about the possibility of being impotent following surgery.

   _____

   _____

RELATING TO THE NURSING PROCESS

Write the step of the nursing process that is related to each nursing assistant action.

Nursing Assistant Action	Nursing Process Step
1. The nursing assistant reports to the nurse that the patient is complaining of itching and has a watery vaginal discharge.	_____
2. The nursing assistant checks the bed at the patient's back for bleeding after the patient has had a mastectomy.	_____
3. The nursing assistant informs the nurse of the grief and frustrations the postoperative mastectomy patient is expressing.	_____
4. The nursing assistant inserts the douche nozzle slowly, while the fluid is flowing, in an upward and backward motion.	_____
5. The nursing assistant carefully notes and reports color and amount of drainage from all areas for the patient who has had a prostatectomy.	_____

DEVELOPING GREATER INSIGHT

1. Think about how you would feel if you found a lump in your breast or testes. What if it turned out to be malignant?

2. Discuss reasons people tend to be particularly sensitive when there is disease or injury involving the reproductive organs.

3. Think about why it is important to use standard precautions when caring for patients who have sexually transmitted diseases.

© 2022 Cengage Learning. All Rights Reserved. May not be scanned, copied or duplicated, or posted to a publicly accessible website, in whole or in part.

Expanded Role of the Nursing Assistant

CHAPTER **47**

Caring for the Patient with Cancer

OBJECTIVES

After completing this chapter, you will be able to:

47-1 Spell and define terms.

47-2 List methods of reducing the risk of cancer.

47-3 Explain the importance of good nutrition in cancer prevention and treatment.

47-4 List seven signs and symptoms of cancer.

47-5 Describe three types of cancer treatment.

47-6 Describe nursing assistant responsibilities when caring for patients with cancer.

© 2022 Cengage Learning. All Rights Reserved. May not be scanned, copied or duplicated, or posted to a publicly accessible website, in whole or in part.

VOCABULARY BUILDER

Definitions

Define the following terms.

1. alopecia _____

2. anorexia _____

3. benign _____

4. cancer _____

5. carcinogen _____

6. chemotherapy _____

7. dosimeter _____

8. immunotherapy _____

9. malignant _____

10. metastasis _____

11. palliative care _____

12. radiology precautions sign _____

13. radiation therapy _____

CHAPTER REVIEW

Fill-in-the-Blank

Complete the following statements in the spaces provided.

1. Cancer is a disease in which the normal mechanisms of _____ are disturbed.

2. Cancer cells use the _____ and _____ targeted for normal cells.

3. Cancers that stay in one location and do not spread are _____.

4. Some types of cancer cells _____, or spread to other parts of the body through the blood and lymphatic systems.

5. Cancers that spread to other parts of the body are _____.

6. A(n) _____ such as tobacco is a cancer-causing substance.

7. People with _____ warning signs of cancer should see a doctor right away.

8. Women should perform breast self-examination _____.

9. Men should perform _____ self-examination _____.

10. A(n) _____ is a minor surgery that is sometimes done to remove tissue to diagnose cancer.

11 _____ involves the use of medications or drugs to destroy the cancer.

12. The nursing assistant should never _____, _____, or _____ in an area where chemotherapy is being prepared.

© 2022 Cengage Learning. All Rights Reserved. May not be scanned, copied or duplicated, or posted to a publicly accessible website, in whole or in part.

3. Waste products from some patients who are receiving chemotherapy require special _____.

14. _____ involves the use of high-energy, ionizing beams aimed at the site of the cancer.

15. _____ is a cancer treatment that alters the patient's immune response to eliminate the cancer.

16. Cancer patients' pain should be treated before it becomes _____.

Short Answer

Complete the assessment in the space provided.

1. List eight risk factors for cancer.

   a. _____

   b. _____

   c. _____

   d. _____

   e. _____

   f. _____

   g. _____

   h. _____

2. List four dietary guidelines that will help prevent cancer.

   a. _____

   b. _____

   c. _____

   d. _____

3. List seven lifestyle changes that will help prevent cancer.

   a. _____

   b. _____

   c. _____

   d. _____

   e. _____

   f. _____

   g. _____

4. Complete the following chart listing signs and symptoms of cancer.

   C = _____

   A = _____

   U = _____

   T = _____

   I = _____

   O = _____

   N = _____

© 2022 Cengage Learning. All Rights Reserved. May not be scanned, copied or duplicated, or posted to a publicly accessible website, in whole or in part.

5. List eight side effects of the drugs used to treat cancer.

a. _____

b. _____

c. _____

d. _____

e. _____

f. _____

g. _____

h. _____

6. List at least seven observations that should be reported to the nurse about patients who are receiving chemotherapy.

a. _____

b. _____

c. _____

d. _____

e. _____

f. _____

g. _____

7. List nine side effects of radiation therapy that should be reported promptly to the nurse.

a. _____

b. _____

c. _____

d. _____

e. _____

f. _____

g. _____

h. _____

i. _____

8. List five measures to take to protect yourself from exposure to radiation.

a. _____

b. _____

c. _____

d. _____

e. _____

© 2022 Cengage Learning. All Rights Reserved. May not be scanned, copied or duplicated, or posted to a publicly accessible website, in whole or in part.

9. List seven observations of the patient who is receiving immunotherapy to report to the nurse.

a. _____

b. _____

c. _____

d. _____

e. _____

f. _____

g. _____

10. List eight ways in which the nursing assistant can help meet patients' emotional needs.

a. _____

b. _____

c. _____

d. _____

e. _____

f. _____

g. _____

h. _____

True/False

Mark the following true or false by circling T or F.

1. T F Breast cancer, ovarian cancer, and pancreatic cancer seem to have a hereditary component.

2. T F Most cancers occur in individuals over the age of 45.

3. T F Obesity is associated with cancer of the brain and lungs.

4. T F Salt from all food sources should not exceed three teaspoons a day.

5. T F Surgery is sometimes done as a means of cancer prevention.

6. T F Although a cure may not be possible, chemotherapy is sometimes done to control and slow the growth of cancer to prolong the patient's life.

7. T F Wash your hands well if you contact a chemotherapy drug.

8. T F Side effects of some cancer treatments are life-threatening.

9. T F Good nutrition and hydration are not particularly important in cancer patients.

10. T F Hair loss is very upsetting to most people.

11. T F Shave the area surrounding the patient's radiation treatment field each day.

12. T F Vital signs should be closely monitored when immunotherapy is used.

13. T F Cancer treatment may be painful for the patient.

14. T F Cancer patients have a high incidence of addiction to narcotic pain-relieving drugs.

© 2022 Cengage Learning. All Rights Reserved. May not be scanned, copied or duplicated, or posted to a publicly accessible website, in whole or in part.

15. T   F   The nursing assistant should always try to instill hope in the patient.

16. T   F   Providing compassionate care; listening; and giving sincere, solid emotional support will help patients and family members cope with cancer.

17. T   F   Many cancer patients fear dying.

18. T   F   Patients with cancer should be evaluated for pain regularly.

19. T   F   Itching is a side effect of immunotherapy.

20. T   F   Always take a rectal temperature for patients who are receiving chemotherapy.

21. T   F   Patients with cancer may go through the grieving process.

22. T   F   Monitor the chemotherapy patient for bleeding, bruising, and abnormal skin lesions.

23. T   F   Following radiation treatments, scrub the markings off the patient's body.

24. T   F   Palliative care is an aggressive cancer treatment.

25. T   F   All cancer patients have "do not resuscitate" orders.

CERTIFICATION REVIEW

Complete the following multiple-choice assessments.

1. What is key to survival for cancer?

    a. Regular screening

    b. Avoiding infections

    c. Getting regular exercise

    d. Achieving a normal body weight

2. What is the role of hormone therapy in the treatment of cancer?

    a. It has no role.

    b. It will be used as the last resort.

    c. It will be used as palliative care.

    d. It may be started before other treatments.

3. Which body cells are commonly affected by chemotherapy?

    a. Hair

    b. Skin

    c. Bone

    d. Muscle

4. Which item should be avoided in a patient who is at risk from bleeding after receiving treatment for cancer?

    a. Gauze pads

    b. Razor blade to shave

    c. Soft-bristled toothbrush

    d. Non-alcohol-based mouthwash

© 2022 Cengage Learning. All Rights Reserved. May not be scanned, copied or duplicated, or posted to a publicly accessible website, in whole or in part.

5. Which action should be taken when caring for a patient with radiation markings?

    a. Apply ice to the area.

    b. Wash the affected skin with lukewarm water.

    c. Rub the skin area with lotion.

    d. Apply a bandage over the area.

6. What does a masking tape marking on the floor of a patient receiving implanted radiation therapy mean?

    a. Patient is not permitted to cross the line.

    b. Place where the biohazard trash is to be placed.

    c. Safe location to be near the patient and the bed.

    d. Location where the room chair should be placed.

7. For which reason would a nursing assistant avoid entering the room of a patient receiving brachytherapy?

    a. Could be pregnant

    b. Has a history of allergies

    c. Is assigned to care for older patients

    d. Is allergic to some of the patient's medications

8. Where should a radioactive-labeled container be placed in a patient's room?

    a. In the bathroom

    b. Near the room door

    c. On the bedside stand

    d. Under the patient's bed

9. What should be done if a radioactive seed is found in the bed when changing the linens?

    a. Notify the nurse.

    b. Drop it to the floor.

    c. Pick it up and place it in the trash.

    d. Pick it up and place it on the bedside stand.

10. What should be expected when a patient is receiving palliative care?

    a. Patient should not receive meal trays.

    b. Patient should have limited oral fluids.

    c. Patient should have limited pain medications.

    d. Patient should not receive cardiopulmonary resuscitation.

© 2022 Cengage Learning. All Rights Reserved. May not be scanned, copied or duplicated, or posted to a publicly accessible website, in whole or in part.

CHAPTER APPLICATION

Differentiation

Determine the type of diet associated with the type of cancer.

Type of Cancer	Type of Diet				
	High Fat	Low Fiber	High Salt	Low Fruit and Vegetables	Low Complex Carbohydrates
Breast					
Prostate					
Colon					
Esophagus					
Bladder					
Stomach					
Larynx					
Lung					

RELATING TO THE NURSING PROCESS

Write the step of the nursing process that is related to each nursing assistant action.

Nursing Assistant Action   **Nursing Process Step**

1. The nursing assistant reports to the nurse that
   Mrs. Lichtenstein, the chemotherapy patient in Room 222,
   is vomiting and has refused her supper tray.   _____

2. The nursing assistant reports in care conference
   that Lashanda Mauro, the cancer patient in Room 233-A,
   uses aromatherapy to help relieve her nausea.   _____

3. The nursing assistant informs the nurse that Mr. Ferraro's
   temperature is 102.6°F.   _____

4. The nursing assistant reports that the injection relieved
   the patient's pain.   _____

5. The nursing assistant followed the nurse's instructions
   to sit with the patient and listen to her until she calmed
   down.   _____

DEVELOPING GREATER INSIGHT

1. Ask a representative of the American Cancer Society or a cancer survivor to speak to the class.

2. Discuss with a group how you would feel if you were given a terminal cancer diagnosis today.

© 2022 Cengage Learning. All Rights Reserved. May not be scanned, copied or duplicated, or posted to a publicly accessible website, in whole or in part.

CHAPTER 48

Rehabilitation and Restorative Services

OBJECTIVES

After completing this chapter, you will be able to:

48-1 Spell and define terms.

48-2 Compare and contrast rehabilitation and restorative nursing care.

48-3 Describe the role of the nursing assistant in rehabilitation and restorative care.

48-4 Describe the principles of rehabilitation.

48-5 List the elements of successful rehabilitation/restorative care.

48-6 List six complications resulting from inactivity.

48-7 Identify four perceptual deficits.

48-8 Describe four approaches used for restorative programs.

48-9 List guidelines for providing restorative care.

48-10 Describe monitoring of the resident's response to care.

VOCABULARY BUILDER

Fill-in-the-Blank

Write the correct term for each definition provided.

1. A physician who specializes in rehabilitation is called _____.

2. Ordinary items that are modified for a specific patient are called _____.

3. The process that assists a patient to reach an optimal level of ability is termed _____.

4. The impairment that affects the person's ability to perform an activity that a person of that age would usually be able to do is called _____.

5. Personal hygiene and self-care tasks that are done throughout life are _____.

6. Another term for walking is _____.

© 2022 Cengage Learning. All Rights Reserved. May not be scanned, copied or duplicated, or posted to a publicly accessible website, in whole or in part.

7. A restorative program that helps a person regain voluntary control of urine and stool is _____ _____.

8. Care of the elderly is _____.

9. Moving from one place to another is _____.

10. _____ occur because of damage to the brain from disease or injury.

11. _____ is a process in which a person is assisted to reach an optimal level of physical, mental, and emotional health.

12. Helping a person learn the use of functional skills needed each day is called _____.

13. The inability to complete any activity of daily living is called a _____.

CHAPTER REVIEW

Fill-in-the-Blank

Complete the following statements in the spaces provided. Select the proper terms from the list provided.

care	disability	disease or injury	handicap
influence	optimum level of performance	problems	rehabilitation
retraining	same approach	self-care deficit	strength

1. Rehabilitation refers to a process in which the patient strives for the _____.

2. A person with paralysis suffers from a(n) _____.

3. A person who has been in bed for a long time because of heart disease may require _____.

4. All the different disciplines that take part in rehabilitation work together to resolve _____ and plan _____.

5. Any activity a patient is capable of doing is considered a(n) _____.

6. Patients and family _____ the emotional and mental health of patients who are being rehabilitated.

7. A patient who cannot complete any or all of the ADLs independently is said to have a _____.

8. Damage to the brain usually occurs because of _____.

9. Restorative programs are sometimes referred to as _____ programs.

10. It is important that everyone working with a patient in restorative care use the _____.

Short Answer

Complete the assessment in the space provided.

1. State activities that are included in the activities of daily living (ADLs).

   a. _____

   b. _____

© 2022 Cengage Learning. All Rights Reserved. May not be scanned, copied or duplicated, or posted to a publicly accessible website, in whole or in part.

    c. _____

    d. _____

    e. _____

    f. _____

    g. _____

2. List three interdisciplinary rehabilitation goals for a person with a disability.

    a. _____

    b. _____

    c. _____

3. Name five professionals, other than nurses and physicians, who are involved in the rehabilitative process.

    a. _____

    b. _____

    c. _____

    d. _____

    e. _____

4. List six rehabilitation activities in which the nursing assistant will assist.

    a. _____

    b. _____

    c. _____

    d. _____

    e. _____

5. Write the four principles that form the foundation for successful rehabilitation or restorative care.

    a. _____

    b. _____

    c. _____

    d. _____

6. State three examples of conditions that limit a person's ability to do self-care.

    a. _____

    b. _____

    c. _____

7. List six examples of perceptual deficits.

    a. _____

    b. _____

    c. _____

    d. _____

    e. _____

    f. _____

© 2022 Cengage Learning. All Rights Reserved. May not be scanned, copied or duplicated, or posted to a publicly accessible website, in whole or in part.

8. Name four approaches used in restorative programs.

   a. _____

   b. _____

   c. _____

   d. _____

9. Describe the type of environment that benefits patients and promotes success in a restorative program.

   a. _____

   b. _____

   c. _____

   d. _____

Complete the Chart

Complete the chart by placing an X in the appropriate column.

Mr. Cochran is admitted for rehabilitation. Mr. Ward is admitted to the same skilled care facility, but his goal is restoration. How does rehabilitation differ from restoration?

Activity	Rehabilitation	Restoration
a. OBRA rules require all skilled care facilities to provide this service	_____	_____
b. Goal is to increase the patient's quality of life	_____	_____
c. May be provided in a general acute care hospital	_____	_____
d. Usually more aggressive and intense	_____	_____
e. Slower therapies over weeks, months, or indefinitely	_____	_____
f. Requires the skills of many different therapists	_____	_____
g. Primarily a nursing responsibility, with consultation	_____	_____
h. Patient must make rapid, substantial improvement to qualify for ongoing participation	_____	_____
i. Maintenance and prevention of decline are acceptable goals	_____	_____

CERTIFICATION REVIEW

Complete the following multiple-choice assessments.

1. Which health professional works with a patient to relearn activities of daily living?

   a. Speech therapist

   b. Nursing assistant

   c. Physical therapist

   d. Occupational therapist

© 2022 Cengage Learning. All Rights Reserved. May not be scanned, copied or duplicated, or posted to a publicly accessible website, in whole or in part.

2. Which is a characteristic of restorative nursing care?

    a. Not paid for by private insurance

    b. Is aggressive and intensive

    c. Requires a physician's order

    d. Goal is to improve abilities

3. What is a skeletal complication of immobility?

    a. Blood clots

    b. Pressure injuries

    c. Indigestion and heartburn

    d. Loss of calcium from the bones

4. What is a mental change associated with immobility?

    a. Lethargy

    b. Alertness

    c. Insomnia

    d. Hyperactivity

5. Which activity of daily living will be lost first?

    a. Eating

    b. Bathing

    c. Transfers

    d. Bed mobility

6. What is the inability to use a common item called?

    a. Apraxia

    b. Aphasia

    c. Confusion

    d. Disorientation

7. Which is true about goals when supporting a patient relearn activities of daily living?

    a. Goals are not used.

    b. Goals are long term.

    c. Goals are very small.

    d. Goals are not achievable.

8. Which should be done first when assisting a patient relearn an activity?

    a. Setup

    b. Verbal cues

    c. Demonstration

    d. Hand-over-hand technique

© 2022 Cengage Learning. All Rights Reserved. May not be scanned, copied or duplicated, or posted to a publicly accessible website, in whole or in part.

9. Which adaptive device helps with putting on shoes?

   a. Cane

   b. Crutch

   c. Long-handled sponge

   d. Long-handled shoehorn

10. What should be done if a patient resists participating in a restorative care activity?

    a. Nothing

    b. Offer a snack.

    c. Report it to the nurse.

    d. Sit and talk with the patient.

CHAPTER APPLICATION

Clinical Situations

Briefly describe how a nursing assistant should react to the following situations.

1. Mr. Fronzoni is very frustrated as the nursing assistant explains how to put his socks on before his shoes.

   _____

   _____

2. Mr. Tracy has a roommate who repeatedly interrupts as the nursing assistant tries to help Mr. Tracy hold his glass. _____

   _____

3. Mrs. Davis is frustrated this morning and says that her progress is "just too slow."

   _____

   _____

4. The nursing assistant is assigned for the first time this morning to care for Mrs. Washington, who needs help with her self-feeding program. _____

   _____

   _____

5. Mr. Smythe is left-handed and has an adaptive device for his left hand. The device is on his bedside table as he attempts to brush his teeth. _____

   _____

6. Mrs. Missel is unable to gather the necessary equipment to give herself a bath and then carry out the procedure.

   _____

7. Mrs. Wexford has difficulty manipulating her clothing when she uses the toilet. She is able to stand and sit independently._____

   _____

© 2022 Cengage Learning. All Rights Reserved. May not be scanned, copied or duplicated, or posted to a publicly accessible website, in whole or in part.

8. Mr. Surgernt can hold his toothbrush and put it in his mouth, but then just holds it there.

_____

_____

9. Mrs. Malone is in a restorative program in the skilled care facility, but seems bored and restless between activity sessions. _____

_____

RELATING TO THE NURSING PROCESS

Write the step of the nursing process that is related to each nursing assistant action.

Nursing Assistant Action	Nursing Process Step
1. The nursing assistant begins passive exercises and positioning for Mrs. Burton, who is stable after a right-sided stroke.	_____
2. The nursing assistant encourages Mr. Jackson, who has poor strength in his dominant right hand, as he tries to feed himself with his left hand.	_____
3. The nursing assistant participates in team care conferences.	_____
4. The nursing assistant reports that Mrs. Parson is able to move her hands but is unable to select and hold items.	_____

DEVELOPING GREATER INSIGHT

1. With a classmate acting as a nursing assistant, practice trying to use your nondominant hand to eat, secure your shoes, and put on your clothes. Discuss how it makes you feel.

2. When first waking in the morning, lie in bed and think how frustrating it would be not to be able to carry out your morning hygiene routine.

3. Borrow a wheelchair and try to navigate around your community, home, and school campus. Discuss the problems you encounter when you cannot use your legs to walk.

© 2022 Cengage Learning. All Rights Reserved. May not be scanned, copied or duplicated, or posted to a publicly accessible website, in whole or in part.

Obstetrical Patients and Neonates

OBJECTIVES

After completing this chapter, you will be able to:

49-1 Spell and define terms.

49-2 Identify the role and responsibilities of the doula as a member of the childbirth team.

49-3 Assist in care of the normal postpartum patient.

49-4 Properly change a perineal pad.

49-5 Recognize reportable observations of patients in the postpartum period.

49-6 Assist in care of the normal newborn.

49-7 Demonstrate three methods of safely holding a baby.

49-8 Describe nursing assistant actions and observations related to the care of the newborn infant.

49-9 List measures to prevent inadvertent switching, misidentification, and abduction of infants.

49-10 Assist in carrying out the discharge procedures for mother and infant.

49-11 Demonstrate the following procedures:

- Procedure 108: Changing a Diaper (Expand Your Skills)
- Procedure 109: Weighing an Infant (Expand Your Skills)
- Procedure 110: Measuring an Infant (Expand Your Skills)
- Procedure 111: Bathing an Infant (Expand Your Skills)
- Procedure 112: Bottle-Feeding an Infant (Expand Your Skills)
- Procedure 113: Assisting with Breastfeeding (Expand Your Skills)
- Procedure 114: Burping an Infant (Expand Your Skills)

© 2022 Cengage Learning. All Rights Reserved. May not be scanned, copied or duplicated, or posted to a publicly accessible website, in whole or in part.

VOCABULARY BUILDER

Spelling

Each line has four different spellings of a word. Circle the correctly spelled word.

1. lokia   lochia   lokeya   lochea

2. neonat   nionat   nionate   neonate

3. fetis   feetes   fetus   feitas

4. doola   duela   doula   doolle

5. umbalical   umbilicale   umbilical   umbelical

6. isolette   eyesolet   isoullette   aecollet

7. arreala   airiola   aerealla   areola

8. preenatul   prenatal   preanatul   prenattel

Definitions

Define the following terms.

1. amniotic sac _____

2. umbilical cord _____

3. postpartum _____

4. lactation _____

5. neonate _____

6. placenta _____

CHAPTER REVIEW

Fill-in-the-Blank

Complete the following statements in the spaces provided.

1. After the baby is born, the placenta, amniotic sac, and remaining cord are expelled as the
   _____.

2. When taking the vital signs in the first few hours after a woman gives birth, position the mother
   _____.

3. Position the mother _____ if spinal anesthesia was used.

4. Immediately after birth, monitor the mother's vital signs every _____ for
   _____.

5. Lift the peri pad away from the body from _____ to _____.

6. The lochia is initially _____ in color.

7. _____ occurs when the uterus begins to return to normal size.

8. Instruct the mother to _____ before flushing the toilet.

© 2022 Cengage Learning. All Rights Reserved. May not be scanned, copied or duplicated, or posted to a publicly accessible website, in whole or in part.

9. Foul-smelling lochia is a sign of _____.

10. Teach the mother to use anesthetic spray _____ cleansing the perineum.

11. The part of the mother's milk that carries important, protective antibodies to the infant is called _____.

12. While weighing a baby, never turn your _____ to the scale, and keep one _____ over the baby at all times.

13. If it is necessary to carry the infant in your arms, always _____ through a doorway.

14. Be sure to wash hands _____ and _____ handling each child and after each _____ change.

15. A circumcision should be checked _____.

16. _____, also known as the flow of milk, does not begin until the _____.

17. A new mother should be encouraged to void within the first _____ hours postpartum.

18. Teach the mother to handle the peri pad only _____.

19. When removing a soiled perineal pad, the nursing assistant must always wear _____, fold the soiled side of the pad _____, and wrap the pad in a(n) _____.

20. Never dispose of soiled perineal pads in the _____.

21. Mothers who are breastfeeding should be instructed to wash their breasts using a(n) _____ motion from _____ to outward.

22. The Apgar score is an evaluation of the _____ which is made at _____ minute and _____ minutes after birth.

23. An Apgar score of 9 indicates that the neonate is in _____ condition.

24. The baby must be kept warm until their _____ stabilizes.

25. In the nursery, the _____, weight, and vital signs are measured.

26. The infant can lose a great deal of body heat through the _____.

27. The _____ is responsible for supporting and comforting the mother and enhancing communication between the mother and medical professionals.

Short Answer

Complete the assessment in the space provided.

1. What is the primary value of colostrum to the baby?

   _____

2. What is the purpose of Apgar scoring? _____

3. List five ways of caring for the breast of the nursing mother.

   a. _____

   b. _____

   c. _____

   d. _____

   e. _____

© 2022 Cengage Learning. All Rights Reserved. May not be scanned, copied or duplicated, or posted to a publicly accessible website, in whole or in part.

4. How should the baby be lifted from the crib?

   a. _____

   b. _____

CERTIFICATION REVIEW

Complete the following multiple-choice assessments.

1. For which reason would a baby be delivered through a cesarean section?

   a. Fetal distress

   b. Patient request

   c. Length of labor

   d. Extensive labor pain

2. What should be done if a postpartum patient has a heavy flow of lochia after lying in bed for a long time?

   a. Assist with bathing.

   b. Report it to the nurse.

   c. Provide patient with another perineal pad.

   d. Encourage to walk to the bathroom.

3. What should be done to reduce edema and discomfort of the perineum after giving birth?

   a. Provide an ice pack.

   b. Report the finding to the nurse.

   c. Encourage to bathe in warm water.

   d. Assist to lie in a comfortable position in bed.

4. Which technique should be used to measure the newborn's temperature?

   a. Oral

   b. Rectal

   c. Axillae

   d. Temporal artery

5. Which position should be avoided when placing a newborn in the crib after a feeding?

   a. Prone

   b. Supine

   c. Left Sims'

   d. Right Sims'

6. What is the color of the newborn's first stool?

   a. Dark

   b. Green

   c. Yellow

   d. Brown-yellow

© 2022 Cengage Learning. All Rights Reserved. May not be scanned, copied or duplicated, or posted to a publicly accessible website, in whole or in part.

7. What needs to be done when measuring the length of an infant?

    a. Use a tape measure.

    b. Place on the abdomen.

    c. Measure in increments.

    d. Have another person assist.

8. Which body area is cleansed first when bathing an infant?

    a. Ears

    b. Eyes

    c. Neck

    d. Hands

9. Which announcement indicates that an infant has been abducted?

    a. Code Red

    b. Code Pink

    c. Code Blue

    d. Code Green

10. What should be done first after feeding a newborn?

    a. Burp the infant.

    b. Place in the crib.

    c. Weigh the infant.

    d. Change the diaper.

CHAPTER APPLICATION

Clinical Situations

Briefly explain how the nursing assistant should react to the following situations.

1. The new mother is very uncomfortable when she tries to sit. _____

2. The new mother has returned to your care in the postpartum area.

    a. _____

    b. _____

    c. _____

    d. _____

    e. _____

© 2022 Cengage Learning. All Rights Reserved. May not be scanned, copied or duplicated, or posted to a publicly accessible website, in whole or in part.

Identification

1. Write the names of the parts or structures indicated in the spaces provided.

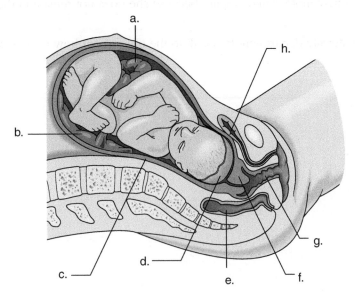

a. _____

b. _____

c. _____

d. _____

e. _____

f. _____

g. _____

h. _____

RELATING TO THE NURSING PROCESS

Write the step of the nursing process that is related to each nursing assistant action.

Nursing Assistant Action	Nursing Process Step
1. The nursing assistant helps other staff members transfer the mother who has just given birth from stretcher to bed.	_____
2. The nursing assistant checks the mother's vital signs as ordered following a cesarean section.	_____
3. The nursing assistant measures and records the first postpartum voiding.	_____
4. The nursing assistant instructs the mother to stand up before flushing the toilet.	_____

© 2022 Cengage Learning. All Rights Reserved. May not be scanned, copied or duplicated, or posted to a publicly accessible website, in whole or in part.

DEVELOPING GREATER INSIGHT

1. Identify what special help a new mother may require because she does not remain in the hospital very long for care.

2. Invite someone from the maternity department to speak to the class about how to prevent infant abduction.

© 2022 Cengage Learning. All Rights Reserved. May not be scanned, copied or duplicated, or posted to a publicly accessible website, in whole or in part.

Pediatric Patients

OBJECTIVES

After completing this chapter, you will be able to:

50-1 Spell and define terms.

50-2 Describe how to foster the growth and development of hospitalized pediatric patients.

50-3 Describe how to maintain a safe environment for the pediatric patient.

50-4 Discuss the problem of childhood obesity and identify special problems and complications that occur as a result of this condition.

50-5 Discuss the role of parents and siblings of the hospitalized pediatric patient.

50-6 Describe Munchausen by proxy syndrome (MBPS).

50-7 List signs and symptoms of physical, emotional, and sexual abuse and neglect.

50-8 Demonstrate the following procedures:

- Procedure 115: Admitting a Pediatric Patient (Expand Your Skills)
- Procedure 116: Weighing the Toddler to Adolescent (Expand Your Skills)
- Procedure 117: Changing Crib Linens (Expand Your Skills)
- Procedure 118: Changing Crib Linens (Infant in Crib) (Expand Your Skills)
- Procedure 119: Measuring Temperature (Expand Your Skills)
- Procedure 120: Determining Heart Rate (Pulse) (Expand Your Skills)
- Procedure 121: Counting Respiratory Rate (Expand Your Skills)
- Procedure 122: Measuring Blood Pressure (Expand Your Skills)
- Procedure 123: Collecting a Urine Specimen from an Infant (Expand Your Skills)

© 2022 Cengage Learning. All Rights Reserved. May not be scanned, copied or duplicated, or posted to a publicly accessible website, in whole or in part.

VOCABULARY BUILDER

Matching

Match each term with the correct definition.

1. _____ to promote
2. _____ magical thinking
3. _____ to move backward
4. _____ brothers and sisters
5. _____ pertaining to children
6. _____ to move away from center
7. _____ a child from birth to 1 year
8. _____ children from 5 to 12 years
9. _____ children from 12 to 20 years
10. _____ able to make choices independently
11. _____ intellectual, social, and emotional tasks that must be accomplished at a certain age level

a. fantasies
b. foster
c. siblings
d. regress
f. deviate
e. infant
g. school-age
h. adolescent
i. pediatric
j. autonomy
k. developmental (tasks)

CHAPTER REVIEW

Short Answer

Complete the assessment in the space provided.

1. What are two ways pediatric departments are usually organized?

    a. _____

    b. _____

2. Who provides the medical and social history when the patient is a child?

    _____

    _____

3. How will the infant change in the first year of life?

    a. _____

    b. _____

4. What is meant by the infant's "developmental milestones"?

    _____

    _____

5. What is the primary psychosocial development task for the infant?

    _____

    _____

© 2022 Cengage Learning. All Rights Reserved. May not be scanned, copied or duplicated, or posted to a publicly accessible website, in whole or in part.

6. How might you foster achievement of the infant's developmental task?

_____

_____

7. How should the care of an infant be organized?

_____

_____

8. What three factors would increase the infant's heart rate and respirations?

   a. _____

   b. _____

   c. _____

9. How might an infant's sucking needs be met when they cannot eat?

_____

_____

10. If a toddler is toilet trained, what information would be helpful for you to know?

_____

_____

11. What is a major fear of the preschooler?

_____

_____

12. Because preschoolers have a limited concept of time, how should you explain when something will occur?

_____

_____

13. How could you foster a school-age child's need for accomplishment?

_____

_____

14. How may an adolescent view the nursing assistant and other caregivers?

_____

_____

15. Who are the most important people to the adolescent?

_____

_____

16. When using a tympanic thermometer to take an infant or child's temperature, what should the nursing assistant do to ensure an accurate reading?

_____

_____

© 2022 Cengage Learning. All Rights Reserved. May not be scanned, copied or duplicated, or posted to a publicly accessible website, in whole or in part.

17. How would you obtain a urine specimen from a 6-month-old infant who wears a diaper and has good skin integrity?

_____

_____

18. List five outcomes of child abuse.

    a. _____

    b. _____

    c. _____

    d. _____

    e. _____

19. Describe Munchausen by proxy syndrome (MBPS).

_____

_____

20. How does the caregiver treat a child with Munchausen by proxy syndrome (MBPS)?

_____

_____

21. Altered appearance upsets teenagers' feelings about their _____.

22. The abused child lives in an _____ world and feels constant

    _____.

True/False

Mark the following true or false by circling T or F.

1. T   F   When a child is hospitalized, caregivers may assume the role of substitute mother.

2. T   F   A 6-month-old infant is able to sit well and pull himself or herself into a standing position.

3. T   F   Infants do not normally respond to the voices, faces, or touch of strangers.

4. T   F   The radial pulse is used for counting the pulse in an infant.

5. T   F   Blood pressure is not routinely taken in infants and small children.

6. T   F   A sterile bottle, nipple, and formula are necessary when feeding an infant.

7. T   F   It is not necessary to burp an infant until the infant has consumed the entire bottle.

8. T   F   It is best to restrain toddlers by keeping them in bed to prevent injury.

9. T   F   The caregiver always advocates for the child in cases of MBPS.

10. T   F   MSBP caregivers derive self-esteem and satisfaction by misleading health care providers whom they consider to be much more important and powerful than themselves.

11. T   F   As a rule, the MSBP caregiver is unable to deceive health care professionals.

12. T   F   The mother is responsible for causing MSBP in 47 percent of all cases.

13. T   F   Toddlers are too immature to need autonomy.

14. T   F   Toddlers usually do not handle separation from the mother well.

15. T   F   Finger painting is a good activity for toddlers.

© 2022 Cengage Learning. All Rights Reserved. May not be scanned, copied or duplicated, or posted to a publicly accessible website, in whole or in part.

16. T F   Allow a 6-year-old to do as much of their own care as possible.

17. T F   It is not necessary to explain procedures to school-age children.

18. T F   School-age children do not need privacy during personal care procedures.

19. T F   Games are a good activity for the school-age child.

20. T F   Body image is not important to adolescents.

21. T F   A safe environment is not a concern for adolescent patients.

22. T F   Allow adolescents to have as much control over their routines as possible.

CERTIFICATION REVIEW

Complete the following multiple-choice assessments.

1. Which action will be taken when caring for a baby?

   a. Stay silent.

   b. Talk to the baby.

   c. Talk to the mother.

   d. Ask the mother what to do.

2. What should be done with a baby while the crib sheets are being changed?

   a. Hold the baby.

   b. Keep the baby in the crib.

   c. Place the baby in a playpen.

   d. Place the baby on a blanket on a chair.

3. What should be done when asked to take a rectal temperature on a baby?

   a. Hold the baby like a football.

   b. Ask the nurse if the rectum is patent.

   c. Place the baby on the abdomen in the crib.

   d. Ask the mother to measure the temperature.

4. In which way should a baby's pulse be determined?

   a. Palpate the radial artery.

   b. Palpate the femoral artery.

   c. Count the apical heart rate.

   d. Count the pulsations on the carotid artery.

5. What should be done when using a collection device to obtain a urine specimen from a baby?

   a. Rub lotion over the perineum.

   b. Apply baby powder over the perineum.

   c. Hold the device in place until the baby voids.

   d. Remove the backing from the tape and apply to the perineum.

© 2022 Cengage Learning. All Rights Reserved. May not be scanned, copied or duplicated, or posted to a publicly accessible website, in whole or in part.

6. Which action should be avoided when feeding a baby?

   a. Hold the infant.

   b. Prop the bottle in the baby's mouth.

   c. Burp the baby during and after the feeding.

   d. Position on the back after the feeding is completed.

7. Which type of device should be used in the hospital if a toddler sleeps in a bed at home?

   a. A cot

   b. A crib

   c. An air mattress

   d. An adult hospital bed with side rails

8. Where should a child receive a medical procedure when hospitalized?

   a. Playroom

   b. Child's room

   c. Nurse's station

   d. Treatment room

9. What should be done if the sister of a hospitalized toddler wants to visit the sibling in the hospital?

   a. Explain that it cannot be permitted.

   b. Take the sibling to the hospital to visit the toddler.

   c. Have the children connect through a Zoom meeting.

   d. Have the children talk to each other over the telephone.

10. What should be done if an adolescent patient is seen vaping in the bathroom?

    a. Provide privacy.

    b. Report the finding to the nurse.

    c. Ask the patient what type they use.

    d. Suggest that they go outside to vape.

CHAPTER APPLICATION

Clinical Situations

Briefly describe how a nursing assistant should react to the following situations.

1. The toddler who is weaned cries for a bottle. _____

_____

_____

2. The toddler is having a temper tantrum _____

_____

_____

© 2022 Cengage Learning. All Rights Reserved. May not be scanned, copied or duplicated, or posted to a publicly accessible website, in whole or in part.

3. The teenager does not want to go to sleep after the television has been shut off.

_____

_____

_____

RELATING TO THE NURSING PROCESS

Write the step of the nursing process that is related to each nursing assistant action.

Nursing Assistant Action   **Nursing Process Step**

1. The nursing assistant measures and weighs the child
   during admission to the pediatric unit.   _____

2. The nursing assistant helps stabilize the preschooler's arm
   while offering comforting support during blood withdrawal.   _____

3. The nursing assistant finds ways to occupy a roommate
   when a school-age patient is visited by a tutor.   _____

4. The nursing assistant always keeps the crib sides up when
   the toddler is in the crib.   _____

5. The nursing assistant discusses with the nurse activities
   for the recuperating toddler in their care.   _____

DEVELOPING GREATER INSIGHT

1. Describe as many different types of "family units" as you can.

2. Discuss reasons teens join gangs. How would you feel about caring for a teen who was injured in a gang fight?

© 2022 Cengage Learning. All Rights Reserved. May not be scanned, copied or duplicated, or posted to a publicly accessible website, in whole or in part.

Response to Basic Emergencies

CHAPTER 51

Response to Basic Emergencies

OBJECTIVES

After completing this chapter, you will be able to:

51-1 Spell and define terms.

51-2 Recognize emergency situations that require urgent care.

51-3 Evaluate situations and determine the sequence of appropriate actions to be taken.

51-4 Describe the 11 standardized types of codes.

51-5 Describe how to maintain the patient's airway and breathing during respiratory failure and respiratory arrest.

51-6 Recognize the need for CPR.

51-7 List the benefits of early defibrillation.

51-8 Identify the signs, symptoms, and treatment of common emergency situations such as:

- Brain attack (stroke)
- Seizure
- Vomiting and aspiration
- Thermal injuries
- Poisoning
- Known or suspected head injury

© 2022 Cengage Learning. All Rights Reserved. May not be scanned, copied or duplicated, or posted to a publicly accessible website, in whole or in part.

VOCABULARY BUILDER

Matching

Match each term with the correct definition.

1. _____ injury

2. _____ to raise

3. _____ stoppage of heartbeat

4. _____ an unintended occurrence

5. _____ loss of large amount of blood

6. _____ emergency cardiac condition

7. _____ sudden loss of consciousness

8. _____ cardiopulmonary resuscitation

9. _____ a situation that develops rapidly and unexpectedly

10. _____ disturbance of oxygen supply to the tissues and return of blood to heart

a. trauma

b. arrest

c. fainting

d. incident

e. emergency

f. heart attack

g. shock

h. elevate

i. CPR

j. hemorrhage

CHAPTER REVIEW

Fill-in-the-Blanks

Complete the statements in the spaces provided.

1. Your actions should never place a victim in additional _____.

2. First aid techniques are taught as a specific course by the _____.

3. Certification in CPR is provided in courses by the _____ and the American Red Cross.

4. When you provide first aid, you must deal with the victim's _____ as well as the victim's physical injuries.

5. The first step when arriving at the scene of an accident is to _____ the situation.

6. If you are in a medical facility when an accident occurs, you should _____ for help and keep the patient _____.

7. The national number for emergency help is _____.

8. The most common cause of airway obstruction is _____, so pulling the _____ forward often opens the airway.

9. If oxygen is denied to the body, the most sensitive organ, the _____, may suffer permanent damage.

10. Care that must be given immediately to prevent loss of life is called _____.

11. A disturbance of the oxygen supply to the tissues and return of blood to the heart is defined as _____.

12. A victim who is in shock should be kept _____ down.

13. The loss of heart function is called _____.

© 2022 Cengage Learning. All Rights Reserved. May not be scanned, copied or duplicated, or posted to a publicly accessible website, in whole or in part.

14. Seizures do not always follow the same _____.

15. In a generalized tonic-clonic (grand mal) seizure, the patient must be protected against _____.

16. Following a generalized tonic-clonic (grand mal) seizure, the patient may be _____ and _____ for a time and feel very tired.

17. A good way to move a victim of electric shock away from the source of electricity is to use something made of _____.

Short Answer

Complete the assessment in the space provided.

1. What four basic actions should be taken in all emergency situations?

   a. _____

   b. _____

   c. _____

   d. _____

2. What five facts should be included when calling the emergency number?

   a. _____

   b. _____

   c. _____

   d. _____

   e. _____

3. What two types of care are included in first aid?

   a. _____

   b. _____

4. What are three ways to summon help for an accident victim in a health care facility?

   a. _____

   b. _____

   c. _____

5. How should you check for breathing activity?

   a. _____

   b. _____

6. What order of victim's responses should be checked when providing urgent care?

   a. _____

   b. _____

   c. _____

7. How would you describe the distress signals of choking? _____

© 2022 Cengage Learning. All Rights Reserved. May not be scanned, copied or duplicated, or posted to a publicly accessible website, in whole or in part.

8. What six steps should you follow to prevent additional blood loss in a bleeding victim?

   a. _____

   b. _____

   c. _____

   d. _____

   e. _____

   f. _____

9. What are the five early signs of shock?

   a. _____

   b. _____

   c. _____

   d. _____

   e. _____

10. What five signs and symptoms might indicate that a victim is having a heart attack?

   a. _____

   b. _____

   c. _____

   d. _____

   e. _____

CERTIFICATION REVIEW

Complete the following multiple-choice assessments.

1. Which action should be taken first when a patient is found in an emergency situation?

   a. Assess airway.

   b. Palpate a pulse.

   c. Look for bleeding.

   d. Check for breathing.

2. What does Code Silver indicate?

   a. Fire

   b. Cardiac arrest

   c. Infant abduction

   d. Geriatric patient missing

3. Which action should be taken to open the airway of a patient with a suspected neck injury?

   a. Jaw-thrust maneuver

   b. Hyperextend the neck

   c. Turning the head to either side

   d. Head-tilt, chin-lift maneuver

© 2022 Cengage Learning. All Rights Reserved. May not be scanned, copied or duplicated, or posted to a publicly accessible website, in whole or in part.

4. Which position is the recovery position?

    a. Supine

    b. Prone

    c. Mid-Fowler's

    d. Modified lateral

5. When will an automatic external defibrillator be used?

    a. Patient is short of breath.

    b. Patient has an occluded oral airway.

    c. Patient is cyanotic with crushing chest pain.

    d. Patient is unresponsive, not breathing, and pulseless.

6. What should be done if a patient is coughing vigorously?

    a. Check the airway.

    b. Encourage continued coughing.

    c. Perform the Heimlich maneuver.

    d. Sweep the mouth with an index finger.

7. What contributes to the development of shock in a patient who is bleeding?

    a. Fatigue

    b. Anxiety

    c. Lethargy

    d. Confusion

8. Which action should be taken after a patient who is fainting is in a safe position?

    a. Provide water.

    b. Loosen tight clothing.

    c. Encourage deep breaths.

    d. Locate a blood pressure cuff.

9. Which action should be taken if a patient begins to seize?

    a. Protect the patient's head.

    b. Restrain the patient's arms.

    c. Measure the blood pressure.

    d. Insert an airway in the patient's mouth.

10. What should be done first if a piece of electrical equipment shocks a patient?

    a. Call for help.

    b. Turn off the electricity.

    c. Remove the device from the patient.

    d. Check the patient for an airway and a pulse.

© 2022 Cengage Learning. All Rights Reserved. May not be scanned, copied or duplicated, or posted to a publicly accessible website, in whole or in part.

CHAPTER APPLICATION

Clinical Situations

Briefly describe how a nursing assistant should react to the following situations.

1. You are the first person on the scene of an auto accident. One person has been thrown out of the car and is lying beside the car, which is on fire. Describe your first action.

   _____

   _____

   _____

2. You discover the husband of your home client on the floor of the basement near a frayed electrical wire. What is your first action?

   _____

   _____

   _____

3. You are in a dining area when an ambulatory patient grasps their throat and is unable to speak.

   _____

   _____

   _____

RELATING TO THE NURSING PROCESS

Write the step of the nursing process that is related to each nursing assistant action.

Nursing Assistant Action	Nursing Process Step
1. The nursing assistant, finding a patient on the floor, first checks for consciousness.	_____
2. The nursing assistant finds an unconscious patient and immediately signals for help.	_____
3. The patient stumbles, injuring their knee, which begins to bleed. The nursing assistant applies direct pressure with their gloved hand.	_____
4. The nursing assistant encourages the patient to rest quietly after a seizure.	_____
5. After summoning help for the heart attack victim, the nursing assistant remains with the patient to offer emotional support.	_____

DEVELOPING GREATER INSIGHT

1. Ensure that each student has been certified in cardiopulmonary resuscitation.

2. Provide an opportunity for the students to practice using an automatic cardiac defibrillator.

3. Invite emergency medical personnel to class to discuss their role in providing care to victims in the community.

4. Ask the students if any have assisted in providing emergency care in the community. Have the students share their experiences with the entire class.

© 2022 Cengage Learning. All Rights Reserved. May not be scanned, copied or duplicated, or posted to a publicly accessible website, in whole or in part.

Moving Forward

C H A P T E R **52**

Employment Opportunities and Career Growth

OBJECTIVES

After completing this chapter, you will be able to:

52-1 Spell and define terms.

52-2 List nine objectives to be met in obtaining and maintaining employment.

52-3 Discuss a process for self-appraisal.

52-4 Name sources of employment for nursing assistants.

52-5 Prepare a résumé.

52-6 Prepare a letter of resignation.

52-7 List the steps for a successful interview.

52-8 List the requirements that must be met when accepting employment.

52-9 List steps for continuing development in your career.

© 2022 Cengage Learning. All Rights Reserved. May not be scanned, copied or duplicated, or posted to a publicly accessible website, in whole or in part.

VOCABULARY BUILDER

Definitions

Define the following terms.

1. résumé _____

   _____

2. networking _____

   _____

3. interview _____

   _____

4. reference _____

   _____

CHAPTER REVIEW

Fill-in-the-Blank

Complete the following statements in the spaces provided.

1. One of the first steps in self-appraisal is to list all your _____ and _____.

2. It is important to think through possible _____ to any limitations to employment.

3. Preference for caring for a particular type of patient could influence your _____ options.

4. Home _____ and transportation are factors that might limit employment.

5. Talking with friends and colleagues about opportunities is called _____.

6. A written summary of work history is called a _____.

7. Always obtain _____ before giving a person's name as a reference.

8. Persons who are listed as references should know you well, but not be _____.

9. Clothing should be _____ and _____ for an interview.

10. It is important to be on _____ for an interview.

11. In a new work situation, there is much to learn from the examples of _____ staff workers.

12. When it is necessary to resign, do so in a _____ manner.

Short Answer

Complete the assessment in the space provided.

1. What will you specifically look for when seeking employment through classified ads?

   a. _____

   b. _____

   c. _____

   d. _____

© 2022 Cengage Learning. All Rights Reserved. May not be scanned, copied or duplicated, or posted to a publicly accessible website, in whole or in part.

2. What information should not be included in a résumé?

a. _____

b. _____

c. _____

d. _____

e. _____

True/False

Mark the following true or false by circling T or F.

1. T   F   You should wait to be invited before sitting at an interview.
2. T   F   Body language is very important in conveying your interest in employment.
3. T   F   Ask for a job description to be sure you are qualified for the position being offered.
4. T   F   Mail your résumé after the interview.
5. T   F   Always thank the interviewer at the end of the interview.
6. T   F   View every interview as a learning experience, even if it doesn't go well.
7. T   F   Nursing and medical literature are good sources of information about patient conditions.
8. T   F   Always give a two-week notice before leaving a job.
9. T   F   Be positive in a resignation even if you are leaving a position because something upsetting has happened.
10. T   F   Always date and sign a letter of resignation

CERTIFICATION REVIEW

Complete the following multiple-choice assessments.

1. Which characteristic is not a part of a self-appraisal?

   a. Assets

   b. Income

   c. Solutions

   d. Limitations

2. In which way should finding employment be approached?

   a. As a chore

   b. As a full-time job

   c. As an activity to do while watching television

   d. As something to do after completing housework

3. What should be done after preparing a résumé?

   a. Make several copies.

   b. Store it in a desk at home.

   c. Save the file on your computer.

   d. Mail it after having an interview.

© 2022 Cengage Learning. All Rights Reserved. May not be scanned, copied or duplicated, or posted to a publicly accessible website, in whole or in part.

4. Which person should be deleted as a reference?

    a. Older sister who is a nurse

    b. Next door neighbor who is a paramedic

    c. Physician that you worked for part-time

    d. School nurse that you helped one summer

5. Which should be done when completing a job application?

    a. Keep blank areas that do not apply.

    b. Write "see résumé" on specific areas.

    c. Use a pen to complete the application.

    d. Include health-related employment only.

6. What should be done during an interview?

    a. Share personal information freely.

    b. Offer the interviewer a mouth mint.

    c. Ask for clarification for any question.

    d. Avoid eye contact with the interviewer.

7. What needs to be done after accepting a position?

    a. Discuss when vacation can be taken.

    b. Ask when salary adjustments are made.

    c. Explain the days and hours you will work.

    d. Provide social security number and picture ID.

8. Which action ensures continuous employment?

    a. Arrive late for a scheduled shift.

    b. Follow policies and procedures.

    c. Call off every weekend you are scheduled to work.

    d. Sit with a patient to avoid helping someone else.

9. Which action demonstrates growth throughout a career?

    a. Request to be laid off.

    b. Take additional education courses.

    c. Work to maintain a specific lifestyle.

    d. Take large breaks between employers.

10. Which action should be taken if an employer asks for your resignation?

    a. Write on a sheet of paper "I quit."

    b. Clean out your locker and go home.

    c. Ask for the reason for the termination.

    d. Write a letter thanking them for the opportunity.

© 2022 Cengage Learning. All Rights Reserved. May not be scanned, copied or duplicated, or posted to a publicly accessible website, in whole or in part.

CHAPTER APPLICATION

Clinical Situations

Briefly describe the actions the nursing assistant might take in the following situations.

1. A classmate who is new to the area asks where nursing assistants can find employment in your community.

   _____

   _____

   _____

2. A family member asks what sources of information you will use as you begin your employment search.

   _____

   _____

3. Your teacher asks you to describe the practices you must keep in mind regarding a résumé.

   a. _____

   b. _____

   c. _____

   d. _____

   e. _____

   f. _____

4. List three things you will do when preparing for an interview.

   a. _____

   b. _____

   c. _____

5. A classmate asks you to explain how you can make a new position more secure.

   a. _____

   b. _____

   c. _____

   d. _____

   e. _____

6. A classmate asks you for six ways to enhance your knowledge and education after certification.

   a. _____

   b. _____

   c. _____

   d. _____

   e. _____

   f. _____

© 2022 Cengage Learning. All Rights Reserved. May not be scanned, copied or duplicated, or posted to a publicly accessible website, in whole or in part.

Complete the form

Practice writing a résumé. When you have finished, check it against the list of areas to be covered.

    a. your name, address, and telephone number

    b. your educational background

    c. your work history

    d. other experiences you have had

    e. references

    f. personal information about interests and activities

Practice Résumé

© 2022 Cengage Learning. All Rights Reserved. May not be scanned, copied or duplicated, or posted to a publicly accessible website, in whole or in part.

Complete the form

Using your résumé, complete the employment application in the following figure.

GENERAL HOSPITAL
Application for Employment

1. Full Name: _____

          Last   First   Middle   Maiden

          Street and Number or Rural Route

          City, State. and ZIP Code

          County   Telephone

          Social Security Number _____

2. Person to notify in case of emergency:
   Name _____
   Address _____

   _____
   Telephone _____
   Relationship _____

3. Education: List in this order—High School, College. You must give complete addresses. Also, please note if you did not graduate from high school and whether or not you have a GED certificate.

School	Address	City	State	Year

4. Work or Vocational Experience: Mention the most recent first.

Name of the Institution or Company	Complete Address	Type of Work	Dates

5. Have you ever been arrested for anything other than minor traffic violations? Yes ___ No ___
6. Are you now or have you been addicted to the use of alcohol or habit-forming drugs? Yes___ No___
7. References: Name three people who know your qualifications or who know your character. They must not be related to you.

   Name _____
   Address _____ Telephone _____

   Name _____
   Address _____ Telephone _____

   Name _____
   Address _____ Telephone _____

8. What are your reasons for wishing to work at this facility? Please answer this question in paragraph form on the back of this application.

© 2022 Cengage Learning. All Rights Reserved. May not be scanned, copied or duplicated, or posted to a publicly accessible website, in whole or in part.

n the following space, practice writing a letter of resignation by filling in the spaces provided.

_____

(date)

Dear _____:

It is necessary for me to leave my position as _____

(position)

as of _____. Working here at _____

(effective date of resignation)   (facility name)

has given me an opportunity to _____.

I find I must leave because _____.

(reason for leaving)

Thank you for your understanding of my situation.

Sincerely,

_____

(your name)

DEVELOPING GREATER INSIGHT

1. Invite a human resource manager to the class to discuss the interview process.

2. Divide the class into pairs. Have the students review each other's résumés, sample application, and sample letter of resignation.

© 2022 Cengage Learning. All Rights Reserved. May not be scanned, copied or duplicated, or posted to a publicly accessible website, in whole or in part.

PART 2

Student Performance Record

© 2022 Cengage Learning. All Rights Reserved. May not be scanned, copied or duplicated, or posted to a publicly accessible website, in whole or in part.

STUDENT PERFORMANCE RECORD

Your instructor will evaluate each procedure you learn and perform, but it will be helpful if you also keep a record so you will know which experiences you still must master.

PROCEDURE	Date	Satisfactory	Unsatisfactory
Chapter 13 Infection Control			
Procedure 1: Handwashing			
Procedure 2: Putting on a Mask			
Procedure 3: Putting on a Gown			
Procedure 4: Putting on Gloves			
Procedure 5: Removing Contaminated Gloves			
Procedure 6: Removing Contaminated Gloves, Eye Protection, Gown, and Mask			
Procedure 7: Serving a Meal in an Isolation Unit			
Procedure 8: Measuring Vital Signs in an Isolation Unit			
Procedure 9: Transferring Nondisposable Equipment Outside of the Isolation Unit			
Procedure 10: Specimen Collection from a Patient in an Isolation Unit			
Procedure 11: Caring for Linens in an Isolation Unit			
Procedure 12: Transporting a Patient to and from the Isolation Unit			
Procedure 13: Opening a Sterile Package			
Chapter 15 Patient Safety and Positioning			
Procedure 14: Turning the Patient Toward You			
Procedure 15: Turning the Patient Away from You			
Procedure 16: Moving a Patient to the Head of the Bed			
Procedure 17: Logrolling the Patient			
Chapter 16 The Patient's Mobility: Transfer Skills			
Procedure 18: Applying a Transfer Belt			
Procedure 19: Transferring the Patient from Bed to Chair—One Assistant			
Procedure 20: Transferring the Patient from Bed to Chair—Two Assistants			
Procedure 21: Sliding-Board Transfer from Bed to Wheelchair			

© 2022 Cengage Learning. All Rights Reserved. May not be scanned, copied or duplicated, or posted to a publicly accessible website, in whole or in part.

PROCEDURE	Date	Satisfactory	Unsatisfactory
Procedure 22: Transferring the Patient from Chair to Bed—One Assistant			
Procedure 23: Transferring the Patient from Chair to Bed—Two Assistants			
Procedure 24: Transferring the Patient from Bed to Stretcher			
Procedure 25: Transferring the Patient from Stretcher to Bed			
Procedure 26: Transferring the Patient with a Mechanical Lift			
Procedure 27: Transferring the Patient onto and off the Toilet			
Chapter 17 The Patient's Mobility: Ambulation			
Procedure 28: Assisting the Patient to Walk with a Cane and Three-Point Gait			
Procedure 29: Assisting the Patient to Walk with a Walker and Three-Point Gait			
Procedure 30: Assisting the Falling Patient			
Chapter 18 Body Temperature			
Procedure 31: Measuring an Oral Temperature (Electronic Thermometer)			
Procedure 32: Measuring a Rectal Temperature (Electronic Thermometer)			
Procedure 33: Measuring an Axillary Temperature (Electronic Thermometer)			
Procedure 34: Measuring a Tympanic Temperature			
Procedure 35: Measuring a Temporal Artery Temperature (Electronic Thermometer)			
Chapter 19 Pulse and Respiration			
Procedure 36: Counting the Radial Pulse			
Procedure 37: Counting the Apical–Radial Pulse			
Procedure 38: Counting Respirations			
Procedure 39: Using a Pulse Oximeter			
Chapter 20 Blood Pressure			
Procedure 40: Taking Blood Pressure			
Procedure 41: Taking Blood Pressure with an Electronic Blood Pressure Apparatus			

© 2022 Cengage Learning. All Rights Reserved. May not be scanned, copied or duplicated, or posted to a publicly accessible website, in whole or in part.

PROCEDURE	Date	Satisfactory	Unsatisfactory
Chapter 21 Measuring Height and Weight			
Procedure 42: Weighing and Measuring the Patient Using an Upright Scale			
Procedure 43: Weighing the Patient on a Chair Scale			
Procedure 44: Measuring Weight with an Electronic Wheelchair Scale			
Procedure 45: Measuring and Weighing the Patient in Bed			
Chapter 22 Admission, Transfer, and Discharge			
Procedure 46: Admitting the Patient			
Procedure 47: Transferring the Patient			
Procedure 48: Discharging the Patient			
Chapter 23 Bedmaking			
Procedure 49: Making a Closed Bed			
Procedure 50: Making an Occupied Bed			
Chapter 24 Patient Bathing			
Procedure 51: Assisting with the Tub Bath or Shower			
Procedure 52: Bed Bath			
Procedure 53: Changing the Patient's Gown			
Procedure 54: Waterless Bed Bath			
Procedure 55: Partial Bath			
Procedure 56: Female Perineal Care			
Procedure 57: Male Perineal Care			
Procedure 58: Hand and Fingernail Care			
Procedure 59: Foot and Toenail Care			
Procedure 60: Bed Shampoo			
Procedure 61: Dressing and Undressing the Patient			
Chapter 25 General Comfort Measures			
Procedure 62: Assisting with Routine Oral Hygiene			
Procedure 63: Assisting with Special Oral Hygiene— Dependent and Unconscious Patients			
Procedure 64: Assisting the Patient to Floss and Brush Teeth			
Procedure 65: Caring for Dentures			
Procedure 66: Providing Backrubs			

© 2022 Cengage Learning. All Rights Reserved. May not be scanned, copied or duplicated, or posted to a publicly accessible website, in whole or in part.

PROCEDURE	Date	Satisfactory	Unsatisfactory
Procedure 67: Shaving a Male Patient			
Procedure 68: Providing Daily Hair Care			
Procedure 69: Giving and Receiving the Bedpan			
Procedure 70: Giving and Receiving the Urinal			
Procedure 71: Assisting with Use of the Bedside Commode			
Chapter 26 Nutritional Needs and Diet Modifications			
Procedure 72: Assisting the Patient Who Can Feed Self			
Procedure 73: Feeding the Dependent Patient			
Procedure 74: Abdominal Thrusts—Heimlich Maneuver			
Chapter 27 Warm and Cold Applications			
Procedure 75: Applying an Ice Bag or Gel Pack			
Procedure 76: Applying a Disposable Cold Pack			
Procedure 77: Giving a Sitz Bath			
Chapter 29 The Surgical Patient			
Procedure 78: Assisting the Patient to Deep Breathe and Cough			
Procedure 79: Applying Elasticized Stockings			
Procedure 80: Applying an Elastic Bandage			
Procedure 81: Assisting the Patient to Dangle			
Chapter 32 Death and Dying			
Procedure 82: Giving Postmortem Care			
Chapter 36 Subacute Care			
Procedure 83: Applying and Removing Sterile Gloves			
Procedure 84: Applying a Dry Sterile Dressing			
Chapter 38 Integumentary System			
Procedure 85: Changing a Clean Dressing and Applying a Bandage			
Chapter 39 Respiratory System			
Procedure 86: Collecting a Sputum Specimen			
Chapter 41 Musculoskeletal System			
Procedure 87: Performing Range-of-Motion Exercises (Passive)			

© 2022 Cengage Learning. All Rights Reserved. May not be scanned, copied or duplicated, or posted to a publicly accessible website, in whole or in part.

PROCEDURE	Date	Satisfactory	Unsatisfactory
Chapter 42 Endocrine System			
Procedure 88: Obtaining a Fingerstick Blood Sugar			
Chapter 44 Gastrointestinal System			
Procedure 89: Collecting a Stool Specimen			
Procedure 90: Testing for Occult Blood Using Hemoccult and Developer			
Procedure 91: Inserting a Rectal Suppository			
Procedure 92: Giving a Soap-Solution Enema			
Procedure 93: Giving a Commercially Prepared Enema			
Procedure 94: Giving Routine Stoma Care (Colostomy)			
Procedure 95: Giving Routine Care of an Ileostomy (with Patient in Bed)			
Chapter 45 Urinary System			
Procedure 96: Collecting a Routine Urine Specimen			
Procedure 97: Collecting a Clean-Catch Urine Specimen			
Procedure 98: Collecting a 24-Hour Urine Specimen			
Procedure 99: Collecting a Urine Specimen Through a Drainage Port			
Procedure 100: Routine Drainage Check			
Procedure 101: Giving Indwelling Catheter Care			
Procedure 102: Emptying a Urinary Drainage Unit			
Procedure 103: Disconnecting the Catheter			
Procedure 104: Connecting a Catheter to a Leg Bag			
Procedure 105: Emptying a Leg Bag			
Procedure 106: Removing an Indwelling Catheter			
Procedure 106: Removing an Indwelling Catheter			
Procedure 107: Ultrasound Bladder Scan			
Chapter 49 Obstetrical Patients and Neonates			
Procedure 108: Changing a Diaper			
Procedure 109: Weighing an Infant			
Procedure 110: Measuring an Infant			
Procedure 111: Bathing an Infant			
Procedure 112: Bottle Feeding an Infant			
Procedure 113: Assisting with Breastfeeding			
Procedure 114: Burping an Infant			

© 2022 Cengage Learning. All Rights Reserved. May not be scanned, copied or duplicated, or posted to a publicly accessible website, in whole or in part.

PROCEDURE	Date	Satisfactory	Unsatisfactory
Chapter 50 Pediatric Patients			
Procedure 115: Admitting a Pediatric Patient			
Procedure 116: Weighing the Toddler to Adolescent			
Procedure 117: Changing Crib Linens			
Procedure 118: Changing Crib Linens (Infant in Crib)			
Procedure 119: Measuring Temperature			
Procedure 120: Determining Heart Rate (Pulse)			
Procedure 121: Counting Respiratory Rate			
Procedure 122: Measuring Blood Pressure			
Procedure 123: Collecting a Urine Specimen from an Infant			

© 2022 Cengage Learning. All Rights Reserved. May not be scanned, copied or duplicated, or posted to a publicly accessible website, in whole or in part.

Nursing Assistant Written State Test Overview

© 2022 Cengage Learning. All Rights Reserved. May not be scanned, copied or duplicated, or posted to a publicly accessible website, in whole or in part.

VOCABULARY

standardized testing

state test content

taking a multiple-choice test

study skills

taking the test

miscellaneous testing concerns

the skills examination

after the test

STANDARDIZED TESTING

The state certification test you will be taking is a **standardized test**. This means it was conceived in a way that will be fair to everyone who takes the test. A test becomes standardized only after having been piloted, used, revised, and used again until it shows consistent results. The purpose of a standardized test is to establish an average score, or *norm*. This allows one person's scores to be compared with the scores of many others across the state or country. A standardized test must be given in the same way each time. This is done by using the same plan and the same directions. The examiner is allowed to give only certain kinds of help. The conditions at all test sites should be similar, and each answer is scored according to definite rules.

The written state test is designed to ensure that you have the knowledge necessary to function safely as an entry-level (beginning) nursing assistant. The test varies in each state. For most states, the test has between 50 and 120 questions. You will be given approximately 2 hours to complete the written test, depending on the length. The test may include approximately 10 extra questions that are not scored. These are in the process of being standardized for use in future tests. You will not know which questions are scored and which are unscored. The time allowed for completing the test is fairly generous. The test examiner will call time near the end of the test to warn you that the end of the allotted time is near.

The written test questions are all in multiple-choice format. Although some questions are difficult, there are no trick questions. Questions are developed by experienced nursing assistant educators and are designed to measure the competency of an average learner. They are not designed to punish slow learners or reward faster learners. Various terms may be used to describe the person giving care. For testing purposes, the term *nurse aide* is commonly used to describe the caregiver, but other terms, such as *nurse assistant* and *nursing assistant*, may be used in your state. The word **client** is commonly used to describe the person receiving care, but the terms *patient* and *resident* may also be used. Your examiner will inform you of the proper terms for these individuals. The questions on the test will be arranged randomly and will not be grouped together by specific category or subject.

Many states have a practice test and candidate handbook available. Ask your instructor if these tools are available in your state. They will be extremely valuable in preparing for your state test. Many practice state tests are available online at http://www.prometric.com/, https://www.tests.com/practice/nursing-assistant-practice-exam-sample, and https://uniontestprep.com/cna/practice-test. Some state nursing assistant registries also maintain websites. If your state registry is online, you may wish to check its website for information about the state test.

STATE TEST CONTENT

The National Nurse Aide Assessment Program (NNAAP) forms the basis for the examination questions. The purpose of the NNAAP Written (or Oral) Examination is to make sure that you understand the responsibilities and can safely perform the job duties of an entry-level nursing assistant. The OBRA law of 1987 was designed to improve the quality of care in long-term care facilities and to establish training and examination standards for nursing assistants. Each state is responsible for following the terms of this federal law. The examination is a measure of the knowledge, skills, and abilities related to nursing assisting. There are two parts to the examination: written and skills. Both parts are usually given on the same day.

© 2022 Cengage Learning. All Rights Reserved. May not be scanned, copied or duplicated, or posted to a publicly accessible website, in whole or in part.

The nursing assistant state written test covers the main content areas that you studied in class. These are listed as follows:

Physical Care Skills

- Activities of daily living (ADLs)/Promotion of health and safety

  ◦ Hygiene

  ◦ Dressing and grooming

  ◦ Nutrition and hydration

  ◦ Elimination

  ◦ Comfort, rest, and sleep

Basic Nursing Skills

- Infection control

- Safety and emergency procedures

- Therapeutic and technical procedures, such as bedmaking, specimen collection, measurement of height and weight, and use of restraints

- Observation, reporting, and data collection

Restorative Nursing Care Skills/Promotion of Function and Health

- Preventive health care, such as contracture and pressure ulcer prevention

- Promotion of client self-care and independence

Psychosocial Care Skills/Specialized Care

- Emotional and mental health needs

  ◦ Behavior management

  ◦ Needs of the dying client

  ◦ Sexuality needs

  ◦ Cultural and spiritual needs

Roles and Responsibilities of the Nursing Assistant

- Communication

  ◦ Verbal communication

  ◦ Nonverbal communication

  ◦ Listening

  ◦ Clients with special communication problems

- Resident rights (long-term care)

- Legal and ethical behavior

- Responsibilities as a member of the health care team

- Knowledge of medical terminology and abbreviations

© 2022 Cengage Learning. All Rights Reserved. May not be scanned, copied or duplicated, or posted to a publicly accessible website, in whole or in part.

TAKING A MULTIPLE-CHOICE TEST

Most standardized tests use multiple-choice items. This is because multiple-choice items can measure a variety of learning outcomes, from simple to complex. They also provide the most consistent results. Each multiple-choice item consists of a **stem**, which presents a problem situation, and four possible choices called **alternatives**. The alternatives include the correct answer and several wrong answers called **distractors**. The stem may be a question or incomplete statement as shown:

Question form:

Q. Which person is responsible for taking care of a client?

    a. janitor

    b. administrator

    c. nursing assistant

    d. social worker

Incomplete statement form:

Q. The care of a client is the responsibility of a (n):

    a. janitor

    b. administrator

    c. nursing assistant

    d. social worker

Although worded differently, both stems present the same problem. The alternatives in the examples contain only one correct answer. All distractors are clearly incorrect.

Another type of multiple-choice item is the best-answer format. In this format, all the alternatives *are correct*, but one is clearly better than the others. Look at the following example:

Best-answer form:

Q. Which of the following ethical behaviors is the MOST important?

    a. Maintain a positive attitude.

    b. Act as a responsible employee.

    c. Be courteous to visitors.

    d. Promote quality of life for each client.

Other variations of the best-answer form may ask you "What is the first thing to do," what is the "most helpful action," what is the "best response" or "best answer," or a similar kind of question. Whether the correct-answer form or best-answer form is used depends on the information given.

Each multiple-choice question lists four answers. The chance of guessing correctly is only one in four, or 25 percent. Each test question has only one correct answer. Do not mark more than one answer per item, or the item will be marked wrong. Do not leave answers blank.

STUDY SKILLS

No matter what type of test you take, you must first master the material. Using index cards is an excellent way to do this. You may wish to prepare index cards listing vocabulary terms, abbreviations, or questions from your workbook or text. Using index cards to create study cards or flashcards will enable you to test your ability to recognize and retrieve important information.

© 2022 Cengage Learning. All Rights Reserved. May not be scanned, copied or duplicated, or posted to a publicly accessible website, in whole or in part.

To study, read the front of the card and try to answer the question. Turn the card over to see if you are correct. After going through all the cards once, you may wish to shuffle them and review them again. Make sure you know the information and can answer questions in any order.

As you review the cards, begin to sort them into two piles. One pile is for those you know well; the other pile is for those you are having trouble remembering. Once you have two piles, try to learn the most difficult information. Continue reviewing the cards until you have mastered the material. Review the cards several times a day during the time before the exam.

There are several advantages to using the card system. First, sorting the cards and preparing extra cards is a good learning experience. Second, the cards are easy and convenient to carry with you in a purse or pocket. You can study them during spare moments throughout the day. Another advantage is that you can use the cards with a friend to quiz each other.

Other Helpful Study Skills

1. Block out a specific time for study. Examine your biorhythms to find the time of day when you are functioning at your peak level of performance.

2. Get plenty of sleep.

3. Begin studying well before the state certification test. Schedule your study sessions so that you can take a break in between. For example, studying for an hour in the morning and an hour in the evening is more effective than studying for two consecutive hours. Trying to study when you are mentally or physically tired is a waste of time.

4. Study the most difficult material when you are most alert.

5. Control your environment. Do whatever it takes to find a quiet place to study. Get up early in the morning, when everyone else is asleep, or find a quiet corner of the library.

6. Become part of a small, dedicated study group of three to five people, or find a study partner.

7. Eat a healthful diet, especially protein and complex carbohydrates.

8. Study key concepts by asking yourself, "What are the four different ways this idea could be tested?"

9. Learn the rationale behind each issue. Write a brief statement of the rationale on the back of each index card with the answer. Study all of the information included in the rationale on your study cards. Ask yourself how the information could be tested. Make sure you can apply the principles and rationale to similar situations.

10. You may also create study checklists. Identify all the material for which you are accountable. Break it down into manageably sized lists of steps, notes, and procedures for each item. For example, write down the steps of a nursing procedure. Create a separate column for supplies needed and any special information you need to know.

11. Record your notes or study questions on an audiotape or any other recording device such as your smartphone. You may play the recording at home or when you are commuting.

12. Many excellent tools and resources for studying are available online at https://focusme.com/blog/tools-to-make-your-revision-and-study-time-more-productive/.

Stress and Test Anxiety

You may be surprised to learn that stress is normal. A certain amount of stress can be good. Almost everyone has some test anxiety. Studies have shown that mild stress actually improves performance by athletes, entertainers, public speakers, and test takers! "Butterflies" in the stomach, breathing faster, sweating, and other symptoms are automatic body responses to stressful situations. Stress can sharpen your attention, keep you alert, and give you greater energy. Remember, it is not the stress that is harmful, but your reaction to it. Learn and practice how to control stress. Some stress cannot be avoided, but you will know the date of this exam well in advance. Try to avoid other stressful situations immediately before the test. Prepare yourself physically and mentally.

© 2022 Cengage Learning. All Rights Reserved. May not be scanned, copied or duplicated, or posted to a publicly accessible website, in whole or in part.

If you feel stressed immediately before or during the exam, try a deep-breathing activity recommended by stress management experts. Breathe slowly and deeply from the diaphragm. Do not move the chest and shoulders. You should feel your abdominal muscles expand when you inhale and relax when you exhale. As you breathe out, your diaphragm and rib muscles seem to relax and your body may seem to sink down into the chair. This helps promote relaxation. Sixty seconds of controlled deep breathing helps relieve stress.

Factors that increase stress and test anxiety are negative thoughts and self-doubt. Perhaps you have thought, "I am going to fail this exam. What will my family or co-workers think if I do not pass?" You must control your reaction to this stress and stop thinking these thoughts. Instead, say to yourself, "I have done this job successfully. I know this material, and I did well in class. I am going to pass this examination." View the exam as an opportunity to show what you know and can do. Positive thinking comes before positive action and positive results. Consciously stop negative thoughts and force them out by using positive ones instead.

TAKING THE TEST

To do well on a test, you should be at your best when you start. Eat a good breakfast or lunch. Try to avoid anything that will cause stress. Dress appropriately, according to exam center requirements. Candidates who are not properly attired may be denied admission.

Be on time. If you are late, you may not be admitted. If you miss the test, your testing fees may not be refundable, and you will lose your money. If weather conditions are unsafe, the test may be cancelled and rescheduled. If you are absent because of a valid emergency, you must promptly submit proof of this emergency to the testing service (usually within 30 days). Examples of acceptable excuses are a death in the immediate family, a disabling traffic accident, you or an immediate family member falling ill jury duty, a court appearance, or military duty. A service fee may be charged if you miss the test, even if you have proof of an acceptable excuse.

Leave for the test site early enough to arrive on time. Allow a little extra time for minor delays. In some states, you may be required to arrive up to 30 minutes early to allow time for registration, processing, verification of identification, and sign-in.

Take a watch and several (two or three) sharpened black lead number 2 pencils with erasers. If your state issues an admission letter, bring it with you and present it to the examiner. Most states have a list of supplies or identification that you must bring to be admitted to the test. Most require a photo identification, and some require you to produce your original social security card, or to furnish a copy of that card. Your photo identification should be a government-issued document, such as a driver's license, state identification card, or passport. The name on the photo identification should be the same as the name used to register for the test, including suffixes such as "Jr.," "III," and the like. The photo identification card must also bear your signature. Each state has a list of acceptable identification that is given to candidates when they register for the test. If you do not have proper photo identification, contact the testing service well in advance to make arrangements for using an alternate means of identification. Some states require two different forms of identification. Learn the requirements in advance and be prepared to meet them. In addition, some states require fingerprinting by a law enforcement agency prior to testing. It is the applicant's responsibility to see that this has been done in a timely manner and to pay all associated fees. You may be required to bring the official (completed) fingerprint card with you at the time of testing. If you are late or fail to bring the required identification or supplies, you may not be admitted, so follow directions carefully.

You will not be permitted to bring audio or video recording devices or personal communication devices, such as pagers and cell phones, into the test site. Likewise, you may not bring children, visitors, or pets. (Service animals are not considered pets and will be admitted.) Do not bring valuables or weapons. You probably will not be permitted to bring personal items other than your keys into the exam room. Leave purses, backpacks, books, notes, and other items in your vehicle. You will not be permitted to eat, drink, or smoke during the examination. Students who display disruptive behavior will be removed and their exam scores recorded as a failure. If necessary, the skills examiner will call law enforcement authorities to remove or manage a disruptive candidate.

When you arrive at the test site, do not let another person's last-minute questions or comments upset you. Do not talk about the test with other students, if possible. Anxiety is contagious. Follow these general rules for taking the test:

1. Choose a good spot to sit. Make sure you have enough space. Maintain good posture and do not slouch. Be comfortable but alert. Stay relaxed and confident.

© 2022 Cengage Learning. All Rights Reserved. May not be scanned, copied or duplicated, or posted to a publicly accessible website, in whole or in part.

2. Remind yourself that you are well-prepared and are going to do well. If you become anxious, take several slow, deep breaths to relax.

3. You will be given verbal instructions and be asked to complete an information form. Pay close attention to the examiner's instructions. They will read the directions. The examiner may not be permitted to answer questions.

4. Take several more deep breaths and try to relax. If you become anxious during the test, close your eyes for a few seconds and practice slow, deep breathing. Remaining relaxed and positive are keys to success. Remind yourself that you have studied well and are prepared to take the test. Think positive.

5. When you receive your test booklet, review the written directions and look at any sample questions. Make sure you understand how to mark your answers. Follow directions carefully. Most state tests are scored by a computer, and stray marks may cause otherwise correct answers to be marked wrong. Write only on your answer sheet. Answers written in the exam book will not be counted.

6. Work at a steady pace.

7. Take the questions at face value. Do not read anything into them. Avoid thinking, "what if?" Answer the question based on the information given. Do not look for trick questions or hidden meanings. Do not add or subtract information.

8. Read the stem of the question. Think of the answer in your own words before reading the answers. Then read all of the answers given. Search for the correct alternative, and then select the option that most closely matches your answer. If necessary, read the stem with each option. If you are still not sure, treat each option as a true/false question, and choose the "most true."

9. It may be helpful to cross out unnecessary words in the question. Distracting information has been crossed out in this example:

   Q. A client ~~who~~ is HIV positive ~~understands that the nurse aide will not talk about this information outside the facility because~~ this information is

      a. legal.

      b. confidential.

      c. negligent.

      d. cultural.

10. If you do not know the answer to a question, circle the number and move on. Come back to it later. You may remember the answer later, or may find a clue to the answer in another question. Do not waste time struggling with questions you are unsure of. This increases your stress and test anxiety. Continuing with the test is best.

11. Be alert to words such as *not* and *except* that may completely change the intent of the question. Pay close attention to words that are *italicized*, are CAPITALIZED, or are within "quotation marks" or (parentheses). Words such as *first*, *last*, *most*, *least*, *best*, and *except* often hold the key to the answer. Read carefully. These words are usually very important.

12. Avoid unfamiliar choices. Information that you are unfamiliar with is probably incorrect.

13. If you do not know the answer, try to identify answers that are not correct. Cross out answers that you know or think are incorrect. If you have crossed out two answers, you have a 50 percent chance of guessing correctly. Other suggestions for eliminating incorrect answers are to cross out:

   a. question options that grammatically do not fit with the stem;

   b. question options that are completely unfamiliar to you; and

   c. question options that contain negative or absolute words, such as those listed in number 11 above.

© 2022 Cengage Learning. All Rights Reserved. May not be scanned, copied or duplicated, or posted to a publicly accessible website, in whole or in part.

Some other strategies may also be useful:

   a. Substitute a qualified term for the absolute one, such as *frequently* instead of *always.* This may help you eliminate another incorrect answer.

   b. If two answers seem correct, compare them for differences, and then refer to the stem to find your best answer.

   c. Use hints from questions you know to help you answer questions that you are not sure of.

14. Look at the shortest and longest of the remaining answers. The correct answer may be shorter or longer than the others.

15. There is no penalty for guessing. If you cannot figure out the answer, guessing is better than leaving a question blank.

16. Do not become upset or nervous if some individuals finish the test early and get up to leave. Some people read more quickly than others. Studies have shown that those who finish first do not necessarily get the best scores.

17. When you get to the end of the test, go back and complete the items you skipped.

18. Do not change your answers without a good reason. Your first answer is more likely to be correct. Change the answer if you misread or misunderstood the question, or if you are absolutely certain that the first answer is wrong.

19. Before turning the test in, check it to make sure you marked every answer. Check the circles or boxes to be sure they are completely marked on the computer scoring sheet. Erase all stray marks.

MISCELLANEOUS TESTING CONCERNS

- In some states, the written test is given on a computer. If you are taking a computerized test, you will be given several practice questions to make sure you know how to use the computer. Complete the practice questions. If you have difficulty in using the computer, speak with the skills examiner.

- Most states administer oral examinations if special circumstances exist. Some states give examinations in languages other than English. These special examinations must be requested from your state testing agency when you register to take the test. If you think you need an oral examination or non-English version of the test, contact your instructor or state testing service for information and instructions. The oral examinations are typically recorded. You will listen to the recording with a headset. Typically, each question is read twice in a neutral manner. You will also be furnished with a written test booklet so that you can review the printed words while listening to the tape. You will answer the question by marking in the answer sheet. However, to be a nursing assistant, you must be able to read and write in English. Even if you take an oral or non-English examination, you will be given a series of reading comprehension questions, typically 10. You must pass this portion of the examination, showing your understanding of the English language, in order to pass the exam as a whole. The time limits for oral testing are usually the same as the time limits for the written test.

- Your state will accommodate individuals with certain disabilities during the test. Contact your state testing agency well in advance for information on requesting accommodations. You cannot wait until the day of the test to request a special accommodation.

- Your state will have a skills (manual competency) examination portion of the state certification test. You must pass both portions of the test before being entered into the nursing assistant registry. Contact your instructor or state testing agency for information.

- *Do not bring personal communication devices, such as pagers, cell phones, tablets, or other electronic devices, to the test site.* Use of these items is not permitted, and you will not be allowed to take them into the test site.

© 2022 Cengage Learning. All Rights Reserved. May not be scanned, copied or duplicated, or posted to a publicly accessible website, in whole or in part.

Test Security

- Do not give help to anyone or receive help from anyone during the test. If the examiner suspects a candidate of cheating on the examination, the candidate's test materials will be seized and they will be asked to leave the testing site. The score will be recorded as a failure. The examiner reports individuals who cheat on the test to the state nursing assistant registry.

- When you have finished testing, turn all paper materials in. You may not remove the examination booklet, notes, or papers from the room.

- Individuals caught removing a test from the testing site may be prosecuted. Copying, displaying, or distributing a copyrighted examination is illegal.

THE SKILLS EXAMINATION

Part of the state test is a skills examination. This examination is administered slightly differently in each state. Usually, a nurse who has no affiliation with your school or educational program administers the examination. You will be tested on the number of skills required by your state. Your skills will be chosen at random from the required skills list for your state. The number of skills to be tested depends upon the state.

Reporting to the nurse, documenting, and doing basic calculations are parts of some skills. For example, if you weigh a patient, you must calculate the total value from the upper and lower bars of the scale correctly. If you take a rectal or axillary temperature, you must show the skills examiner that you know how to record it correctly by placing an "R" or "A" after the temperature reading. If you count the pulse or respirations for 30 seconds, you must calculate and document the full-minute value correctly. If a value is abnormal, such as a temperature of 103.6°F (R), you must recognize that the value is abnormal and report it to the nurse or proper person. (In this case, inform the skills examiner of the abnormal value and state that you would report it to the nurse. If you are taking the test on a real patient, notify the nurse promptly as soon as the exam has ended, or ask the examiner's permission to leave briefly to report.) If you empty a catheter bag or measure intake and output, you must use a graduated cylinder and measure, calculate, add, and document the total(s) correctly. This also applies to estimating meal intake and other measurements and calculations on the examination. If you are concerned about your math skills, ask your instructor if you will be permitted to use a calculator. If so, take one with you to the exam.

The passing rate for the skills component of the exam will vary with your state. The number of skills to pass also depends upon your state. You may not need to complete each skill perfectly. Certain steps are designated as critical points in the skill. If you perform these correctly, you will pass the skill, even if you make a mistake. In some states, this testing is done in the skills laboratory using other students as patient volunteers. The examiner reads the student volunteer a statement and gives instructions on what is expected in playing the role of the patient. Treat the student volunteer exactly as you would a patient. Some skills, such as perineal care, may be done on a manikin. Pretend the manikin is a patient, and treat it with the same courtesy and precautions as you would use for a patient. All equipment and supplies will be available to perform the skill, but you must know what you need and gather it before beginning. Ask questions before you begin testing on the skill. Once the test begins, the nurse examiner will be unable to answer questions.

Some states do the state skills test only on residents in a nursing facility. Some states time the skills examination. For example, you may be given 35 minutes in which to complete this portion of the test. Some states require you to pass the written test first, before you will be permitted to take the skills exam. In other states, the opposite is true: You must pass the skills examination before you will be permitted to take the written test. Although foreign-language options are available for the written test, the skills examination is given only in English.

Preparing for the Skills Examination

The only way to adequately prepare for the skills examination is to practice each procedure in sequence. If you practice, the skills will become automatic. The skills that you will be tested on are randomly selected from the procedures you learned in class. If your nursing assistant class has a review day or mock skills examination before you take the test, be sure to attend. This will be very helpful to you in preparing for the test.

© 2022 Cengage Learning. All Rights Reserved. May not be scanned, copied or duplicated, or posted to a publicly accessible website, in whole or in part.

You should also review your vocabulary terms so that you are familiar with the various names for the procedures. For example, the skills examiner may direct you to "ambulate the patient." From your review of the vocabulary, you know that *ambulate* means to walk. If the examiner instructs you to do range-of-motion exercises on the lower *extremities*, you must know that these are the *legs*. Practice your skills with other students or with your family, and use your procedure checklists or forms provided by your state.

When reviewing the procedures, pay close attention to the list of supplies and equipment you will need to gather before you perform the procedure. It is essential that you collect the right supplies at the time of the skills test, or you may be unable to complete a procedure.

There is no way to study for the skills examination other than reviewing and practicing the procedures you learned in class. The skills examiner will watch for certain things during the examination. Some of these observations are very important and may be the deciding factor on whether you pass or fail a particular skill on the examination.

Observations Made During the Skills Examination

Gather all the supplies you will need before beginning each section of the test. If you will be making the bed, stack the linen in order of use. The test will go more smoothly if you are well organized.

Direct Care

Most of the skills examination consists of **direct care activities**. Direct patient care activities assist patients in meeting basic human needs, such as feeding, drinking, positioning, ambulating, grooming, toileting, and dressing. They may involve collecting, recording, and reporting information.

Indirect Care

Certain skills are part of every procedure that you perform. These are usually called **indirect care skills**. Indirect activities focus on maintaining the environment and the systems in which nursing care is delivered. They assist in providing a clean, efficient, safe, comfortable, respectful patient care environment. An indirect care skill is an important part of the procedure, but does not necessarily affect the outcome. Data collection, documentation, consultation with other health care providers, and reporting of information are indirect care skills. Examples of indirect care tasks are communication, comfort, patient rights, safety, and infection control. The skills examiner will look closely at (and score) your indirect care skills in each and every procedure. Doing these things each and every time is critical to your success. Indirect care skills on which you will be tested include the following essential elements:

- The skills examiner will observe **handwashing**. Your handwashing technique will be monitored, so be sure that you follow accepted standards and procedures. Wash your hands before and after caring for each patient, and more often as necessary. This skill will not be prompted by the examiner, meaning that you will not be told or reminded to do it. Nursing assistants are expected to know when and how to wash their hands. Use the proper technique. Each handwashing should last a minimum of 15–20 seconds, or according to your state rules. You may be permitted to use alcohol-based hand cleaner unless your hands are soiled. Consult your instructor about this in advance. However, the skills examiner may still request you to do at least one handwash at the sink so that your ability to wash hands correctly can be observed.

- **Infection control** is another area on which you are evaluated. The skills examiner observes your technique in patient care, and the use of standard precautions and medical asepsis. The examiner will also observe if you wear gloves and other personal protective equipment (PPE) when necessary. You will be evaluated on whether you wash your hands before applying and removing gloves, as well as whether you use proper technique in applying and removing the gloves themselves. Other important considerations are keeping clean and soiled items separated, disposing of soiled articles correctly, and preventing environmental contamination from used gloves and equipment.

- The examiner will observe how well you **communicate** with each patient. You must introduce yourself and the skills examiner. Explain what you are going to do, even if the patient is confused. Inform the patient before each step, such as "Now I am going to turn you over on your side." You may also be evaluated on whether you speak with the patient throughout the procedure.

© 2022 Cengage Learning. All Rights Reserved. May not be scanned, copied or duplicated, or posted to a publicly accessible website, in whole or in part.

- The skills examiner will observe how well you practice **safety**. In fact, many safety violations constitute automatic test failures, such as leaving the bedside with the bed in the high position and side rails down. Another example is failure to lock the wheelchair brakes before transferring the patient. These are potentially serious problems that could result in patient injuries, so the skills examiners take them very seriously. Protect patient safety throughout the procedure. When you have finished the procedure, make sure the patient is left safe, with the call signal within reach. Do not leave the room if the patient is in an unsafe location or position, or if the ordered side rails or restraints are not in place.

- Protecting and honoring **patient rights** is also very important. Be sure to knock on doors and wait for permission to enter. Use the bath blanket for modesty when the patient's body will be exposed, such as during bathing and perineal care. Pull the privacy curtain, close the window curtains, and close the door to the room. Speak with the patient in a dignified manner. Avoid terms such as *honey, dear, granny,* and *sweetie*. Although facility staff may call patients by endearing names, the skills examiner will consider it undignified and unprofessional. Treat patients with the utmost respect. The nurse examiner will monitor your attention to the patient's dignity, privacy, and safety.

- Patient **comfort** is an important consideration. You must ensure patients' comfort by doing things such as handling patients gently, asking about their comfort, supporting the arm when taking blood pressure, positioning patients in good body alignment, and leaving each patient in a comfortable position upon completion of the skill.

Critical Points

Critical points are things that could potentially harm a patient. If you skip a critical point on your state skills examination, you will fail the skill. If your state or program uses skills checklists with key or critical points listed, pay close attention to them. For example, in many states, failure to balance the scale before weighing a patient is a critical (automatic failure) point.

Studying the critical points for each skill will be very helpful to you. Because these things could potentially harm a patient, you will feel more confident in providing care on the nursing units. Learning the critical points for each skill creates a win–win situation for both you and the patients. The following is an example of an actual skills test from one state. The underlined steps are the critical skills or automatic failure points.

Handwashing

1. Turns on water.

2. Wets hands.

3. Applies skin cleanser or soap to hands.

4. Rubs hands together for at least 15–20 seconds in a circular motion.

5. Washes all surfaces of the hands at least up to the wrist.

6. Rinses hands thoroughly from wrist to fingertips; cleans under fingernails, if needed, fingers down, under running water.

7. Dries hands on clean paper towel/warm air dryer.

8. Turns off faucet with paper towel and/or avoids contact with sink or other dirty surfaces during rinsing and drying of the hands.

9. Discards wet towel appropriately.

When taking the skills test, think through each task that is asked of you. If the nurse examiner tells you that your patient has had a stroke with right-side paralysis, and then instructs you to get the patient out of bed, think about which side the patient will transfer to, where you will position the wheelchair, how you will keep the patient safe, and whether another assistant is needed to help. Critical points for this skill will include locking the wheelchair brakes and using a transfer belt (unless contraindicated).

© 2022 Cengage Learning. All Rights Reserved. May not be scanned, copied or duplicated, or posted to a publicly accessible website, in whole or in part.

Other Mistakes

If you think you have made a mistake or forgot to do something during the skills examination, inform the skills examiner immediately. They may allow you to go back and correct the problem. This depends on the nature of the error and when you notify the examiner. If you inform the examiner of the error in a timely manner, you may be permitted to go back and begin again at the point where the error was made. The skills examiner will not correct you if you make an error and will not answer questions about the procedure during the test. If you have questions, ask them before testing begins. The skills examiner will not assist you or intervene during the test unless an unsafe patient condition develops.

AFTER THE TEST

After the test, you will breathe a sigh of relief. Listen carefully to the examiner's instructions for returning test materials. Information may also be provided about how and when you will find out the test results. In many states, you get preliminary results the same day. You will not be given a percentage or letter grade. Preliminary scores are listed as either "pass" or "fail." The results are considered preliminary until they are validated by the testing agency in its offices. After the tests are validated, you will be given a more complete explanation of your score. You should receive a report in the mail in approximately two weeks. If you have not received the results within 30 days, contact the examination service.

If you have passed the written and skills examinations, your name will be entered into your state nursing assistant registry. This may take several weeks. In some states, the criminal background and fingerprint checks must also be completed and cleared before you are entered into the registry.

In some states, the nurse examiner will fax your answer sheet for scoring as soon as you finish the exam. You will receive an official score report before leaving the test center. The report will indicate whether you have passed or failed the written (or oral) exam.

You will be issued a wallet card to show as proof of your certification. Protect your wallet card and do not lose it. Never give your employer or a prospective employer the original. If someone needs a copy, make a photocopy and keep the original in a safe place. If you lose your card, your state will issue a duplicate, but there is usually a fee for this service. Your certification must be current for the state to issue a duplicate card. Do not alter your card in any way. Altering the card may result in loss of certification.

The test is fair and most candidates pass the first time. If you did not pass the test, you will have at least two more opportunities to retest. You have three opportunities to pass each part of the examination. However, there is a fee for each retesting. Your instructor may have to register you for the retest. All testing fees must be submitted to the testing service at the time of registration. Meet with your instructor to find out what to study to increase your chances of successfully passing the retest.

You must keep your state nursing assistant registry informed of any changes in your name or address. If you move or change your name, notify the state registry promptly in writing. Provide your state registration number or social security number so that the information can be listed for the proper person. (More than one person may have the same name.) Many states have forms for change of name or address available on their websites.

Your nursing assistant certification will expire in 24 months. To renew it, you must meet your state continuing education requirements. To remain active, you must submit a form verifying that you have provided paid nursing assistant services during the renewal period. The number of hours you are required to work to maintain your certification varies with each state.

© 2022 Cengage Learning. All Rights Reserved. May not be scanned, copied or duplicated, or posted to a publicly accessible website, in whole or in part.

PART 4

Flashcards

© 2022 Cengage Learning. All Rights Reserved. May not be scanned, copied or duplicated, or posted to a publicly accessible website, in whole or in part.

© 2022 Cengage Learning. All Rights Reserved. May not be scanned, copied or duplicated, or posted to a publicly accessible website, in whole or in part.

abdomin/o	cephal/o
aden/o	cerebr/o
	chol/e
angi/o	
arteri/o	col/o
arthr/o	
bronch/o	crani/o
card, cardi/o	cyst/o

© 2022 Cengage Learning. All Rights Reserved. May not be scanned, copied or duplicated, or posted to a publicly accessible website, in whole or in part.

head	abdomen
brain	gland
bile	
e	vessel
colon, large intestine	artery
	joint
skull	bronchus, bronchi
bladder, cyst	heart

© 2022 Cengage Learning. All Rights Reserved. May not be scanned, copied or duplicated, or posted to a publicly accessible website, in whole or in part.

cyt/o	gloss/o
dent/o	hem/o
dermat/o	
encephal/o	hepat/o
enter/o	hyster/o
erythr/o	
gastr/o	lapar/o
geront/o	laryng/o

© 2022 Cengage Learning. All Rights Reserved. May not be scanned, copied or duplicated, or posted to a publicly accessible website, in whole or in part.

tongue	cell
blood	tooth
	skin
liver	brain
uterus	small intestine
	red
abdomen, loin, flank	stomach
larynx	elderly

© 2022 Cengage Learning. All Rights Reserved. May not be scanned, copied or duplicated, or posted to a publicly accessible website, in whole or in part.

mamm/o	
mast/o	ophthalm/o
men/o	oste/o
my/o	ot/o
myel/o	pharyng/o
nephr/o	phleb/o
neur/o	pneum/o
ocul/o	proct/o

© 2022 Cengage Learning. All Rights Reserved. May not be scanned, copied or duplicated, or posted to a publicly accessible website, in whole or in part.

	breast
eye	breast
bone	menstruation
ear	muscle
pharynx, throat	spinal cord, bone marrow
vein	kidney
lung, air, gas	nerve
rectum	eye

© 2022 Cengage Learning. All Rights Reserved. May not be scanned, copied or duplicated, or posted to a publicly accessible website, in whole or in part.

psych/o	thorac/o
pulm/o	
rect/o	
rhin/o	trache/o, trache/i
	ur/o
splen/o	urethr/o
stern/o	urin/o
	uter/o

© 2022 Cengage Learning. All Rights Reserved. May not be scanned, copied or duplicated, or posted to a publicly accessible website, in whole or in part.

chest	mind
	lung
	rectum
trachea	nose
urine, urinary tract, urination	
urethra	spleen
urine	sternum
uterus	

© 2022 Cengage Learning. All Rights Reserved. May not be scanned, copied or duplicated, or posted to a publicly accessible website, in whole or in part.

ven/o	thromb/o
fibr/o	tox/o, toxic/o
glyc/o	a—
gynec/o	
hydr/o	
lith/o	
ped/o	brady—
py/o	

© 2022 Cengage Learning. All Rights Reserved. May not be scanned, copied or duplicated, or posted to a publicly accessible website, in whole or in part.

clot	vein
poison	fiber
without	sugar
	female
	water
	stone
slow	child
	pus

© 2022 Cengage Learning. All Rights Reserved. May not be scanned, copied or duplicated, or posted to a publicly accessible website, in whole or in part.

dys—	poly—
hyper—	pre—
hypo—	post—
	retro—
	tachy—
	—algia
	—ectomy
	—emia

© 2022 Cengage Learning. All Rights Reserved. May not be scanned, copied or duplicated, or posted to a publicly accessible website, in whole or in part.

pan—	—gram
	—itis
	—logy
many	pain or difficulty
before	above, excessive
after	low, deficient
behind, backward	
fast	

© 2022 Cengage Learning. All Rights Reserved. May not be scanned, copied or duplicated, or posted to a publicly accessible website, in whole or in part.

pain	
removal of	
blood	
record	all
inflammation	
study of	
—oma	
—otomy	—scope

© 2022 Cengage Learning. All Rights Reserved. May not be scanned, copied or duplicated, or posted to a publicly accessible website, in whole or in part.

	—scopy
—plegia	
—pnea	
	—tumor
examination instrument	incision
examination using a scope	
	paralysis
	breathing, respiration

© 2022 Cengage Learning. All Rights Reserved. May not be scanned, copied or duplicated, or posted to a publicly accessible website, in whole or in part.